AF772019

Safe Motherhood Initiatives: Critical Issues

Edited by
Marge Berer
and
TK Sundari Ravindran

Blackwell Science

Reproductive Health Matters

Published by Blackwell Science Limited for
Reproductive Health Matters, 1999

A catalogue record for this book is available in
the British Library.

ISBN 0 9531210 1 1

Typeset by Boldface, London

Design by Mark Nelson and Boldface

Printed in Great Britain by Spider Web, London

The views expressed in this book are those of the individual authors.

For

Erica Royston

who put

Safe Motherhood

on the map

Contents

PREVENTING MATERNAL DEATHS THROUGH EFFECTIVE POLICIES AND PROGRAMMES

RESOURCES

Acknowledgements

The editors have benefited immeasurably from the knowledge and advice of many experienced and committed people in the reproductive health field. We would like to express our gratitude for the generosity with information and time and the willingness to respond to so many editorial demands and questions, on the part of all the authors and peer reviewers and others who have contributed so much to this book.

Above all, we acknowledge the unstinting support of four women, all of whom have been leaders in making safe motherhood a focus of international attention. Each of them not only peer reviewed and wrote or contributed to a number of papers in this book and gave advice on others; they also helped us to find papers, provided data, editorial advice and personal support throughout the time we have been working on it. To all of them, our heartfelt thanks:

Carla AbouZahr
Judith Fortney
Deborah Maine
Erica Royston

We are also grateful to the following equally distinguished leaders in safe motherhood work and contributors to reproductive and sexual health work more broadly, for good advice, valuable peer reviews, and the willingness to follow up reviews personally with authors when asked. For peer reviews of three or more papers each:

Barbara Kwast
Jerker Liljestrand
Gaynor Maclean
Della R Sherratt
Godfrey Walker

and for peer reviews of one to two papers each:

Sulochana Abraham
Lawrence Adeokun
Barbara Bradby
Peter Brocklehurst
Nahid Chowdhury
Susan Crane
Veronique Felippi
Andres de Francisco
Adrienne Germain
Sally Girvin
Wendy Graham
Manisha Gupte
G Justus Hofmeyr
Marge Koblinsky
Anu Kumar
Ana Langer
Saramma Mathai
Suman Mehta
Mala Ramanathan
Sunanda Ray
Carine Ronsmans
Sheela Shenoy
Sidney Ruth Schuler
Cindy Stanton
Farhang Tahzib
Anne Thompson
Lewis Wall

Lastly, our thanks to the UK Department for International Development (DFID) and the World Bank for their financial support for this book; to Sally Barber for researching photographs; and to Mark Nelson, Carol Brickley and Paul Crittenden for support and assistance with design and production.

We believe the future of Safe Motherhood depends on the mobilisation of women, of expertise, information and resources, and most importantly of action at community, policy and health service levels in all countries, on the part of women themselves, women's health activists, researchers, health professionals and policymakers. This book is an acknowledgement of their efforts and experiences.

Contributors

Carla AbouZahr is a social statistician and technical officer with the Department of Reproductive Health and Research, World Health Organization. She formerly worked for the UK Government and for the Statistical Office of the European Communities. She is responsible for advocacy and information activities and has authored many articles and documents on measurement of maternal mortality.

Pascale Allotey is a lecturer with the Key Centre for Women's Health, a World Health Organization Collaborating Centre, at the University of Melbourne, Australia. She has extensive experience in public health nursing and midwifery in West Africa and in research on migrant women in Australia. She is currently on the WHO Tropical Diseases Research Task Force for Gender Sensitive Interventions.

Maggie Bangser is an affiliate at the Harvard Center for Population and Development Studies, Cambridge USA, and the director of the Women's Dignity Project, a regional VVF programme in East Africa. She was project advisor to the Bugando Medical Centre VVF Project. **Balthazar Gumodoka** is a consultant obstetrician/gynaecologist and head of the Department of Obstetrics and Gynaecology at Bugando Medical Centre in Mwanza, Tanzania, and director of the VVF Project. **Zachary Berege** is director of Bugando Medical Centre and a consultant obstetrician/gynaecologist at the hospital, and was formerly the regional obstetrician/gynaecologist in Arusha, Tanzania.

Marge Berer is editor of *Reproductive Health Matters*, editor/author of *Women and HIV/AIDS: An International Resource Book*, and chair of the Gender Advisory Panel, UNDP/UNFPA/WHO/World Bank Special Programme of Research Development and Research Training in Human Reproduction, Geneva. She has been campaigning for women's reproductive rights and safe, legal abortion since the 1970s.

Oona Campbell currently heads an international research programme on 'Effective Services in Maternal Health' at the London School of Hygiene and Tropical Medicine, London, UK. She is a reproductive epidemiologist interested in maternal health, abortion, contraceptive safety, female mortality, and breastfeeding.

Kim Dickson-Tetteh is a physician, clinical director of the Reproductive Health Research Unit, Johannesburg, and co-ordinator of the National Abortion Care Programme in South Africa. **Helen Rees** is a physician, executive director of the Reproductive Health Research Unit, chairperson of the National Termination of Pregnancy Advisory Group, chairperson of the South African Medicines Control Council and president of the Planned Parenthood Association of South Africa.

Do Thi Ngoc Nga trained in English literature and sociology in Vietnam and India and worked at the Institute of Sociology, National Centre for Social Sciences and Humanities, Hanoi. She is now teaching English at the Department of Foreign Languages, Hanoi University of Science, Vietnam. **Martha Morrow** is international programmes director at the Key Centre for Women's Health in Society, University of Melbourne, Australia. She travels frequently to Asia to conduct workshops on research methods and undertake collaborative research on nutrition, breastfeeding, smoking and gender, and adolescent health needs.

Emily Fatula graduated with a Master's of Health Science from the Johns Hopkins University School of Hygiene and Public Health in May 1997. She now works at the Economic and Social Research Institute, a small non-profit health policy research firm in Washington DC, USA.

Judith Fortney is a reproductive epidemiologist with Family Health International and a professor in the Departments of Epidemiology and Maternal and Child Health at the University of North Carolina (UNC) at Chapel Hill, USA. **Jason B Smith** is a behavioural scientist specialising in reproductive health, a senior research associate at Family Health International and adjunct assistant professor of health behaviour and health education at the UNC School of Public Health.

Coeli J Geefhuysen is an honorary research consultant at the Australian Centre for

International and Tropical Health, University of Brisbane, Australia. She has taught epidemiology, maternal and child health and infectious diseases in university public health courses in Australia, Indonesia and South Africa, and was a paediatrician in Soweto for 25 years.

Wendy Graham is a reproductive epidemiologist and demographer with a particular interest in the measurement of health outcomes, especially maternal mortality. She is the director of the Dugald Baird Centre for Research on Women's Health, Department of Obstetrics and Gynaecology, University of Aberdeen, UK. **Susan F Murray** is a social scientist and midwife, lecturer in international maternal health and coordinator of the Safer Motherhood and Newborn Care Group, at the Institute of Child Health, University College London, UK. **Clare Taylor** is a reproductive health researcher working as an associate professional officer for the Department for International Development (UK) Eastern Africa in Nairobi, coordinating DFID's involvement in the Safe Motherhood initiative in Kenya.

Zahidul A Huque is a public health physician specialising in reproductive health and population. He was the senior technical advisor for MotherCare in the USA while this article was written and is now UNFPA Representative for the Sudan. **Margaret Leppard** is a public health nurse who has worked extensively in rural Bangladesh and is currently a PhD student, London School of Hygiene and Tropical Medicine, UK. **Dileep Mavalankar** is a public health physician specialising in public sector health policy and management. He was team leader of the Bangladesh Maternal Health Assessment 1997 and is currently chairman, Department of Public System Group, Indian Institute of Management, Ahamedabad, India. **Halida Hanum Akhter** is a public health physician specialising in reproductive health and population and director of Bangladesh Institute of Research for Promotion of Essential and Reproductive Health and Technologies, Dhaka, Bangladesh. **TA Chowdhury** is a professor of obstetrics and gynaecology, formerly director of the Institute of Post-Graduate Medicine, Dhaka, and currently senior obstetric consultant, Bangladesh Institute of Research and Rehabilitation for Diabetes, Endocrine and Metabolic Disorders, Dhaka.

Ana Langer is regional director for the Population Council in Mexico City. A physician, her main areas of interest are maternal health/mortality, sexually transmitted diseases, quality of reproductive health care, psychosocial aspects, and linkages between research and policy. She has published extensively and provides technical assistance to governments and NGOs throughout Latin America and the Caribbean. **Bernardo Hernández** is the head of nutrition and health at the National Institute of Public Health-Mexico and a social psychologist with interests in maternal mortality and adolescent health. **Cecilia García-Barrios** is a physician and epidemiologist who has conducted research on reproductive health and maternal mortality with governmental organisations and NGOs in Mexico, including with the National Safe Motherhood Committee of Mexico. **Gloria Luz Saldaña-Uranga** has trained in communications and has contributed to the coordination of research projects in public health, including reproductive health, at the Ministry of Health, National Institute of Public Health and National Safe Motherhood Committee of Mexico.

Deborah Maine, an epidemiologist with a background in anthropology, is a professor at the Center for Population and Family Health, Columbia University, New York, USA. She was director of the Prevention of Maternal Mortality programme from 1987 to 1996, and is now director of a new programme, Averting Maternal Deaths and Disability, at the Centre. **Tessa Wardlaw** is an epidemiologist and works as a Technical Advisor in Statistics and Monitoring in the Division of Evaluation, Policy and Planning at UNICEF, New York. She has previously worked with UNFPA, the Demographic and Health Surveys, and Contraceptive Prevalence Surveys programmes.

Vinaya Pendse has worked for more than three decades as an obstetrician-gynaecologist in teaching hospitals in Rajasthan, India. She has been the chair of the maternal mortality subcommittee, Udaipur Ob-Gyn Society, organised several seminars on maternal mortality at the state and national levels, and published numerous reports, articles and booklets on maternal deaths.

Susanna Rance lives in La Paz, does research on gender and health, and co-ordinates three regional Working Groups on Unwanted Pregnancy and Abortion. From 1997-98 she worked on a project with the Bolivian Ministry of Health, researching medical discourses on abortion, which is the topic of her PhD dissertation at Trinity College, University of Dublin.

TK Sundari Ravindran is an activist-researcher on women's health and reproductive health and rights. She is honorary executive director of the Rural Women's Social Education Centre, Chengalpattu, India and was co-editor of *Reproductive Health Matters* from 1993-1998. **R Savitri** is a statistician-demographer, and deputy director in the Department of Health and Family Welfare, Government of India, New Delhi. **A Bhavani** is the co-ordinator of RUWSEC's community-based women's health programme.

Helen Schneider is a medical doctor and community health specialist and is currently director of the Centre for Health Policy, University of Witwatersrand, Johannesburg, South Africa. **Lucy Gilson** is a senior lecturer at the London School of Hygiene and Tropical Medicine and deputy director, Centre for Health Policy, Johannesburg, where she is presently based.

Dora J Shehu is the co-ordinator of the Prevention of Maternal Mortality Programme, Usmanu Danfodiyo University, Sokoto, Nigeria.

Della R Sherratt is a midwife with expertise in midwifery education in the UK and South East Asia, and has undertaken a number of short-term consultancies for WHO. She is currently working in development studies, specialising in reproductive health and safe motherhood at the Centre For Development Studies, School of Social Sciences & International Development, University of Wales, Swansea, UK.

Eva Weissman is an international health economist based in New York. **Olive Sentumbwe-Mugisa**, an obstetrician-gynaecologist, is the Uganda National Safe Motherhood Programme coordinator, based in Kampala, and also serves as family health and population desk officer with WHO, Kampala. **AK Mbonye** is demographer and principal medical officer, Reproductive Health Division, Uganda Ministry of Health, Kampala. **Craig Lissner** is a technical officer covering economics and financial matters, Department of Reproductive Health and Research, World Health Organization, Geneva.

Vivian Taam Wong is an academic obstetrician turned health service manager. She has been involved in international health as a public health specialist for the World Bank, advisor and consultant to the World Health Organization, and chair of the Safe Motherhood Initiative of the International Federation of Gynecology and Obstetrics. **Jerker Liljestrand** is an obstetrician-gynecologist with experience of work and research in reproductive health and public health in several countries. He is currently with the Department of Reproductive Health and Research, World Health Organization, Geneva.

Introduction

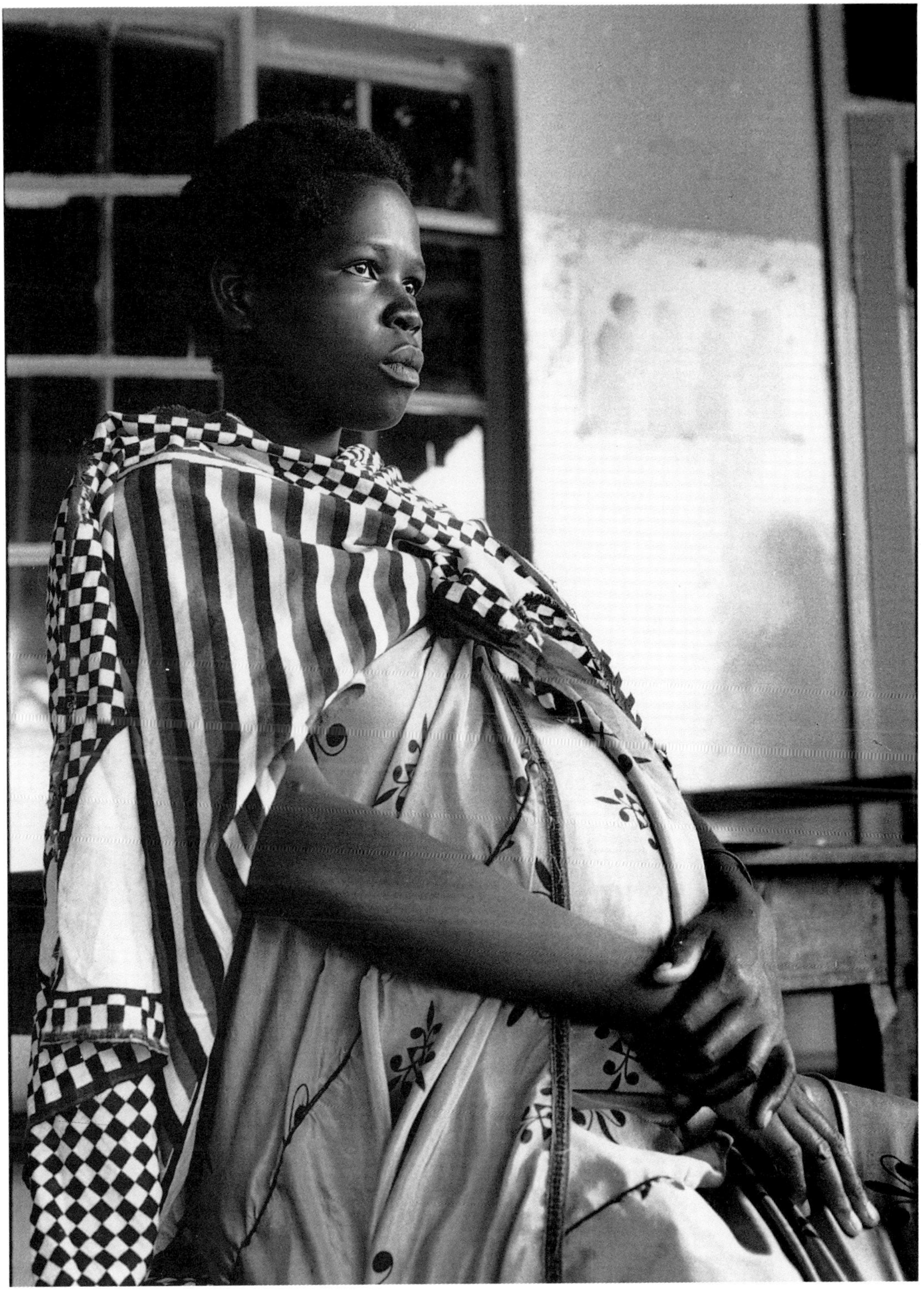

JENNY MATTHEWS

Preventing Maternal Mortality: Evidence, Resources, Leadership, Action

Marge Berer, TK Sundari Ravindran

> *'...Not simply because these are women in the prime of their lives.... Not simply because a maternal death is one of the most terrible ways to die.... But above all because almost every maternal death is an event that could have been avoided, and should never have been allowed to happen.'*[1]

A new millennium is starting, and pregnancy, childbirth and abortion continue to be unnecessarily hazardous for the majority of the world's women. In spite of a century of accumulated knowledge about why maternal deaths occur and what needs to be done to avert them, nearly 600,000 women are still dying each year in developing countries, and preventing these deaths seems to be as elusive as ever in many countries.

This lack of progress is not puzzling at the end of a century in which growing wealth and growing poverty, advanced education and lack of education, superhighways and impassable mud roads, complex technology and lack of clean water, advances in health care and lack of access to health care – all exist side by side. But it is not excusable either.

Maternal mortality in Norway, Sweden, Italy, Denmark and Netherlands had already dropped by the first decade of the 20th century to between 200 and 300 deaths per 100,000 live births. Long before the last decade of the century, maternal deaths had become rare events throughout the developed world. There are many reasons for this decline, including decreasing levels of poverty; improved living conditions; better nutrition; greater autonomy among women; improved standards and practice of midwifery and obstetric care based on evidence from research; aseptic practices in assisting deliveries; drugs to combat sepsis, eclampsia and haemorrhage; lower fertility rates with the use of modern birth control; improvements in the safety of procedures such as caesarean section; legalisation of abortion and provision of safe abortion services; leadership on the part of midwives and obstetrician-gynaecologists for better training and services, and procedures to identify avoidable causes of deaths such as maternal death audits.[1-5]

In 1987, unbeknownst to each other at first, two independent initiatives drew attention to the continuing high levels of maternal mortality and morbidity in developing countries. The better known of these, the Safe Motherhood Initiative, was launched at an international consultation of UN agencies, governments, donors and large NGOs in Nairobi, Kenya, in 1987.[6] The second was the International Day of Action for Women's Health on 28 May 1988, launched by the Women's Global Network for Reproductive Rights and the Latin American and Caribbean Women's Health Network through a 'Call to Women for Action to Prevent Maternal Mortality', which had been endorsed by participants at the 5th International Women and Health Meeting in 1987 in San José, Costa Rica.[7]

More countries have now made a commitment to Safe Motherhood than ever before – through the Programme of Action of the International Conference on Population and Development (ICPD) in Cairo in 1994, the Technical Consultation on Safe Motherhood in Colombo, Sri Lanka in 1997[8] and the ICPD+5 review process in New York in 1999. At the ICPD in 1994, all governments agreed to reduce maternal mortality by one half of the 1990 levels by the year 2000, and by a further half by 2015. The Colombo meeting in 1997 brought together the lessons learnt in the previous decade and called on governments and donors to contribute more to these efforts.[9]

Together, these initiatives created widespread awareness that maternal mortality merits high priority for action. Since 1987, much more information is available from research on the dimensions and causes of maternal mortality. National Safe Motherhood policies and programmes, as well as local projects and services, have been developed and undertaken by governments,[10] donors and non-governmental organisations (NGOs) alike. National and community-based women's groups have incorporated advocacy, community education and mobilisation in their activities as well.[11]

However, since 1987 global attention to maternal mortality has waxed and waned several times. After the 1994 ICPD, the newly agreed reproductive and sexual health agenda, with its equivocal paragraph on unsafe abortion, seemed for a time to have 'displaced' the Safe Motherhood agenda, or at least put into question the priority it was to be given. The annual International Day of Action for Women's Health and the attention of many in the international women's health movement also ceased to focus on maternal mortality at around that time. Then, with economic crises and government and donor spending cuts in the mid-1990s, there was a deterioration in the functioning of health systems and investment in the health sector dropped, especially in the poorest countries.

Despite this, the ICPD+5 review at the UN Special Session in 1999 reaffirmed international commitment to Safe Motherhood, setting out the kinds of strategic action needed. It was agreed that reduction of maternal mortality should be prominent in and used as an indicator of efforts to strengthen health systems.[9]

This book provides an overview of the problems and challenges raised by this work and examples of some of the efforts towards achieving Safe Motherhood in developing countries in the past decade. It contains papers by different authors, covering the following issues:

- the values and limitations of different forms of measurement of maternal mortality and morbidity;
- reviews and summaries of what has been planned and achieved in national policies and programmes, and what remains to be done;
- case studies of the causes of maternal deaths and morbidity; and
- how deaths can be prevented through effective, evidence-based policies and programmes.

It takes both a public health and a social justice perspective on these issues.

What has changed in the past decade and where are the stumbling blocks?

Ten years ago, there was a lack of knowledge and agreement internationally on which interventions were the most important and should be carried out first. This affected progress considerably. Today, there is both more information and greater consensus on what needs to be done, reflected in the papers in this book.

Improvements may appear to be slow in taking place, but there is always a time-lag between carrying out research, understanding and disseminating the results, developing nationally agreed policies and programmes, putting them into practice, reviewing progress and so on. Budgets and programmes are devised for periods of three to five years in advance. If an intervention has no impact in a five-year period, expectations as well as training and the deployment of staff and resources may all have to be revised accordingly. Furthermore, solutions must take account of the wide diversity of problems in different countries and regions; hence, they must be country-specific and based on good evidence. From this point of view, a decade is a very short time indeed.

At the Sri Lanka Consultation some decried the 'too-broad' approach to Safe Motherhood that is now being recommended – saying it would result in programmes that are too ambitious and expensive for governments and donors to take on.[12] What should countries be advised to do, then?

Setting priorities

Many inter-related factors contribute to maternal mortality. Women's low status and lack of decision-making power are important underlying factors. Women and their families need information in order to recognise the signs of complications; they need to be able to access care when complications develop and the resources to reach an appropriate care facility in time. The short period of time from the development of a serious complication to death means care must be available close to women's homes, or reachable further away by a quick and affordable means of transport. Nor can the importance of functioning health care facilities with well-trained providers in place be overstated.

Is there a definite sequence of what to do and who to work with first and next? Is it correct to start by putting good quality health facilities in place, and only then work with women and the community to get them to use these facilities? The answer is not so simple. There often needs to be pressure from the community on policymakers in the first place, as the women's health movement and many NGOs have shown in the past, for any substantial investment to be made. Furthermore, if quality of care means to meet women's needs, then community awareness on one side and accountability to the community on the other are required from the time that facilities are set up. At the same time, the health sector needs to improve the clinical skills and managerial capabilities of those providing care. Policymakers need to be involved in the planning of programmes which they have agreed to support, and leadership and commitment on the part of health professionals is a crucial element too. Thus, although the criticism made in Sri Lanka is understandable, there are good reasons to tackle the problem from all these different angles.

In the past, isolated, single-focus and sometimes competing projects have been set up, with little or no joint planning or co-operation. Institutions and organisations not uncommonly went their own way and acted as if they alone were doing the right thing – or felt they needed to work alone to justify their funding. This is clearly not the best way of achieving international goals. The way forward lies in partnerships among all potential stakeholders – health professionals, researchers, government ministries, policymakers and donors, women, communities, women's health advocates and health and development NGOs.

Addressing different aspects of the problem through integrated projects within limited geographical areas – rather than tackling only one aspect on a macro-scale – would also appear to be a more effective way to proceed. First, however, cohesive national strategies need to be evolved, so that each group of actors has an agreed role to play in addressing different facets of the problem. Priorities and goals need to be clearly defined, based on evidence of where the problems lie, using interventions that are focused and effective, and implemented in an incremental fashion.

Key lessons of the past decade

Some of the key lessons learned from important efforts in developing countries in the past decade have been:

- The 'risk' approach does not help to predict which women will develop complications and which women will not. It is necessary to start from the premise that complications can develop during or after any pregnancy.[13,14]
- Use of family planning methods by women who do not wish to become pregnant will reduce the number of women with unwanted pregnancies, and the deaths that might result from these, and resources must continue to be invested in the provision of contraceptive information and methods for both women and men. However, contraception does nothing to reduce the risk of complications and death once a woman is pregnant, whether her pregnancy is wanted or not.
- Training of traditional birth attendants (TBAs) and of community-based health workers with limited midwifery skills has not reduced maternal mortality.[15] The decision to work with TBAs arose in response to situations where health systems were weak, literacy levels among women were low, and there were few women with the requisite schooling to be trained as midwives. Traditional birth attendants should never have been expected to save women's lives in cases of obstetric emergency. They were not trained for this, but only to use safe birth kits, prevent sepsis and refer women to a higher level of care when complications arose or seemed imminent.
- The limited procedures carried out in the name of antenatal and post-partum (or post-natal) care have had little impact in lowering maternal mortality and morbidity. In many cases, this is because the services being provided are more for the benefit of infants than of women. Both women and infants

are important, but the interventions required for each are not identical and cannot be substituted one for the other. New paradigms are necessary to avoid turning two sets of distinct and legitimate needs into competing demands for appropriate care and attention.

- More resources have been put into antenatal care in developing countries than into delivery and immediate post-partum care, emergency obstetric care and safe abortions. Yet the vast majority of complications and deaths arise during and after delivery and in the first hours and days post-partum,[16] and from unsafe abortions.
- Operational difficulties owing to the poor functioning of health systems as a whole can make emergency obstetric care ineffective, even where facilities exist.[17]
- The values and limitations of different forms of measurement of levels and trends in maternal mortality have only recently become clear. Rather than trying to measure maternal mortality ratios more accurately, diagnostic, action-oriented means of gathering information on where, how and why deaths are occurring, and what kinds of action are needed and have been taken, are now recommended.

The unfinished agenda: making every maternal death count

An important basis for progress in the coming years has been a greater understanding of what works and what does not – and what still needs to be done. The most important items on this unfinished agenda include:

- ***Improving and upgrading of emergency obstetric services, providing in-service training for better diagnosis and treatment within referral facilities, improving management to reduce delays, and instituting mechanisms for audit/review of all maternal deaths, to support better practice.***

For midwives and doctors who have spent a lifetime fighting to improve the quality of midwifery and obstetric care in clinics and hospitals, it is a source of terrible frustration and dismay that many women arrive too late for their lives to be saved. Traditional birth attendants too, trained or not, feel helpless when women under their care die. On the other side, who can blame women and their families for delaying or deciding against attending health facilities when they have not recognised the seriousness of a complication or do not have the money or transport to access care anyway?

There has been much talk about women dying in childbirth because they did not come to a health facility. It is time to acknowledge how many women die despite reaching a health facility. Where problems such as a lack of essential drugs and equipment, a lack of competent staff, and professional delays and errors in diagnosis and treatment have been tackled head-on, the results have been swift and rewarding. Under the leadership of committed physicians and midwives, better management of resources, improvements in staff skills through on-the-job training, systematic reviews of all maternal deaths and near-miss events, adherence to standard treatment protocols, and promotion of professional responsibility can achieve a great deal in the space of several years. In addition, if all maternal deaths were classified as immediately and compulsorily notifiable to district health authorities, they could be investigated by maternal mortality committees.

- ***Training of professionally recognised, community- and facility-based midwives.***

We are still a long way from having skilled professionals providing care to all pregnant women in normal deliveries, handling basic obstetric emergencies using life-saving skills within their level of competency, and making referrals upwards for the rest. Midwives need to be accessible to every community, either as independent practitioners or attached to a primary health facility that provides pregnancy/delivery care.

Although WHO recommends at least one post-partum contact with a health worker during the first three days following delivery,[18] post-partum care does not feature as an essential part of maternal health care in developing countries, if at all. Yet there can be no greater tragedy than a woman going all the way to a district hospital to deliver and being discharged within a few hours or a day because of the shortage of beds, only to go home and die without medical help days or even hours later.

Further, there are legal restrictions in many countries which limit midwives' ability to respond to obstetric emergencies adequately, e.g. to administer oxytocins to stop bleeding in case of haemorrhage. Removal of such restrictions and more midwifery training should be important items on the agenda of all Safe Motherhood initiatives.

- ***Provision of safe, legal abortion services.***

Unsafe abortions continue to be a major cause of maternal death, accounting for about one in six of all maternal deaths globally, and a much higher proportion in some parts of the world. Yet some of the most vocal champions of Safe Motherhood are still walking tip-toe around this issue, in deference to the anti-abortion politics of a powerful minority. The plea for 'safe services for pregnancy termination where it is not against the law'[19] ignores the reality of why women are forced to undergo and die from dangerous abortions in the first place. These abortions are being self-induced or carried out by unskilled health workers and TBAs, using procedures which are outdated or carry a high risk.

Abortion by trained providers is a simple, safe, low-cost, life-saving intervention, which is needed by women worldwide. Treatment for abortion complications following unsafe procedures is better than letting women die untreated, but it is not an acceptable substitute for the legitimate provision of proper abortion services. Abortion law reform and training for midwives to provide medical and vacuum aspiration abortions is called for.

- ***Strengthening of primary care to improve women's general health and provide beneficial antenatal care, post-partum follow-up, family planning, health education on pregnancy and its complications.***

There are many situations where women arrive at a referral hospital from far away but cannot be saved because they received no first-level care. Many women are suffering from anaemia, parasitic infections and communicable diseases such as HIV, malaria and hepatitis, which compromise their general health and put their lives at risk. These problems call for strengthened public health activities at primary care level. Antenatal care should be redirected to these activities, and to giving health education to women, their families and communities on the signs of obstetric complications and how quickly these can lead to death, and making contingency plans with women to access emergency care if required.

- ***Giving professionally recognised midwives the responsibility to train and incorporate TBAs into the work of primary care facilities and the health system, and gradually to replace TBAs with midwives in the community.***

Training of traditional birth attendants and multi-purpose health workers in isolation has been shown time and again to be inadequate, yet such training goes on in some places as if nothing has been learned. In other quarters, in contrast, there is haste to do away with even this amount of training before an effective alternative exists to take its place.

Documentation of the work of TBAs in many settings has created awareness of their greater accessibility and interpersonal and culturally sensitive skills, which make them popular with women. This needs to be better understood by professionals. Programmes could integrate the strengths brought by TBAs, and where possible TBAs themselves, into the provision of services, in recognition of the fact that women will not automatically switch to trained midwives and hospitals overnight. The aim should be, however, to replace TBAs with trained midwives as soon as possible.

- ***The dimensions of chronic maternal morbidity as they affect women's lives need to be better documented in order to design interventions to address them.***

Millions of women suffer from acute and chronic morbidities such as poor repair of episiotomy and perineal tears, vesico-vaginal fistula and utero-vaginal prolapse, which can have a devastating effect on their ability to work, and on sexual relations and personal life generally. Although medical attention to all of these are badly needed, this will not alleviate the consequences of social and economic realities such as too early marriage, too frequent childbearing, poor obstetric practice and women being forced to resume heavy household work before they have recovered from childbirth.

- ***New clinical problems and dilemmas have also emerged which need to be recognised and taken account of.***

The presence of HIV infection in a large segment (as high as 20-30 per cent) of the antenatal population in a growing number of countries, especially in sub-Saharan Africa, has serious implications for increased maternal mortality and morbidity as well as infant deaths.

Further, there are practices such as symphysiotomy for dealing with obstructed labour which are no longer necessary in health systems with good maternity care. These still have a place when the standard of maternity care is poor and where the risk of death from complications of emergency caesarean section is high. This is an example of a highly technical issue which mainly concerns obstetricians in developing countries, but it is really about the level of development of tertiary-level care and whether doctors in the poorest countries are learning such skills today.

This book addresses all of these issues.

Needed: evidence, resources, leadership and action

Meeting the international development target for maternal mortality will be a tough challenge; indeed, the year 2000 will have come and gone long before the first target set in 1994 has been reached.[9] Young and poor women constitute the majority of women dying of pregnancy-related causes. Hence, what is particularly discouraging today is the existence of policies and resource crunches that are forcing all governments to cut health budgets, charge fees for services at the point of use and relinquish responsibility for certain health care services to the private sector. Further, across countries, policymakers are choosing to focus health resources on other pressing needs, such as communicable diseases, and choosing not to invest enough in what are uniquely women's health issues.[20]

Current models used to identify priorities in health sector reform undervalue pregnancy-related deaths and disability.[21] For example, the 'burden of disease' analysis, currently being used by sections of WHO and the World Bank to weight global spending on different aspects of disease and health, has so far under-estimated the magnitude and significance of maternal mortality and morbidity. This is due not only to lack of accurate prevalence data, but to the fact that neither co-morbidities, poor perinatal outcomes nor the knock-on effect within families and communities of maternal deaths and disability are factored in.[20]

These trends all serve to marginalise Safe Motherhood programmes for sufficient resource allocation. Furthermore, health-financing strategies such as user fees and privatisation of care are likely to restrict access to and utilisation of services by those most in need, in spite of good intentions to the contrary. Cuts in welfare spending in general do not augur well for women; they mean less investment in programmes to improve women's status through education and work, and to the social benefits which reduce and alleviate poverty.

Thus, in spite of the expressed support nationally and internationally for Safe Motherhood programmes, it is not yet clear where the substantial investment required to improve health systems, train midwives, strengthen hospitals and upgrade primary and secondary level care is to come from.

This book shows that highly medical, highly technical, and highly social and political aspects of Safe Motherhood exist side by side, all requiring attention. The most difficult issues are probably not the technical ones, but the political and economic ones.

The international community has made a strong commitment to maternal health. Strong and effective global leadership is now required. At the ICPD+5 review, the World Health Organization was charged with this role. While there is a limit to what any agency or individual donor can do on their own, if the international community works together with those at national level, real progress can and will be made.[9]

'Not simply because a maternal death is one of the most terrible ways to die...'[1]

Working to prevent maternal deaths is not an act of benevolence towards women because they are mothers, but the duty of all who respect human rights, which includes the right of women to life.

Acknowledgements

Thanks to Deborah Maine, John Worley, Carole Presern, Anne Tinker and Adrienne Germain for comments on and contributions to this text.

References

1. Fathalla M, 1997. Opening address, Safe Motherhood Technical Consultation, Colombo, Sri Lanka, 18-23 October.
2. Oakley A, 1986. The Captured Womb. Basil Blackwell, Oxford.
3. Loudon I, 1992. *Death in Childbirth. An International Study of Maternal Care and Maternal Mortality 1800-1950.* Clarendon Press, Oxford.
4. van Lerberghe, W, 1997. A historical perspective on maternal mortality reduction. Paper presented at Safe Motherhood Technical Consultation, Colombo, Sri Lanka, 18-23 October.
5. Drife JO, 1998. We know why they die. *BMJ*. 312:1044.
6. Starrs A, 1987. *Preventing the Tragedy of Maternal Deaths. A Report on the International Safe Motherhood Conference, Nairobi, Kenya, February 1987.* World Bank/World Health Organization/UNFPA.
7. Berer M (ed), 1988. *Maternal Mortality: A Call to Women for Action. International Day of Action for Women's Health, 28 May 1988.* WGNRR/LACWHN, Amsterdam and Santiago.
8. Starrs A, Inter-Agency Group for Safe Motherhood, 1997. *The Safe Motherhood Action Agenda: Priorities for the Next Decade. Report on the Safe Motherhood Technical Consultation, 18-23 October 1997, Colombo, Sri Lanka.* UNFPA/UNICEF/ World Bank/WHO/IPPF/Population Council/Family Health International, New York.
9. John Worley, Population and Reproductive Health Specialist, Carole Presern, Senior Health and Population Advisor, and Julia Cleves, Acting Chief - Health and Population Department, UK Department for International Development, Personal communication, August 1999.
10. Tinker A, 1999. *Safe Motherhood and the World Bank: lessons from ten years' experience.* (Draft)
11. Berer M, 1992. *Women's Groups, NGOs and Safe Motherhood.* Maternal Health and Safe Motherhood Programme, Division of Family Health, World Health Organization, Geneva.
12. Inter-Agency Group for Safe Motherhood, 1997. Introduction: The Safe Motherhood Initiative 1987-1997. In: *The Safe Motherhood Action Agenda, Priorities for the Next Decade. Report on the Safe Motherhood Technical Consultation, 18-23 October 1997, Colombo, Sri Lanka.* Inter-Agency Group for Safe Motherhood.
13. Graham W, 1997. Every pregnancy faces risks. In: *The Safe Motherhood Action Agenda, Priorities for the Next Decade. Report on the Safe Motherhood Technical Consultation, 18-23 October 1997, Colombo, Sri Lanka.* Inter-Agency Group for Safe Motherhood.
14. Maine D, Rosenfield A, Wallace M et al, 1987. Prevention of maternal mortality in developing countries: program options and practical considerations. Official background paper for the International Safe Motherhood Conference, Nairobi, February 1987.
15. Kamal IT, 1998. The traditional birth attendant: a reality and a challenge. *International Journal of Gynecology and Obstetrics.* 63(Suppl 1):S48-S52.
16. McDonagh M, 1996. Is antenatal care effective in reducing maternal morbidity and mortality? *Health Policy and Planning.* 11(1):1-15.
17. Le Coeur S, Pictet G, M'Pele P et al, 1998. Direct estimation of maternal mortality in Africa (Letter). *Lancet.* 352 (November 7):1525-26.
18. Inter-Agency Group for Safe Motherhood, 1997. Appendix A: Action Messages for the Tenth Anniversary. In: The Safe Motherhood Action Agenda, Priorities for the Next Decade. Report on the Safe Motherhood Technical Consultation, 18-23 October 1997, Colombo, Sri Lanka. Inter-Agency Group for Safe Motherhood.
19. Abou Zahr C, 1997. Improving access to good quality maternal health services. In: *The Safe Motherhood Action Agenda, Priorities for the Next Decade. Report on the Safe Motherhood Technical Consultation, 18-23 October 1997, Colombo, Sri Lanka.* Inter-Agency Group for Safe Motherhood.
20. Germain A, 1999. A gender perspective on the question: 'Does the DALY approach truly represent global needs?' Presentation at Annual Conference, Global Health Council, 29 June 1999. This paper is a commentary on analyses such as those found in: Murray CLJ, Lopez AD (eds), 1998. *Health Dimensions of Sex and Reproduction.* Global Burden of Disease & Injury Series, Vol 3. Harvard School of Public Health, WHO/World Bank.
21. See discussion of health sector reform in: Cassels A, 1995. Health sector reform: key issues in less developed countries. *Journal of International Development.* 7(4):329-47. Discussed by Germain in [20].

Measurement: its values and limitations

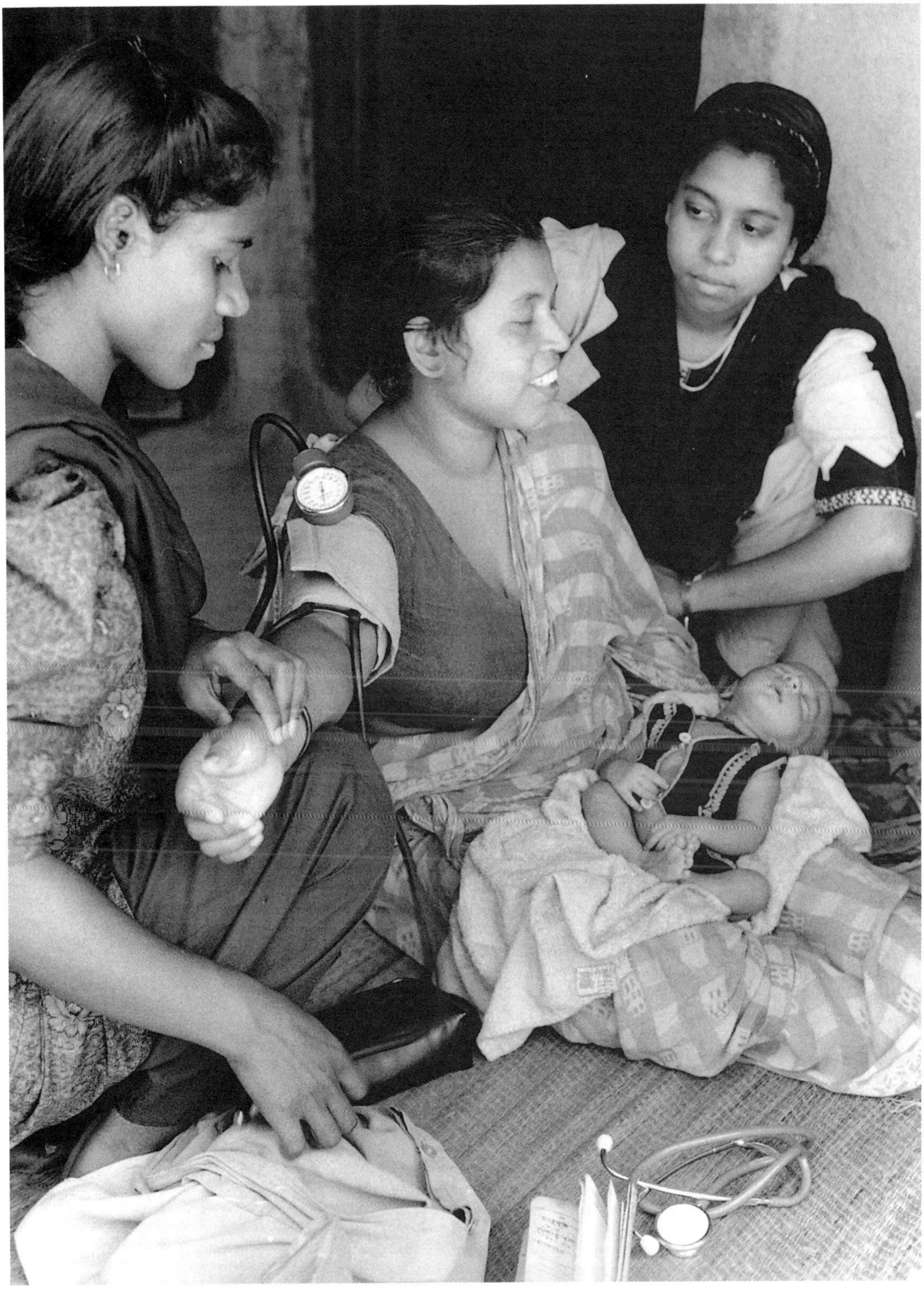

JENNY MATTHEWS

Measuring Maternal Mortality: What Do We Need to Know?

Carla AbouZahr

Knowing the dimensions of a problem is generally regarded as an essential first step in public health action. However, this presupposes that accurate measurement tools are available. Measuring maternal mortality is problematic because the approaches currently available are complex, resource intensive and imprecise, and the results are often misleading. The time has come to shift the focus from measurement to analysis, from trying to determine the size of the problem to seeking to understanding its underlying causes and determinants. Qualitative research techniques, used at local health facility level can provide action-oriented information that is probably more useful to programme managers and planners. Such techniques, starting at local level health care facilities, can answer the questions of why maternal deaths occur and what can be done to avert them.

'YOU don't have to know where you are to be there, but it is helpful to know where you are if you wish to be someplace else.'[1] It is axiomatic in public health that action to address a problem should follow from a knowledge of its dimensions and nature. Maternal mortality was a neglected issue during the 1970s and early 1980s, less because health professionals in developing countries were unaware of the problem than because they lacked the tools to quantify and analyse it. Countries with the ability to measure maternal mortality were precisely those where levels were low and vice versa.

Why measurement of maternal deaths began

During the 1980s, studies in several developing countries drew attention to a problem of some considerable magnitude[2] – not only the issue of maternal mortality but also the methodological challenge of adequately measuring it. This stimulated the establishment of the international Safe Motherhood Initiative in 1987. Early on, it was acknowledged that the most reliable measurement method – comprehensive and accurate registration of deaths coupled with medical certification of cause of death – would not be feasible in most developing countries within the foreseeable future. Attention turned, therefore, to other techniques, some of them adapted from experiences in measuring infant mortality in developing countries.

The 10th anniversary of the Safe Motherhood Initiative was marked by an international technical consultation in Sri Lanka in October 1997.[3] It provided an opportunity to share lessons learned and assess progress both in implementing safe motherhood programmes and in measuring the dimensions of the problem. The latter was the subject of considerable discussion, if not controversy. With the hindsight of over a decade of measurement experience, one might have anticipated a degree of consensus around levels and trends, and on the most appropriate and cost-effective measurement methods for use in different settings. In practice, it was clear that there continue to be important differences in opinion regarding what should be measured, the strengths and weaknesses of different approaches and how the results should be interpreted.[3]

Key measurement issues

The key measurement issues can be summarised as follows. Few developing countries (notable exceptions being Cuba, China, Malaysia, Sri Lanka, and a number of Latin American countries) have a vital registration system of sufficient coverage and quality to enable it to serve as the basis for the assessment of levels and trends in maternal mortality.[4] While household surveys using direct estimation would appear at first sight to provide a promising alternative, and have been used in developing countries such as Indonesia[5] and Ethiopia,[6] in practice they have a number of serious weaknesses. For a start, they are extremely expensive and complex to implement, because large sample sizes are needed to provide a statistically reliable estimate. The most frequently quoted example is the household survey in Addis Ababa, Ethiopia, where it was necessary to interview more than 32,300 households to identify 45 deaths and produce an estimated maternal mortality ratio of 480. At the 95 per cent level of significance this gives a sampling error of about 30 per cent, i.e. the ratio could lie anywhere between 370 and 660.[6]

The problem of wide confidence intervals is not simply that such estimates are imprecise. They may also lead to inappropriate interpretation of the figures. For example, using point estimates for maternal mortality may give the impression that the maternal mortality ratio is significantly different in different settings or at different times. In fact, maternal mortality may in truth be rather similar because the confidence intervals overlap (see Chart 1).[7]

The large costs associated with such household surveys led researchers to develop more cost-efficient alternatives, the most well-known and elegant of which is the Sisterhood method, developed during the late 1980s.[8] It is an indirect measurement technique of the kind frequently used to measure a variety of demographic parameters (such as child or adult mortality), which has been adapted for the measurement of maternal mortality. The method substantially reduces sample size requirements, because it obtains information by interviewing respondents about the survival of all their adult sisters. Respondents are asked four simple questions about how many of their sisters reached adulthood, how many have died and whether those who died were pregnant around the time of death. The term 'indirect' is used because the indicator of interest, the maternal mortality ratio, is not obtained directly. Instead, the risk of death is first obtained from the answers to the questions about the survival of respondents' sisters and subsequently transformed into the ratio through a series of simple mathematical calculations.

The Sisterhood questions can be added to an ongoing study and take very little additional

Chart 1. Are levels of maternal mortality really different in these three settings?

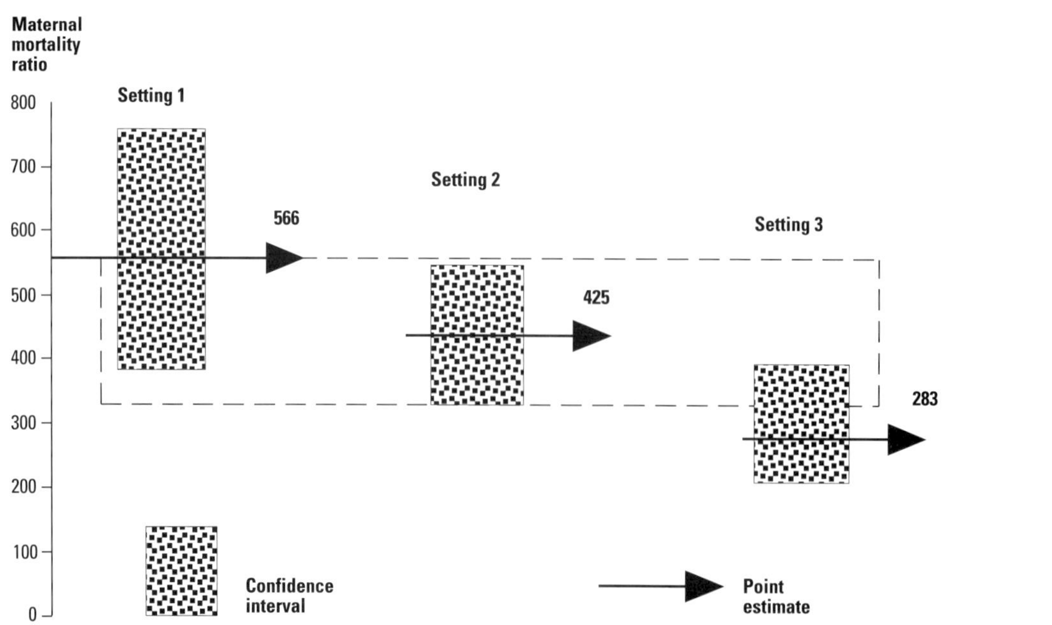

time, so the method is particularly cost-effective. The method relies on a number of assumptions about the relationships between fertility and age-specific maternal mortality. It should not be used, therefore, in settings where levels of fertility are low (Total Fertility Rate below 3), or where there have been recent and marked declines in fertility, or major migration. Because respondents' reports cover deaths occurring over a large interval time, the results generate an overall estimate of maternal mortality for a point centred around 10-12 years before the survey.[9] Studies using this methodology have been undertaken in a range of developing countries.

The Demographic and Health Surveys have been using a variant of the approach, rather confusingly known as the 'direct' Sisterhood method because the maternal mortality ratio is calculated directly from the information obtained from respondents' sister's birth histories.[10] This method involves asking respondents to provide more detailed information about their sisters, including the number reaching adulthood, the number who have died, the age at death, the year in which the death occurred and the years since the death. These questions can also be added to an ongoing survey, but they require more time than the four questions of the original method. Also, because the questions themselves are more complex and time-consuming to administer, additional efforts are needed to train and supervise interviewers and to correct for misreporting.[10] The direct approach relies on fewer assumptions than the original, indirect method, but it requires larger sample sizes and the information generated is considerably more complex to analyse. The direct method does not provide a current estimate of maternal mortality, but the larger sample sizes permit the calculation of a ratio for a more recent period of time. The reference point for a survey based on a reference period of 0-7 years would be 3-4 years prior to the data collection.

Both methods provide estimates of maternal mortality that should be seen as giving orders of magnitude, rather than precise ratios, since both can have large standard errors (that is, wide confidence intervals). Neither method provides a current estimate for the year of the survey. For these reasons, Sisterhood studies cannot be used to monitor changes in maternal mortality nor to assess the impact of safe motherhood programmes in the short term (usually taken as meaning within periods of less than 5 years). Both direct and indirect methods will tend to under-report early pregnancy deaths, particularly those related to abortion or those that occur among unmarried women. These issues will always be difficult to address and under-reporting of abortion-related mortality is common to all currently available methods for measuring maternal mortality.

A direct validation study of the indirect Sisterhood method for data collection on maternal deaths was recently completed in the Matlab area of Bangladesh.[11] This area is unique in having had a Demographic Surveillance System (DSS) in operation since 1966. Reporting of maternal and non-maternal deaths of sisters by respondents was compared with DSS classification of deaths. Of the 384 maternal deaths for which siblings were interviewed, 305 deaths (79 per cent) were correctly reported, 16 (4 per cent) were not reported and 63 (16 per cent) were misreported as non-maternal deaths. Misreporting was most likely for all women when induced abortion was the probable cause of death and for deaths of women who were unmarried when they became pregnant and died. It is probable that deaths related to direct obstetric causes have the best chance of being reported in a Sisterhood survey.[12]

Sisterhood methods are generally used to produce an estimate of the dimensions of the problem rather than an analysis of its causes. For the latter, more in-depth investigations are required. One way of finding out why women died – in settings where deaths often occur outside health care facilities and medical certification of cause of death and autopsy are not available – is through verbal autopsy.[13] This technique uses lay reporters, interviewers and a review panel who, after examining the lay reports (the symptoms leading to the death), assign the cause of death to ICD categories. The reliability of verbal autopsy for identifying maternal deaths has not been established, and there is some evidence that the method may fail to correctly identify some maternal deaths, particularly those associated with abortion complications or occurring some time after the termination of pregnancy, e.g. due to sepsis. All such methods require great care in their application and different interviewers and interviewing techniques can greatly influence the reliability of the results.

As experience with different methodologies has accumulated over the past few years, it has become clear that obtaining comprehensive information about maternal mortality requires the use of a variety of sources of information. The investigation of a group of deaths of women of reproductive age and in-depth study of those identified as maternal is generally known as a Reproductive Age Mortality Study (RAMOS).[14] This involves identifying and investigating the causes of all deaths of women of reproductive age and has been used successfully in countries as different as Egypt,[15] Honduras,[16] and Jamaica.[17] How the deaths are identified differs according to the records and/or the types of knowledgeable informants available. All successful studies use multiple and varied sources of information – civil registers, hospitals and health centres, community leaders, schoolchildren, religious authorities, undertakers, cemetery officials etc. A general finding has been that no single source identifies all the deaths.[18] RAMOS approaches can, when competently handled, provide valuable insights into the circumstances leading up to maternal deaths. They do not always provide good data on levels of maternal mortality, however, because of the difficulties encountered in matching the numerator with an appropriate denominator.

Limitations and difficulties: not unique to this field

It is important to be aware that the difficulties inherent in measuring maternal mortality are not unique to this field. The measurement of cause-specific adult mortality is complex and resource-intensive, whatever the specific cause of death. The situation may change in the near future. Interest in the measurement of adult mortality in general is increasing and may result in further methodological developments. One example is the recent, renewed interest in using the decennial censuses to provide estimates of maternal mortality. A high quality decennial census could include questions on deaths in the household in the last two years, followed by more detailed questions which would permit the identification of maternal deaths (verbal autopsy). The advantages of such an approach are that it would generate both national and sub-national figures and that it would be possible to undertake analysis according to the characteristics of the household. The approach would generate all the major maternal mortality indicators (ratio, rate, lifetime risk and proportionate mortality ratio). Trend analysis would be possible because sampling errors would be eliminated or greatly reduced.

Despite the clear attractions of using the census to generate maternal mortality data, many researchers remain unconvinced that the approach would prove of value in practice. The existing literature on direct and indirect estimation of overall adult mortality via a census in the developing world suggests that enquiries into recent deaths in the household in a census have rarely provided useful information.[19] For example, in the majority of African censuses, 40-50 per cent of deaths may have been omitted. Common problems can be classified as those relating to respondent difficulties (omission of events and poor reporting of age at death); interviewer difficulties (lack of sensitivity and inadequate training); and difficulties relating to household structure and characteristics (omission of reporting or possible double-counting where adults live between more than one household). Nonetheless, a number of countries have used the census to generate maternal mortality figures and work is underway (notably, through the Measure 2 project implemented by Macro Inc) to assess the extent to which such approaches may prove of value in measuring maternal mortality.

What can we conclude following this summary of measurement techniques? Measuring maternal mortality is difficult, not because of the lack of measurement tools – several alternatives are now available – but because the resource requirements needed for accurate measurement are too great. There is an inevitable trade-off that has to be made between a method that provides an accurate and complete estimate of maternal mortality and one that is affordable and feasible in resource-constrained settings. How can we balance the apparently conflicting demands of the need for information with the absence of resources required to generate it? The answer to the conundrum lies in looking again at what we are trying to measure and why. Should we focus on finding out the dimensions of the problem or would we be better off directing a larger share of limited resources into efforts to understand why the problem exists? What balance should we seek between measurement and in-depth understanding? I shall argue in this paper that answering this question will provide the information we need for decision-making on the use of resources and on what should be measured and how. Essentially, the question we should be asking ourselves is why do we need information and what will we do with it once we have it?

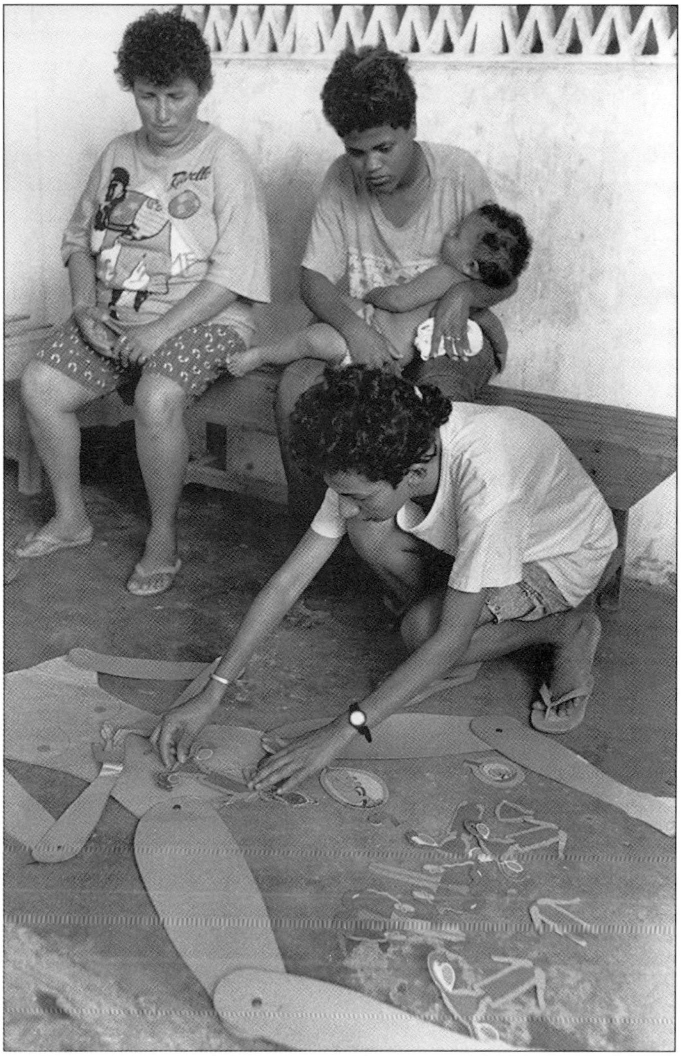

JENNY MATTHEWS

What we are trying to measure and why

Let us look again at what we are trying to measure. Most studies of maternal mortality focus on measuring the maternal mortality ratio, that is, the number of maternal deaths divided by the number of live births in a given population and time period. There are very good reasons for focusing on the ratio. This is, after all, the statistic that best expresses the dangers that women face once pregnant, that is, the obstetric risk. However, the ratio does not reflect the relationship between maternal mortality and fertility and may hide what is really going on rather than illuminate it. For example, it is possible for the ratio to remain unchanged despite decreases in both the maternal mortality rate and in general fertility. On the other hand, a rise in the ratio can be accompanied by falls in both the rate and in total fertility.[20]

There are other problems with the maternal mortality ratio that make measurement particularly difficult. The most obvious is absolute numbers. The maternal mortality ratio is composed of a small number in the numerator (maternal deaths) divided by a comparatively large number in the denominator (live births). This is true even in settings where maternal mortality levels are very high; the number in the denominator is usually at least 100 times larger than the number in the numerator. It is because of this that it is usual to apply an inflation factor of 100,000; the ratio is expressed per 100,000 live births rather than per 1000 (as for infant mortality) or as a percentage.[21] Because the numerator is very small, the maternal mortality ratio can fluctuate widely, particularly where levels are quite low. This makes it difficult to assess progress on a year-on-year basis and it is often necessary to apply moving averages to ascertain the direction of a trend.

Another problem relates to interpretation. The maternal mortality ratio is often used alongside the infant mortality rate. However, this is to invite invidious and inappropriate comparisons. Although the maternal mortality ratio may look like the smaller of the two, women usually face the risk more than once in their lives whereas an infant can only face the risk of infant death once. This has led some researchers to favour the use of the lifetime risk of death which summarises the cumulative risk of pregnancy-related death faced by women across their reproductive lives.

Whatever the problems associated with measuring the maternal mortality ratio, the fact remains that the real challenge lies in the essential first step, the identification of the numerator – maternal deaths themselves. Researchers have argued against using numerator data alone for the very good reason that it is not possible to draw any conclusions about trends or to make meaningful comparisons when using absolute numbers as opposed to ratios or rates. These are compelling arguments if the question that one is trying to answer is 'Where do we stand compared with others?' or 'Has the situation changed over the past few years?'. But if the question that we want to answer is 'Why are maternal deaths happening?', analysis of maternal deaths themselves is more likely to provide the answer than knowledge of ratios or rates.

Answering the 'why' question is more important for programme planners that answering the 'how much' question. In Sri Lanka, there was a consensus that purely quantitative indicators, such as the maternal mortality ratio, have important limitations; they offer no insight into why maternal deaths occur or what programme managers need to do to prevent them. To gather such information, other tools, often qualitative in nature, have to be used.

Using qualitative information to supplement quantitative information is, of course, not new. In many developed countries, quantitative information on levels of maternal mortality is routinely supplemented and its value enhanced by the in-depth analysis of cases of maternal death, through facility-based audits and national-level confidential enquiries. In the UK, for example, the system of confidential enquiries started in 1952 and has served since then as a mechanism for improving the quality of maternal health care.[22] In the USA, the Centers for Disease Control (CDC) uses the term, maternal mortality epidemiological surveillance, to describe the ongoing and systematic study of maternal deaths.[23] Similar approaches are gradually being adopted as an element of maternal health policy in a number of Latin American and Caribbean states.[23] The goal of such surveillance is to obtain information to guide public health efforts to address the problem.

'Collecting data is a mechanism for obtaining information but is not in itself the goal.' [24]

The key point is that counting cases – and calculating the maternal mortality ratio or rate – is not enough.

'The data must lead to information that can, in turn, lead to specific recommendations and actions, as well as to an evaluation of the interventions.' [24]

Using a variety of sources, both quantitative and qualitative

The first step is, of course, the identification of maternal deaths. Methods used to determine which deaths are maternal will vary from country to country. In settings with vital registration, the starting point is usually death certificates for women of reproductive age (generally 15-49 although in some settings the younger age limit can be 12 or 10 years). However, a finding that holds true in all settings is that one cannot assume that vital records by themselves are sufficient for the ascertainment of all maternal deaths. The key to success is active case finding; the degree of completeness of maternal death ascertainment depends critically on the rigour with which active case finding is conducted.

For example, although it is possible to count as maternal all the deaths classified by ICD-9 codes 630 through 676.9, reliance on this source will result in a proportion of maternal deaths being missed. Researchers often find, for example, that death certificates that at first sight appear to record a death unrelated to pregnancy, turn out on closer inspection to contain margin annotations indicating maternal conditions. One way of dealing with this problem is to introduce a check box on all death certificates indicating whether or not the deceased was or had been pregnant in the previous year. This modification in Puerto Rico in 1989 resulted in the identification of an additional 69 per cent of maternal deaths.[25]

Another mechanism for active case-finding is to link death certificates to birth certificates or, in some cases, certificates of other pregnancy outcomes such as fetal deaths. Such linkages resulted in increases in maternal mortality ratios of between 30 per cent and 150 per cent in the USA.[25,26] A recent review of maternal mortality found that in the USA at least six different sources can be used to identify deaths related to pregnancy.[27] These included, in addition to published vital records:

- a manual review of death certificates to identify additional cases in which pregnancy has been indicated on the death certificate;
- using vital record linkage to match death certificates for women of reproductive age to certificates of reportable pregnancy outcomes (live births, stillbirths, fetal deaths and, sometimes, abortion);
- review of autopsy reports;
- review of medical records;
- interviews with family members, health care providers, etc.

Different countries have tried different approaches for identifying all maternal deaths. Some have established task forces to undertake periodic reviews of all deaths of women of reproductive age, with active case-finding of maternal deaths. In France, such a review took place retrospectively and involved an analysis of all death certificates of women aged 15-44 years.[28] An important reason for the failure to identify a maternal death correctly was simple clerical or coding error; 17 of the 41 deaths reported as being related to maternal conditions by the certifying doctor were subsequently miscoded by the coding clerks.

Where death certificates are not sufficiently reliable or widespread to serve as the starting point for maternal death identification, other approaches have to be used. Many researchers advocate community identification of deaths. Clearly, success depends critically on community members being interested in and willing to report maternal deaths, as well as on their ability to correctly identify which deaths are likely to have been pregnancy-related. In some settings local Maternal Mortality Committees visit funeral homes, cemeteries, places of worship and community leaders to follow up reports or rumours of pregnancy-related deaths. In Mexico, for example, a Simplified Surveillance System designed for TBAs and non-literate people contains pictures of signs and symptoms designed to facilitate identification of maternal deaths and their immediate causes.[29]

In practice, community-based death identification is difficult and unlikely to be sustainable. It requires close and continuing relationships of mutual trust and information sharing between local communities and the health authorities, a situation that is often difficult to establish and maintain in circumstances where the demands on health services and providers are multiple and resources extremely limited. Indeed, there is no evidence of community-based identification of maternal deaths having been maintained beyond the life of a study or research project such as a reproductive age mortality study (RAMOS). In Honduras, for example, a RAMOS approach carried out over a 12-month period in 1989-90 stimulated considerable interest and was successful in identifying a large number of previously unrecognised maternal deaths. However, once the study ended and the researchers moved on to other responsibilities, the numbers of maternal deaths reported fell by more than three-quarters.[16]

This raises the question of how sustainable community identification of maternal deaths is likely to be in settings where vital records are not available or inadequate. Identifying maternal deaths, even in a local setting, requires a lot of work and may divert energies and resources away from programme implementation. The answer lies in adapting the method to the specific, local circumstances. A stepwise approach is needed, which may involve initially focusing on areas where the problem is particularly acute, or simply where some information is available to provide a starting point for analysis. Alternatively, it may be possible to start by confining work to pilot areas and extending to cover a larger area once the skills and competences have been built up.

The problems inherent in community-based identification of maternal deaths have led researchers to look again at the most simple approach, namely, focusing on deaths occurring in health care facilities. While it is important to be aware that such deaths are a non-representative sample and should not be used to calculate rates and ratios, there are, nonetheless, important advantages in such an approach. Maternal deaths that occur in a hospital are usually the easiest to identify. Moreover, hospital records often contain valuable information on the medical factors that contributed to the death. This is too valuable a source of information to be ignored despite the problem of non-representativeness. Furthermore, it is possible to supplement the quality of information and to build up a picture of community factors contributing to maternal deaths by extending information-gathering beyond the health facility and into the community itself. This is the approach recommended by WHO in the Maternal Death Review (MDR).[30]

The MDR is a 'qualitative, in-depth investigation of the causes and circumstances surrounding a small number of maternal deaths occurring at selected health facilities.'[30] It involves taking as a starting point a death within the health care facility and using quantitative and qualitative data collection methods to formulate hypotheses about weak points in the maternal health care system and how they might be overcome. The MDR thus goes further than the hospital-based audit because it involves investigating events beyond the health facility, such as those taking place within communities or families. In order for this approach to work, it is necessary to involve communities themselves rather than only facility-based health care providers. Inputs from a multi-disciplinary team composed of formal and informal health care providers, different levels of the health care system, community members, women and families not only serve to improve the quality of the data collected, but also contribute to advocacy and consensus-building around interventions to address the problem. The MDR can become a mechanism for improving the quality of care if the identification of sub-standard care is accompanied by interventions to address the underlying reasons for it. Building a feedback component into the MDR turns it from simply a descriptive tool to a more pro-active, quality enhancing one.

Some researchers feel that despite the undoubted benefits of such in-depth investigations of individual cases, maternal deaths are too infrequent to provide adequate numbers for meaningful analysis (see Chart 2). Several strategies are being tested to try to overcome this problem. One involves broadening the scope to include other adverse pregnancy outcomes as well as maternal deaths. These might include, for example, severe complications or perinatal deaths.

Using perinatal outcomes to increase the number of events available for analysis has been criticised on the grounds that: (a) the causes of perinatal deaths are likely to differ in significant ways from the causes of maternal deaths, and (b) the lessons learned from analysing them will have different implications for the care of mothers and children.[31] There is some validity in these criticisms. A substantial proportion of perinatal mortality is due to inadequate care of the newborn (management of asphyxia, control of hypothermia, management of infections, management of congenital anomalies) and can provide only circumstantial evidence of sub-standard care of the woman herself.

A more promising avenue is the study of severe maternal complications, or 'near-misses'. The concept was originally developed in the UK to monitor the quality of obstetric care at hospital level and the occurrence of life-threatening complications at regional level.[32] A method of defining near-misses in developing country situations is possible but only at the hospital level and only if good hospital records are available.

A collaborative study conducted in 1995-96 developed algorithms to define near-miss cases in the context of inadequate health records and to test them in the main university maternity hospital in Cotonou, Benin.[33] Cases were identified retrospectively through a review of medical records. Over a 12-month period there were

Chart 2. Annual maternal deaths expected at different given levels of maternal mortality

Deliveries		Number of deaths if:		
Weekly	Annually	MMR = 200	MMR = 400	MMR = 600
5	260	<1	1	2
20	1040	2	4	8
40	2080	4	8	17
100	5200	10	21	42

4291 deliveries, 1170 direct obstetric complications, 353 near-misses and 30 maternal deaths. In other words, for every maternal death there were nearly 12 serious, life-threatening complications in which the women survived. Case-fatality rates were highest for puerperal infections (21 per cent), followed by haemorrhage (9 per cent), eclampsia (5 per cent) and dystocia (4 per cent). Analysis of the factors associated with death revealed that the timing of the admission (time, day of the week and season) and prompt treatment were the most significant.

The main methodological problem to be resolved is the development of reproducible and valid case definitions of near-misses. Researchers in developed countries have often defined near-misses as cases admitted to the intensive care ward. The problem with this definition is that many life-threatening complications may never be admitted to the intensive care ward because they are managed in the operating theatre and thereafter sent directly to the recovery ward. Some researchers advocate clinical definitions of near-miss events such as post-partum blood loss of 1,000 ml or more. Others advise definitions based on 'rapid deterioration of clinical signs', and others simply on subjective clinical judgement on the part of the attending health care providers – 'this woman nearly died'. As this is a relatively new area, where such definitions have yet to be agreed upon by the clinical and research community, readers are advised to seek expert advice if this sort of study is being considered.

Qualitative approaches such as those described here can offer a range of benefits. They can:

- help create awareness among health care providers and among communities that maternal deaths are avoidable;
- help create stronger linkages between the health care facility and the community;
- provide actionable data for improving quality of care;
- rationalise routine statistics gathering and reporting;
- stimulate the development of reporting systems that are responsive to changing needs in the health service;
- strengthen linkages between users and collectors of data; and
- provide timely feedback relevant to improving quality of care.

Most important of all, however, they can provide answers to the question 'Why do maternal deaths occur and what can be done to prevent them?'

Conclusions

We have reached a stage in our understanding of maternal mortality at which it is necessary to turn more of our attention towards comprehensive approaches to measurement and information generation, using diagnostic, action-oriented, analytical techniques designed to improve programme implementation. Does this mean that we should stop trying to measure actual levels and indicators such as the MMR, or that the measurement approaches developed over the past decade or so – e.g. Sisterhood surveys, RAMOS – should be abandoned? Clearly not.

Knowing the level of maternal mortality and how it changes over time is an important goal but it is one that can be achieved only in the long term, as countries increase their efforts to develop comprehensive and sustainable systems of vital registration.[34] In the meantime, and despite their limitations, population based measurement approaches remain important tools for use in specific circumstances and settings. The more cost-effective of them – the variants of the Sisterhood method – are particularly valuable tools for policy-makers and health planners who want a rough estimate of maternal mortality. But they do provide just that – an approximate or 'ball park' estimate – and should not be taken as offering precise and accurate information on levels and still less as providing data on trends. For the latter, the use of process indicators which are causally related to maternal health outcomes and responsive to and reflective of change, is recommended.[7]

An excellent example of the value of re-directing efforts towards approaches that help answer 'why' questions is a recently published study from Nepal.[35] Two direct Sisterhood studies in Nepal found levels of maternal mortality ratios of the order of 500-600 per 100,000 live births. Yet what these studies could not provide was information on the underlying reasons for these deaths or pointers for policy direction. Therefore, the Ministry of Health conducted a detailed investigative study into the medical and non-medical causes of death, using a combination of quantitative and qualitative approaches, and bringing together information from both community and facility sources. The resultant study now provides a firm evidence base upon which the Government of Nepal and its partners in the multi-lateral, bilateral and NGO community can build a substantive safe motherhood programme.

What then should our conclusions be? First, the use to which we intend to put information on maternal mortality should drive our data collection efforts and choice of sources and methodologies. Second, no single source of data on maternal mortality offers a complete and reliable picture of the situation. We must use a variety of sources and approaches, depending on the setting and resources available. Third, we should supplement quantitative data with qualitative information. There is much to be learned from examining individual maternal deaths and not just the aggregated statistics. If we can maintain this perspective, our decision-making will be more rational and we will be able to make better use of limited resources.

Correspondence

Carla AbouZahr, Department of Reproductive Health and Research, World Health Organization, Ave Appia, 1211 Geneva 27, Switzerland. Fax 41-22-791-4189. E-mail: abouzahrc@who.ch

Note

The views expressed in this paper are those of the author and do not necessarily represent those of the World Health Organization.

References and Notes

1. Foege WH, 1996. Foreword. In: *The Global Burden of Disease.* Murray CJL, Lopez AD (eds). World Health Organization, Harvard School of Public Health, World Bank.
2. World Health Organization, 1991. *Maternal Mortality Ratios and Rates: A Tabulation of Available Information.* WHO/MCH/MSM/91.6.
3. Starrs A, 1998. The Safe Motherhood Action Agenda: Priorities for the next decade. *Report on the Safe Motherhood Technical Consultation, 18-23 October 1997, Colombo, Sri Lanka.* Family Care International, New York.
4. AbouZahr C, 1998. Maternal mortality overview, In: *Health Dimensions of Sex and Reproduction.* Global Burden of Disease and Injury Series, Murray CJL, Lopez AD (eds). World Health Organization, Harvard School of Public Health, World Bank.
5. Agoestina T, Soejoenoes A, 1989. *Technical report on the study of maternal and perinatal mortality, Central Java Province.* Republic of Indonesia, BKS PENFIN/ Ministry of Health.
6. Kwast BE et al, 1985. Epidemiology of maternal mortality in Addis Ababa: a community-based study. *Ethiopian Medical Journal.* 23:7-16.
7. WHO, UNICEF and UNFPA, 1997. *Guidelines for Monitoring the Availability and Use of Obstetric Services.* WHO, UNICEF and UNFPA.
8. Graham W, Brass W, Snow RW, 1989. Indirect estimation of maternal mortality: the sisterhood method. *Studies in Family Planning.* 20(3):125-35.
9. WHO and UNICEF, 1997. *The Sisterhood Method for Estimating Maternal Mortality: Guidance Notes for Potential Users.* WHO/RHT/97.28 and UNICEF/EPP/97.1.
10. Rutenberg N, Sullivan JM, 1991. *Direct and Indirect Estimates of Maternal Mortality from the Sisterhood Method.* IRD/Macro International Inc, Washington DC.
11. Shahidullah M, 1995. The sisterhood method of estimating maternal mortality: the Matlab experience. *Studies in Family Planning.* 26(2):101-06.
12. Shahidullah M, 1995. A comparison of sisterhood information on causes of maternal death with the registration causes of maternal death in Matlab, Bangladesh. *International Journal of Epidemiology.* 24:937-42.
13. World Health Organization, 1995. *Verbal Autopsies for Maternal Deaths.* WHO/FHE/MSM/95.15, WHO, Geneva
14. World Health Organization, 1987. *Studying Maternal Mortality in Developing Countries: A Guidebook.* WHO/FHE/87.7.
15. Ministry of Health, Child Survival Project, 1994. *National Maternal Mortality Study. Findings and Conclusions. Egypt, 1992-1993.* July. In cooperation with USAID, Egypt.
16. Castellanos M et al, 1990. *Mortalidad materna. Investigación sobre mortalidad de mujeres en edad reproductiva con énfasis en mortalidad materna.* Honduras. SSA.
17. Walker GJ et al, 1986. Maternal

mortality in Jamaica. *Lancet.* 1(8479):486-88.
18. Walker GJA, McCaw-Bins A, Ashley DEC, Bernard GW, 1990. Identifying deaths in developing countries. Experiences from Jamaica. *International Journal of Epidemiology* 19:599-605.
19. Timeaus I, 1987. Estimation of fertility and mortality from WFS household surveys. In: Cleland J, Scott CJ (eds). *The World Fertility Survey: An Assessment.* Oxford, Clarendon Press.
20. Campbell OMR, Graham WJ, 1990. *Measuring Maternal Mortality and Morbidity: Levels and Trends.* Maternal and Child Epidemiology Unit, London School of Hygiene and Tropical Medicine.
21. Early estimates of levels of maternal mortality in Sweden, Netherlands, and England and Wales expressed the ratio in terms of thousands rather than hundreds of thousands. The latter was introduced gradually as levels fell, in order to make some sense of the very low ratios that became common in those countries after World War II.
22. Lewis G, Drife J et al, 1998. *Why Mothers Die: Report on Confidential Enquiries into Maternal Deaths in the United Kingdom 1994-1996.* Department of Health, Welsh Office, Scottish Office, Department of Health and Social Services Northern Ireland. HMSO.
23. Centers for Disease Control and Prevention, 1992. *National Pregnancy Mortality Surveillance Coding Manual.* Atlanta, DHHS PHS.
24. Berg C, Danel I, Mora G, 1996. *Guidelines for Maternal Mortality Epidemiological Surveillance.* Pan American Health Organization, Washington DC.
25. Centers for Disease Control and Prevention,1991. Maternal mortality surveillance – Puerto Rico 1989. *Mortality and Morbidity Weekly Report.* 40:521-23.
26. Centers for Disease Control, 1995. Pregnancy-related mortality Georgia, 1990-1992. *Mortality and Morbidity Weekly Report.* 44:93-96. And: Centers for Disease Control, 1991. Enhanced maternal mortality surveillance – North Carolina, 1988 and 1989. *Mortality and Morbidity Weekly Report.* 40:469-71.
27. Atrash H, Alexander S, Berg C, 1995. Maternal mortality in developed countries: not just a concern of the past. *Obstetrics and Gynecology.* 86(4). (II)
28. Bouvier-Colle et al, 1991. Reasons for the under reporting of maternal mortality in France, as indicated by a survey of all deaths of women of childbearing age. *International Journal of Epidemiology.* 20:717-21.
29. Alvarez Fernandez DL et al, 1994. La productividad de las parteras a traves del sistema de vigilancia epidemiologica simplificada de la partera. In: *La partera traditional en la atención materno-infantil en Mexico.* Programa Nacional de Parteras Tradicionales, Dirección General de Atención Materna.
30. World Health Organization, 1997. Maternal death review guidelines: field testing version. (Unpublished)
31. World Health Organization, 1994. *Indicators to Monitor Maternal Health Goals. Report of a Technical Working Group.* Maternal Health and Safe Motherhood Programme, WHO/FHE/MSM/94.14e.
32. Stones W, Lim W, Al-Azzawai F, Kelly M, 1991. An investigation of maternal morbidity with identification of life-threatening 'near miss' episodes. *Health Trends* 23: 13-15.
33. Filippi V, Alihonou E, Mukantaganda S, Graham W, Ronsmans C, 1998. Near misses: maternal morbidity and mortality. *Lancet* 351:145-46.
34. Vital registration is an important tool for a range of social, economic and political policy development and decision-making, not just for health.
35. Government of Nepal, 1998. *Maternal Mortality and Morbidity Study.* Family Health Division, Department of Health Services, Ministry of Health, Nepal.

Process Indicators for Maternal Mortality Programmes

Tessa Wardlaw, Deborah Maine

In order to monitor progress in the Safe Motherhood Initiative, we must have indicators that can register changes in a relatively short period of time (e.g. 3-5 years). Furthermore, if monitoring is to be an ongoing process, these indicators need to be calculated from data that are relatively inexpensive to gather. 'Impact' indicators, such as the maternal mortality rate and ratio, do not meet these requirements. However, guidelines published by UNICEF, WHO and UNFPA present 'process' indicators that do. These process indicators are for monitoring the availability and utilisation of treatment for life-threatening obstetric complications. We believe that the use of these indicators will help to mobilise governments, agencies and communities to reduce maternal deaths substantially.

GOALS for reducing maternal mortality are often expressed in terms of a percentage reduction in the maternal mortality ratio (MMR), the number of maternal deaths per 100,000 live births. Maternal mortality ratios and rates are called 'impact' indicators, in that they measure the impact that we would like to see programmes have – a decline in maternal deaths. There are, however, a number of important problems with using impact indicators to monitor progress in reducing maternal mortality.[1] In brief, gathering the data necessary to measure changes in maternal mortality is very difficult, or in some circumstances impossible. Furthermore, knowing the level of maternal mortality does not indicate what actions are needed to reduce it.

A promising alternative: process indicators

Since it appears unlikely that changes in maternal mortality can be economically measured directly, an alternative approach to monitoring progress is needed. An alternative approach is to use 'process' indicators, which measure levels and changes in processes that are believed to influence the event of interest. Process indicators are not a new idea. They are used in many other settings. For example, the proportion of children in a population who have been immunised against measles is a process indicator that is used in child health programmes. The use of oral rehydration therapy to treat children with diarrhoea (a process indicator) is more commonly used than is change in diarrhoea-specific mortality among young children (an impact indicator). To monitor reductions in iodine and vitamin A deficiency, we generally focus on the measurement of salt iodisation and coverage of vitamin A supplements, rather than changes in urinary iodine or serum retinol levels, which are much more difficult to measure. The impact indicators are measured much less frequently.

In this paper, we will describe the advantages and limitations of using process indicators in Safe Motherhood programmes. A series of indicators will be presented which were developed by staff at Columbia University and UNICEF, and published by UNICEF, WHO and UNFPA.[2,3] These indicators focus on the availability and use of services for treatment of life-threatening obstetric complications.

Programme relevance: Process indicators have a number of distinct advantages over impact indicators. Most importantly, process indicators provide information on the actions that need to be taken to improve the situation. For example, if a survey showed that the MMR in a given area was 600, what would that tell us? It would tell us that maternal mortality is unacceptably high, but it would not tell us what needs to be done to reduce deaths. In contrast, the indicators discussed below point to specific actions that need to be taken. For example, they may indicate that certain parts of the country do not have sufficient health facilities in which obstetric complications are being treated.

Affordability: Process indicators are generally less expensive to measure than impact indicators. This is especially true when they are composed of data collected in a few locations (e.g. health facilities), rather than data collected in population surveys. Because process indicators are less expensive, they can be measured more frequently. In fact, when using facility-based data, monitoring can be done continuously through routine (e.g. monthly) reports.

Responsiveness: Process indicators can reflect changes immediately, which permits feedback to programme activities in a short period, not years later. This will be demonstrated below, using actual country examples. The process indicators presented here can be used both for an initial situation analysis and subsequently for monitoring of progress.

Why focus on obstetric services?

When using any kind of process indicator, it is important that the processes measured are really linked to the desired outcome, e.g. the reduction of maternal deaths. During the past few years, there has been an increasing clarity about which are the most effective ways to prevent maternal deaths. In theory, there are three main pathways to reduce maternal deaths: (1) reducing the number of pregnancies and births; (2) reducing obstetric complications; and (3) preventing deaths among women who have developed serious obstetric complications.[4]

A woman is not at risk of a maternal death unless she becomes pregnant. Therefore, anything that reduces her chances of becoming pregnant will reduce her chances of maternal death. However, once she becomes pregnant, any woman can develop a complication during pregnancy, labour and the post-partum period. Some complications can be prevented by appropriate management of pregnancy, labour and delivery (for example, clean delivery practices). And some groups of women can be identified as being at higher risk, for example women who have experienced a previous complication. However, in the majority of cases it is not possible to predict who will develop obstetric complications. In fact, most complications occur among low-risk women.

Since any woman can suddenly develop a serious problem during pregnancy, delivery or the post-partum period, maternal deaths cannot be substantially reduced unless all pregnant women have access to treatment of life-threatening complications, or 'essential obstetric care' (EOC). For this reason, the process indicators discussed below focus on the third pathway – that is, reducing deaths among women who develop obstetric complications.

The UNICEF/WHO/UNFPA process indicators

The process indicators proposed here were designed to answer a series of questions about the availability, utilisation and quality of care for women with obstetric complications:

- Are there enough facilities providing EOC?
- Are they well distributed?
- Are enough women using these facilities?
- Are the right women (those with obstetric complications) using these facilities?
- Are sufficient quantities of critical services being provided?
- Is the quality of the services adequate?

How do we assess whether any of the values obtained for these indicators are sufficient? Based on the best available data at this time, UNICEF, WHO and UNFPA have set certain 'acceptable levels'. These levels are necessarily approximate, and should be viewed as guides, not targets.

The basic assumption in developing these acceptable levels is that at least 15 per cent of all pregnant women will develop serious obstetric complications. This estimate is based on the best data available at this time.[5] Therefore, it can be assumed that the minimum proportion of pregnant women who require medical care in order to avoid death or disability is 15 per cent.

In selecting these indicators, our aim was to design a system that is not very complicated or expensive to implement, but would still yield the minimum amount of information needed for programme planners and policy makers (*see* Table 1). While these indicators can point out

Table 1. Process Indicators and Acceptable Levels: A Guide

Indicator	Acceptable level
1. Number of Essential Obstetric Care (EOC) facilities – Basic EOC – Comprehensive EOC	For every 500,000 population: – At least 4 basic EOC facilities – At least 1 comprehensive EOC facility
2. Geographic distribution	Minimum level is met in sub-national areas
3. Percentage births in EOC facilities	At least 15% of all births in the population take place in EOC facilities
4. Met need for EOC	All women with obstetric complications (estimated as 15% of births) are treated in EOC facilities
5. Quantity of critical services – Caesarean section rate	Not less than 5% and not more than 15%, as a proportion of all births in the population, are by caesarean section
6. Quality of care – Case-fatality rate	Not more than 1% of women with obstetric complications admitted to comprehensive EOC facilities die.

problems, additional information may be required at the local level to identify more clearly the nature of the problem and the appropriate solution. These indicators were designed to be useful at different levels, including at the national, regional or local levels.

Indicator No. 1: Number of EOC Facilities

The first indicator in this series requires a count of the facilities in which EOC services are actually being provided. This is different from process indicators which measure the capacity to perform EOC or related services.[6] Unfortunately, as the case studies presented later will show, there are many health facilities in developing countries that should be able to provide EOC (that is, they have the staff and so on), but in fact they do not provide it. That is why these indicators focus on actual functioning, not capability.

How many facilities are required to treat obstetric complications? That depends, of course, on the size and capabilities of these facilities. As the table shows, the minimum acceptable level for this indicator is one Comprehensive and four Basic EOC facilities per 500,000 population.

If the only facilities that were counted were ones where all EOC functions are performed, that would impose unnecessarily strict standards. Moreover, it would impart the wrong message by implying that only hospitals can help in reducing maternal mortality. This is not what is being recommended. In fact, one of the most promising interventions is the upgrading of health centres and other small facilities so that they can perform some, though not all, EOC functions.

In this indicator, two levels of EOC facilities are identified and counted: Basic and Comprehensive EOC facilities. For the purposes of programme monitoring, it is useful to select a few 'signal' functions to use in identifying these different levels of care. These are:

- Basic EOC services: administration of parenteral antibiotics, parenteral oxytocic drugs and parentaral anticonvulsant drugs, manual removal of placenta, removal of retained products, and assisted vaginal delivery.
- Comprehensive EOC services: all basic EOC services, plus surgery (caesarean section) and blood transfusion.

The major difference between Basic and Comprehensive EOC is the capacity to give blood and perform surgery (i.e. caesarean section). It is important to remember that these 'signal functions' do not include all the important functions in an EOC facility. For example, in

Basic EOC facilities it would be extremely helpful to have intravenous fluids available, and in Comprehensive EOC facilities there needs to be anaesthesia in order to perform surgery.

In general, Comprehensive EOC services will be provided in hospitals, and Basic EOC services will be provided in health centres and other peripheral facilities.[7] If Basic EOC services are provided by a midwife who does home deliveries, they would also be counted. In other words, the EOC does not always have to be based in a facility, although in the large majority of cases it will be.

Indicator No. 2: Geographic Distribution of EOC Facilities

If a sufficient number of EOC facilities exist, then the next step is to determine whether they are adequately distributed. One telling indicator is the average travel time to an EOC facility. While this is an informative indicator, the data required are difficult to obtain. In addition, it is sometimes difficult to interpret. A crude but efficient way to assess the distribution of EOC services throughout the country is to calculate the amount of EOC services available in areas smaller than the country as a whole – such as a province or district. Therefore, the minimum acceptable level for Indicator No. 2 is the same as that for Indicator No. 1, but applied to smaller geographic areas. Mapping facilities would be helpful for visualising the geographical distribution of EOC services.

Indicator No. 3: Percentage of Births in EOC Facilities

The next question is: are women using these facilities? If we estimate that at least 15 per cent of women develop obstetric complications, then we can assume that at the very least 15 per cent of all births should take place in EOC facilities. If fewer than 15 per cent of all births are taking place in an EOC facility, we then know that some women who need these services are not receiving care.

Indicator No. 4: Met Need for EOC

Of course, just because 15 per cent of all births are taking place in EOC facilities does not mean that the women with obstetric complications are receiving appropriate care. It might be that most of the births in EOC facilities are normal deliveries. Therefore, we need a more refined measure of the utilisation of EOC services – that is, the proportion of all women with obstetric complications[8] that are being treated in a facility. This has been termed the 'met need' for obstetric care. Note that this indicator can be calculated either as met need or unmet need. In any case, the target would be to achieve 100 per cent coverage for women in need of obstetric care.

While the met need for EOC may be used as a gauge of the level of EOC activity in an area, it cannot describe what needs to be done. If the proportion of need being met is low, it is not possible to distinguish from this statistic alone where the problem lies. It may be in the availability, accessibility or quality of care being provided, or it may lie in utilisation of the services or, most probably, in both. Further investigation is then required. Additional information can be obtained through focus groups in the community, and through maternal death audits or other types of research.

Indicator No. 5: Quantity of Critical Services

Another indicator of whether EOC facilities are, in fact, providing life-saving obstetric services is the number of caesarean sections as a proportion of all births. Of all the procedures used to treat the major obstetric complications, caesarean section is the easiest to study. In many facilities in developing countries, record systems are not complete, and therefore not all EOC procedures are recorded. However, the records regarding surgery (e.g. operating theatre log books) are often the most complete records available.

Despite the practical advantages, using casarean sections as an indicator is somewhat controversial because the procedure is sometimes overused. While certain elective caesarean sections are performed because they are convenient and lucrative for physicians, they can be dangerous and expensive for their patients. Therefore, in setting acceptable levels for caesarean sections, it seems appropriate to set both minimum and maximum levels. In the UNICEF/WHO/UNFPA Guidelines, the lower limit is set at five per cent of all births in the population, which is a relatively conservative lower limit, especially as no attempt is made in this indicator to distinguish between caesarean sections that are done for fetal as opposed to maternal indications. For the upper limit, 15 per cent was used. It is slightly higher than the level in most developed countries, but less than the level in the countries known to have problems with excessive use of this procedure, such as the USA and Brazil.[9]

While data on caesarean sections need to be interpreted with caution, they do have the advantage of being available where information on complications treated is not. In some situations, it will be necessary to use the proportion of births that are delivered by caesarean section as a proxy for met need for EOC, while countries begin to gather information on complications. Certainly, if the national or regional data show that less than 5 per cent of births are by caesarean section, this means that some women with life-threatening complications are not receiving the necessary care.

Indicator No. 6: Quality of Care

The previous indicators have focused on measuring the coverage and utilisation of EOC facilities. The sixth indicator is a rough measure of the quality of services provided. Case-fatality is the number of deaths among women admitted to a facility with a major obstetric complication. The case-fatality rate (CFR) as an indicator of performance has not been used frequently, even though it is relatively easy to calculate. The available data indicate that there is a wide gulf between CFRs in developed and developing countries. Based on the available data, a minimum acceptable level of 1 per cent has been set for case-fatality rates for all major obstetric complications combined. This level falls between the rates from Africa and those from the USA. However, the case-fatality rate is a relatively crude measure of performance and it would be best to supplement this with information from in-depth analyses such as maternal death audits, or other qualitative studies.

It should be noted that case-fatality rates should be calculated for Comprehensive EOC facilities only, because CFRs from Basic EOC facilities are difficult to interpret. This is because women with serious complications may be referred from Basic to Comprehensive EOC facilities, which would make the CFR in the Basic EOC facility artificially low. Even with this stipulation, interpretation of CFRs may also be complicated. For example, a teaching hospital may receive the worst cases. However, if a CFR is high it is an indication that further study is needed to find out why. Are women dying because they have to wait too long after they are admitted before they are treated? Are they arriving at the facility near death because it took too long to get there? Is the quality of care inadequate? Again, different types of data are required to answer these questions.

UNICEF/WHO/UNFPA published a second edition of these indicators in 1997. This document – *Guidelines for Monitoring the Availability and Use of Obstetric Care* – provides information on how to measure and interpret these indicators. It includes detailed data collection forms, as well as suggestions for sampling of facilities should this be necessary. This second edition has also incorporated the results of field tests of the indicators in a number of countries, including, India, Bangladesh, Ghana and Morocco. Copies are available from UNICEF and WHO.

Using process indicators to decide what action is needed

The following are two case studies that illustrate how using these process indicators can point the way to actions that are needed. Once a programme is designed and implemented, these same indicators can be used to monitor progress.

Case Study No. 1: Morocco

This case study illustrates how these indicators can eloquently express the need for better access to EOC, even when complete data are not available. In fact, the information presented below was gathered in a few hours.

In a mountainous province in the north of Morocco, in 1995, there were two hospitals which provided basic EOC. A larger hospital which performs caesarean sections (a Comprehensive EOC facility) was two hours drive away. The province had a population of 600,000 with a crude birth rate of around 33 births per 1000 population, or 20,000 births a year. A review of hospital records showed that from January through March, 28 women were transferred from the two rural hospitals to the larger hospital. Of these, eight women had caesarean sections.

Using the UNICEF/WHO/UNFPA minimum acceptable levels, an estimated 3,000 women in the province would need EOC (15 per cent of

20,000 births) each year, and at least 1,000 would need caesarean sections (5 per cent of 20,000 births). If eight women were referred for caesarean section in a three-month period, that is the equivalent of 32 women a year or about 3 per cent of the minimum acceptable level. So even if many women found their way to the city hospital without going to the local hospital, it is probable that only a fraction of women who needed an emergency caesarean section obtained one.

It should be noted that before this analysis was conducted, the government health officials in this area had no way of assessing the unmet need for EOC in the community. They were surprised and dismayed at what they learned, and were keen to remedy the situation.

Case Study No. 2: Egypt

In this case study, a more extensive needs assessment was conducted, and all the UNICEF/WHO/UNFPA indicators were calculated. This assessment was done in the Akhmiem District of Sohag Governorate in Upper Egypt by UNICEF/Egypt and the Ministry of Health and Population in 1997. It took three weeks to complete and was done using existing records. The assessment involved site visits to the facilities, as well as in-depth interviews with key health officials and staff at the facilities.

Table 2 shows the data required to calculate the indicators, and the results. By comparing the results to the minimum acceptable levels, it becomes clear that while there were enough

Table 2. Akhmiem District, Sohag Governorate, Egypt, 1996

Demographic and obstetric data*	
Population	254,000
Births	7,800
Deliveries in a health facility	258
Complicated cases seen in a health facility	104
Complicated cases expected (minimum)	1,170
Caesarean sections carried out	3
Obstetric deaths in the hospital	7
Basic EOC facilities	1
Comprehensive EOC facilities	1

Indicator	**Current number/ level reached**	**Acceptable?**	**Number/level required to be acceptable**
No. EOC facilities			
– Basic	1	No	At least 2
– Comprehensive	1	Yes	At least 1
Geographic distribution	The Comprehensive EOC facility can also cover an adjoining area of comparable population size		
Births in EOC facility	3.3% (258/7800)	No	At least 15%
Met need for EOC	8.8% (104/1170)	No	100%
Quantity of critical services			
– Caesarean section rate	0.04% (3/7800)	No	At least 5%
Quality of care			
– Case-fatality rate	6.7% (7/104)	No	1%

** Source: UNICEF/Egypt and Ministry of Health and Population, Egypt*

comprehensive facilities in the district, unmet need for EOC services was high. Only 8.8 per cent of women estimated to have serious obstetric complications were treated in EOC facilities. The caesarean section rate was very low, at 0.04 per cent (compared to the minimum acceptable level of 5 per cent) and the CFR was high at 7 per cent (compared to the maxmimum acceptable level of 1 per cent).

To build a more complete picture of why the levels of care were so low, the data were augmented with information obtained during site visits and interviews with health personnel. The results showed that much of the infrastructure needed is already in place, but the functioning needed to be improved. Of the 13 government facilities, only two provided EOC. There was no serious shortage of electricity, water, equipment or supplies. However, there appeared to be poor use of existing resources, as well as inadequate supervision. The low caesarean section rate could partly be explained by the unavailability of anaesthesiologists, either for most of the day or completely. In addition, the training of nurses and obstetricians provided little hands-on experience with normal deliveries, let alone treatment of complications. A variety of activities are underway to address these problems.

Conclusion

In closing, there are a few points which should be made about these indicators. First, these indicators were designed as a series and each indicator needs to be interpreted in the context of all the information gathered. Second, data on complications may be difficult to collect in the beginning, due to poor record-keeping. Consequently, in most places effort will have to be put into improving records of obstetric complications.

We believe that these process indicators can be powerful tools for understanding the reasons why women continue to die of obstetric complications, for determining what action needs to be taken and implementing it, and for monitoring progress in reducing these needless deaths.

Acknowledgements

This article is based on a presentation by Tessa Wardlaw at the conference 'Safe Motherhood Matters: Ten Years of Lessons and Progress', Colombo, Sri Lanka, 18-23 October 1997. We are grateful to our colleagues in the Governments of Morocco and Egypt, and the UNICEF office in Egypt (Leila Bisharat, Amira El-Mallatawy, and Ibrahim El-Kerdany) for the information used in the case studies.

References and Notes

1. Other papers in this book discuss the advantages and disadvantages of impact indicators. For information about maternal mortality ratios etc, see: World Health Organization and UNICEF, 1996. *Revised 1990 Estimates of Maternal Mortality*. April.
2. Maine D, McCarthy J, Ward VM, 1992. *Guidelines for Monitoring Progress in the Reduction of Maternal Mortality: A Work in Progress*. UNICEF, New York, October.
3. Maine D, Wardlaw TM, Ward VM, et al, 1997. *Guidelines for Monitoring the Availability and Use of Obstetric Services*. UNICEF/WHO/UNFPA, New York, September.
4. McCarthy J, Maine D, 1992. A framework for analyzing the determinants of maternal mortality. *Studies in Family Planning*. 23:23-33.
5. Division of Family Health, 1994. WHO *Mother-Baby Package*. WHO, Geneva.
6. Sloan NL, Quimby C, Winikoff B, Schwalbe N, 1995. *Guidelines and Instruments for a Situation Analysis of Obstetric Services*. Population Council, New York.
7. World Health Organization, 1994. *Indicators to Monitor Maternal Health Goals: Report of a Technical Working Group, Geneva, 8-12* November, 1993. Geneva, WHO/FHE/MSM/94.14.
8. A complicated case is defined as a woman who has one or more of the following conditions: haemorrhage, prolonged or obstructed labour, sepsis, complications from abortion, pre-eclampsia or eclampsia, ectopic pregnancy or ruptured uterus.
9. Notzon FC, 1990. International differences in the use of obstetric interventions. *Journal of American Medical Association*. 263: 3286-91.

Measuring Progress in Safe Motherhood Programmes: Uses and Limitations of Health Outcome Indicators

Oona MR Campbell

There is great demand to show that progress is being made as a result of Safe Motherhood programmes to reduce maternal mortality. However, while maternal mortality indicators are intuitive and appealing, they are costly to measure precisely. Measures of maternal morbidity are also problematic. This paper examines the scope for using health outcome indicators for measurement, and the use of both experimental and descriptive study designs. Women's perceptions of obstetric morbidity can be measured using population-based interviews, but they agree poorly with biomedical diagnoses. Underlying (chronic) maternal morbidity, but not direct obstetric morbidity, can be measured via relatively expensive health-examination surveys. Facility-based information on maternal morbidity is a promising alternative to population-based interviews. The impracticality of using health outcome indicators leaves process indicators as the alternative in most settings, possibly supplemented by facility-based data on health outcomes. Considerably more work on process indicators, and documentation of that work, is needed. Study design is a key factor in determining whether change can be attributed to a Safe Motherhood programme intervention. Experimental approaches are definitive, but difficult and costly; hence, descriptive approaches are more likely to be used. Descriptive designs require the use of many process indicators, not just a few global ones, to build a convincing case that change is due to programme interventions. Better record-keeping and more critical use of data are recommended.

INFORMATION that determines whether Safe Motherhood interventions are succeeding could be used to mobilise resources for greater and more appropriate action. Obtaining such information to measure progress presents its own challenges, however, which go beyond the difficulties of implementing a coherent and effective Safe Motherhood programme. These include:

- determining the most desirable indicators,
- understanding whether it is possible to measure mortality and morbidity easily and with sufficient accuracy to show progress (change), and
- knowing if it is possible to attribute any change observed to Safe Motherhood programme interventions.

The literature on indicators makes inconsistent use of a wide variety of terms. One useful categorisation distinguishes between population-based outcome indicators and programme-based performance indicators (which include input, process and output indicators). In Safe Motherhood programmes, the outcome indicators refer to the health outcomes of maternal morbidity and mortality. Inputs refer to human and financial resources, physical facilities, equipment, and operational policies that enable services to be delivered. Process refers to the multiple activities that are carried out to achieve the activities of the programme. It includes what is done and how well it is done. Outputs refer to the results of efforts at the programme level. An output indicator from one programme may be a process indicator for another. Because this paper concentrates on the uses and limitations of health outcome indicators, process and output indicators are grouped together and termed process indicators.[1]

The appeal of health outcome indicators

In order to choose the best indicators, systematic answers to the following four questions are required.

What are the programme goals?

The main goal set for the joint UN Inter-agency Safe Motherhood Initiative is a 50 per cent reduction in maternal mortality, with subsidiary goals of a healthy woman and newborn infant. It therefore seems obvious that the most desirable indicator of this reduction should be a health outcome indicator, namely a maternal mortality indicator. These measure maternal mortality over time in one of the following ways:

- maternal mortality ratio – maternal deaths per 100,000 live births;
- maternal mortality rate – maternal deaths per 100,000 women aged 15-49; or
- lifetime risk – probability of maternal death over reproductive life
- alternatively, another health impact indicator, the prevalence of life-threatening complications, can be monitored.

What is the conceptual framework?

Safe Motherhood programmes are broad and encompass many inputs, which may include clinical training, supplies and equipment, drugs and forms of therapy, and communications and transport, among others. They also encompass many intermediate outputs and outcomes. These suggest that there is broad scope for using many possible indicators of achievement – both process and health outcome indicators.

How efficacious are the inputs?

This is an important consideration; where efficacy is high and largely independent of either the user or the provider, short-cuts can be taken in choosing the outputs and outcomes to measure. For example, immunisation against tetanus with tetanus toxoid and tubal ligation to prevent future pregnancies are highly efficacious procedures, which confer long-lasting protection. Although there is scope for error in carrying out these interventions, it is generally assumed that carrying them out leads to the desired outcomes. Interventions such as these are therefore evaluated according to the numbers of women immunised or sterilised (output measures) rather than according to the numbers of tetanus deaths or rates of unwanted pregnancy (health outcome measures).

This is not the case for other types of interventions (inputs). For example, if the input consists of family planning services, which is a much broader form of intervention, it is not possible to assume that use of the service in itself will give the desired outcome of prevention of unwanted pregnancy. Safe Motherhood programmes are a similarly broad form of intervention. While it is possible to measure the extent of use of antenatal care or professional birth attendants, the degree of protection these confer against morbidity or mortality cannot be determined by their use alone. Hence, process indicators would not necessarily reveal whether a programme is achieving its goals; this argues in favour of using health outcome indicators, especially measures of mortality.

The responses to the first three questions above suggest that the most desirable indicators are of health outcome, that is, of mortality and morbidity. Moreover, planners, policymakers and donors are used to monitoring progress in maternal and child health using increases or decreases in infant mortality and they appear more likely to be convinced by changes in health outcome indicators than process indicators. However, it is in the answer to the fourth question that the desirability of health outcome indicators is diminished.

How easily and accurately can mortality and morbidity be measured?

As described below, health outcome measures (maternal mortality and direct obstetric morbidity) are usually too costly or difficult to obtain with sufficient accuracy to measure progress.

Mortality indicators

Routine methods, primarily vital registration data, but also data from surveillance, whereby an ongoing effort is made to identify all maternal deaths in a defined population, are the best way to monitor maternal mortality. In theory, vital registration data are collected routinely, cover the entire population (and, hence, provide large sample sizes), and provide time trends. However, vital registration in most developing countries suffers from two main problems: low coverage (under-reporting), where not all deaths are recorded, and misclassification, where causes of death are wrongly ascribed, in this case to non-maternal causes.

At the beginning of the 1990s, the UN estimated that less than a third of the world's population lived in areas with complete death registration and medical certification of death.[2] A review of data on adult mortality in Africa concluded that registration of death was far too incomplete to be useful for demographic estimation.[3] Even where deaths are registered, misclassification occurs. Special studies have shown that vital registration in the UK,[4] France[5] and the USA[6] misclassifies 39 per cent, 56 per cent, and over 50 per cent of maternal deaths identified through special studies respectively. Studies in developing countries have typically shown that between 25 and 60 per cent of maternal deaths are missed.[7] These continuing problems limit the use of routinely collected data, even though numerous attempts have been made to improve the quality of vital registration, or to interpret such data creatively.[7,8]

Fortunately, even in the absence of complete and accurate vital registration, there are two relatively inexpensive ways of obtaining a rough national estimate of maternal mortality. One is the sisterhood method, a demographic technique used in surveys, that requires relatively small sample sizes. The method asks adult respondents four questions about the number of sisters they had who reached age 15, how many of these were dead, how many were alive, and how many of those who were dead had died in pregnancy, childbirth or the 42 days after the end of pregnancy. The original, indirect approach[9,10] does not restrict the time period of death, while a more recent derivation used in Demographic and Health Surveys (DHS) adds questions on age at death, year of death, and years since death.[11] This latter approach gives more recent estimates but requires larger sample sizes and takes slightly longer.

The second is the WHO/UNICEF model, which predicts the maternal mortality ratio (MMRatio) based on a country's general fertility rate (GFR) and the percentage of births delivered by a skilled attendant (defined as a doctor or midwife, not a trained traditional birth attendant). These models were built using data from countries with good estimates of maternal mortality[12] and require no additional data collection. They are suitable for the estimated 55-60 countries with no empirically derived estimate of the maternal mortality ratio.

Since there are at least two relatively inexpensive ways to estimate maternal mortality, can this health outcome indicator be used to measure progress? The short answer is 'No'. In the absence of a good, routine system which identifies all maternal deaths, measuring changes in maternal mortality over too short a period of time is too costly, although it may be possible over a longer period. That is, the usual project or programme time scale of three to five years[13] is too short; however, a period of 10 years may be possible.

Neither the sisterhood method nor the WHO/UNICEF models can be used for monitoring change for shorter periods of time, for the following reasons:

- The sisterhood method yields a retrospective estimate (for the past 10-12 years) rather than a current one. Thus, a study in 1998 may yield MMRatio estimates for 1986. Also, unless the sample size is enormous, confidence intervals with the sisterhood method are generally wide. For example, the DHS sisterhood estimate for Malawi, based on a sample size of 4,850, gives an MMRatio which ranges between 497 and 1006. For Indonesia the range is narrower, between 378 and 529, but this is based on a larger sample size of 28,168.[14] The sisterhood method is also sensitive to changes in fertility and migration.
- The WHO/UNICEF models will only show change as a result of changes in the model inputs of GFR and the percentage of births delivered by skilled attendants, rather than by observed changes in MMRatio.

In other words neither of these two approaches is precise enough to show change without large cost. Statistically, maternal mortality is a rare event, even where the risk is high. Moreover, as with other adult deaths it is difficult to sample and is usually under-reported.

Other approaches for measuring maternal mortality include:

- Studies involving identification of deaths, including reproductive age mortality studies (RAMOS), which identify all deaths of women of reproductive age as a source of maternal deaths;[15] facility-based audits, which identify all pregnant or recently delivered women among health-facility deaths; and studies which identify deaths from multiple sources.[16]

- Prospective studies which follow women or pregnant women to identify maternal deaths.[17]
- Direct survey approaches which ask about deaths in the year or two prior to the survey. These are notoriously poor and are to be avoided, in general, as they require very large samples and can miss 40-50 per cent of adult deaths.[18] There are, however, some good examples where the exclusive focus was on maternal deaths.[19]

More recently, Benin, Iran, Laos, and Zimbabwe have used the direct approach in their censuses. This approach is worth considering if census questions on adult deaths are asked.

These latter methods for obtaining accurate population-based estimates are usually costly and research intensive,[7,8] though many have the advantage of providing useful information on avoidable factors and causes of death. For example, a RAMOS-type study conducted in Egypt identified a nationally representative sample of maternal deaths through the vital registration system. These deaths were reviewed by medical specialists at governorate and central level. Results showed that sub-standard care by the obstetrician teams (47 per cent) and delay in seeking care (42 per cent) were among the leading avoidable factors contributing to the deaths, while lack of drugs and equipment played a minor role (2 per cent).[20,21]

Maternal death audits (or confidential enquiries) can be conducted in facilities where deaths take place, as well as in the community. Verbal autopsy tools exist for determining the biomedical causes of death,[22] although reliability may be poor.[23] Determining the processes that contribute to maternal deaths is useful for programme planning and implementation because it may provide valuable clues to access or quality-of-care problems which are amenable to intervention.

Establishing a reliable baseline level of maternal mortality, let alone demonstrating changes, requires a very large sample size and is costly, irrespective of the method used. Except where the vast majority of deaths occur in a country's hospitals, or where vital registration/surveillance is very good, few countries have the means to evaluate their intervention programmes by using maternal mortality as a health outcome indicator. Instead maternal mortality measurement will remain in the domain of special studies. Nevertheless, reducing maternal mortality should continue to be the goal of Safe Motherhood programmes in developing countries, as this maintains the focus on the complications which are killing an estimated 585,000 women globally each year.

Morbidity indicators

Maternal morbidity is more common than maternal mortality. Studies in Ghana, Egypt and Indonesia found 240-333 instances of maternal morbidity per maternal death.[24] For this reason, population-based figures of direct obstetric morbidity have been proposed as alternatives to mortality indicators. However, despite being more common, complications known to lead directly to a maternal death are unlikely to replace maternal mortality for measuring progress. This is because morbidity is difficult to define, interpret and measure.

Interpreting the association between trends in morbidity and programme inputs is not as conceptually straightforward as with mortality. Most Safe Motherhood interventions aim at preventing complications from becoming severe or leading to death (secondary prevention), rather than at preventing complications *per se* (primary prevention). Thus, Safe Motherhood programmes may reduce mortality without reducing the incidence of obstetric morbidity. For example, US data show that the rate of mild pre-eclampsia has remained constant and the rate of severe pre-eclampsia has increased, while the rate of eclampsia and deaths from eclampsia have decreased.[25] Also the obstacles in interpretation of morbidity data are compounded by measurement problems. Death is an unambiguous outcome, while morbidity is not, even to those with medical training. Minor and major illnesses can easily be misclassified.

With maternal morbidity, it is useful to distinguish three types of morbidity: more chronic/indirect conditions (e.g. urinary tract infection, fistula, anaemia and malaria), direct acute obstetric complications (e.g. prolonged labour, haemorrhage, eclampsia and sepsis), and perceived morbidity. Most maternal deaths are due to haemorrhage, sepsis, hypertensive diseases of pregnancy, obstructed labour, unsafe abortion, severe anaemia, malaria and cardiovascular complications; not all types of morbidity are implicated in maternal deaths.

Underlying maternal morbidity such as anaemia, malaria, rheumatic heart disease, syphilis, urinary tract infection (UTI), high blood pressure and long-term disabilities such as uterine prolapse, fistula and female genital mutilation are often chronic or long-lasting conditions. Because they are less acute than direct obstetric complications, they can potentially be measured using population-based health examination survey methods (with clinical, anthropometric and laboratory diagnosis). These approaches are research intensive, and are not likely to play a big role in monitoring progress. Moreover, with the exception of severe anaemia, malaria and rheumatic heart disease, many chronic forms of morbidity are not implicated in maternal death. For example, UTI, hyperemesis, breast abscess, fistula or prolapse are very rarely causes of death.

Direct obstetric complications are usually acute and infrequent so they cannot be captured in health examination surveys. Rather, attempts are made to ask women to recall these morbidities using health interview techniques.

Comparisons of women's self-reports in interviews with their medical records to estimate the population prevalence of prolonged labour, haemorrhage, eclampsia and sepsis, have shown that women's perceptions are not reliable compared to biomedical results.[26-28] For example, data from South Kalimantan, Indonesia, suggested that 13 per cent of the women might have reported excessive bleeding during their most recent birth, even though this may actually have been the case for 5 per cent of them. Other research has shown that household survey approaches to determine the prevalence of induced abortion[29,30] and chronic/indirect conditions[31] are similarly flawed. Estimates of maternal morbidity based on data from in-depth, more focused studies may be more accurate if considerable efforts are made to determine the appropriate wording of questions,[32,33] but these are not likely to be relevant for large-scale efforts to monitor progress.

It is, of course, possible and reasonable to want to measure perceived complications.[34,35] Such questions are perhaps best used in the context of understanding health-care seeking behaviour. Models of behaviour seek to understand the intent to use services in relation to actual use when the perceived need arises. Thus, a woman could be asked, for example, whether a woman with antepartum bleeding should seek care, whether she herself experienced antepartum bleeding in her last pregnancy, and if so, whether she actually sought care for this antepartum bleeding. However, policymakers, donors, service providers and most researchers have remained sceptical of relying on perception and prefer to address biomedical disease. This is partly because perception of disease is known to depend on the characteristics of the respondent. For example, respondents with a high socioeconomic status may report more perceived morbidity despite the fact that clinical and laboratory examinations find they have less morbidity.

One unanswered question with respect to monitoring progress using health outcome indicators is whether facility-based data can be substituted for population-based data collection. The potential for facility- or provider-based records and registers to measure progress in Safe Motherhood activities is greater than for population-based surveys. This is because these records and registers have the potential to provide biomedically valid information about morbidity and mortality (though clinical diagnoses are often wrong compared to laboratory tests and autopsies), and of outcomes following treatment.

In practice, it is often possible to collect useful data on maternal mortality and morbidity from health facilities using facility-based and/or provider-based records and registers and in-depth review of case records. For example, the Prevention of Maternal Mortality Network derived much useful data for problem identification and monitoring using hospital records.[36] In many settings, however, retrospective review of existing facility- or provider-based records and registers is not a practical tool for measuring maternal morbidity.[37] Records are often missing information or have illegible writing. For example, in Assiut, Egypt, among women who had delivered in hospital, 93 per cent, 92 per cent and 95 per cent of patient records listed parity, sex of the infant and presence of abnormalities respectively, but only 20 per cent, 1 per cent and 1 per cent respectively recorded problems with the pregnancy, birth weight of the infant, or APGAR scores.[38] Inconsistent definitions may be used in record-keeping, and interventions such as caesarean section are often recorded without mentioning the medical complication that indicated surgery.

Where facility-based records can be used, complications at the severe end of the morbidity spectrum, such as near-miss death events, have special potential as useful health outcome indicators. A near-miss death event is a severe, life-threatening complication, necessitating an urgent medical intervention in order to prevent the likely death of the mother.[39,40] The advantage of measuring near-miss death events over all complications is that near-misses are a better proxy for maternal deaths, while still occurring in large enough numbers for statistical analysis. Near-misses are also less likely to pose problems of inconsistent definition, double counting of women and types of morbidity, and variable prevalence over time.

Facility-based data are obviously not population-based. However, they can be used to derive an indirect, population-based estimate of the proportion of women with obstetric complications who seek care in a facility. Interpreting such data requires:

- assuming that there is a relatively constant proportion of women with obstetric complications (however these are defined),
- ensuring that there is no, or minimal, double-counting of complications, assuming that the obstetric complications can only be treated in specialised medical facilities under consideration, and
- having a defined catchment area (i.e. being able to define the population served by the facilities under consideration in such a way that all service use by that population is captured and use of the service by other populations is minimal or can be excluded).

These requirements are more likely to be fulfilled if near-misses are used instead of any obstetric complication, if the catchment area chosen is large and if all relevant facilities (including private or mission hospitals) are included. Although in practice all hospitals, maternities, health centres, health posts or clinics can be included in facility-based data collection activities, it is simplest to limit facilities to those where women would go for potentially life-threatening obstetric complications, such as public and private hospitals.

The Prevention of Maternal Mortality Network used the number of women with obstetric complications as one of many indicators for assessing the overall functioning of services.[36] They found this to be extremely useful, although it needed to be interpreted in light of other factors (closure of nearby facilities and/or deteriorating political and economic circumstances). Facility-based data collection should not be under-estimated in terms of time, resources and intensity of programme effort required. Record-keeping is likely to need to be improved before facility-based sources can be used.

Process indicators

There is now considerable understanding of the options for and difficulties of measuring maternal health outcome indicators. Given the difficulties, recognition of the importance of process indicators has increased. Some process indicators, such as where delivery takes place and who attends it, have proved invaluable. However, experience with many other process indicators remains more limited. At this stage, an overall assessment would be that while many process indicators may prove useful, they usually cannot be interpreted on their own, they may need to be disaggregated for various sub-populations, and they may need to be looked at over several points in time.

Can change be attributed to programme interventions?

Showing that progress has occurred because of a Safe Motherhood programme or a specific intervention is even more complicated than showing a change *per se*. An important factor in determining how convincingly progress is attributable to an intervention is the study design. However, design options are restricted, not only because it is hard to measure maternal mortality and morbidity as outcomes, as argued above. It is also because the intervention is usually a comprehensive package or system (rather than a single drug or procedure) and is often delivered to communities not individuals. In practical terms, this limits the study design options and complicates specifying the conceptual framework.

As a result of these obstacles, Safe Motherhood programmes are more likely to use descriptive rather than experimental designs for evaluation, and to rely on process indicators to measure the implementation and use of appropriate services. While these are now seen as the most feasible and likely options, results based on these approaches will always be open to challenge.

Experimental study designs

The 'gold standard' design for testing whether an intervention has an effect is the experimental approach. In health research this is exemplified by the randomised, controlled trial (RCT) or the community randomised trial (CRT). Other design approaches are more widely used in evaluation, but none of these offer as definitive a standard of proof as RCTs or CRTs.

The role of RCTs for evaluating single interventions is indisputable. For example, the RCT of using sulfadoxine-pyrimethamine as malaria prophylaxis for preventing severe anaemia in pregnant women in Kenya showed clearly that this intervention reduced severe anaemia by 39 per cent.[41] The main feature of the RCT is that it randomly allocates individuals to an intervention or a control group, and then measures the outcome of interest in both groups. Random allocation ensures that there are no systematic differences between the group receiving the intervention and the one which is not, and that any differences are due to chance.

If RCTs are 'double blind' then neither the provider/interviewer nor the individual enrolled in the trial is aware of whether the intervention or the placebo is being administered. This removes the potential for reporting bias and bias due to the Hawthorne effect (whereby people behave differently because they are under observation). RCTs have been designed to look at Safe Motherhood service delivery issues. For example, several RCTs in developed countries have assessed outcomes among women randomly allocated to conventional versus alternative places of delivery.[42] However, RCTs are not generally useful for evaluating Safe Motherhood programmes which are aimed at communities rather than individuals.

Where interventions are delivered to communities, CRTs are the most scientific approach. CRTs are large-scale undertakings where a 'community' may be the catchment area of a hospital, or of a health centre. Typically, twelve or more communities will be required for inclusion, divided equally and randomly into intervention and control communities. This scale of operation, and the need for skilled research personnel, makes the cost high.

Other disadvantages of CRTs are:

- Randomised trials of interventions involving service delivery are context-specific and the cost may be prohibitive when measured against the benefit, if the intervention cannot be generalised beyond this immediate context.
- Randomised trials cannot be used to evaluate interventions that have already been put into place, or where the evaluators cannot influence which communities do and do not receive the intervention.
- CRTs are not always fully 'controlled' since it may be difficult to maintain a strict separation between intervention and control communities, particularly when the intervention involves communication strategies (i.e. information, education and communication about danger signs in pregnancy).
- The scale of operation may preclude carrying out a CRT at all. For example, if the intervention includes components targeted at hospitals providing essential obstetric care (EOC) for entire districts, there may not be 12 communities each with a hospital available to randomise.

By contrast, the essential advantage of CRTs (and RCTs) is that they lead to conclusions that remain true even if the complex processes leading to the outcome cannot be fully measured, are not fully understood or do not fully follow their expected path. It is possible to justify a CRT if the results have a commensurate importance to the cost. A CRT is most justified when the results are of general importance and of wide applicability, rather than being context-specific. If maternal mortality is the outcome of interest, then both RCTs and CRTs will require a large sample size. For example in a setting where the maternal mortality ratio is 700/100,000, a sample size of over 58,000 births would be required for an RCT for an intervention that is expected to reduce mortality by 30 per cent.

Non-experimental (descriptive) designs

Countries which currently have low levels of maternal mortality did not design and evaluate their programmes using CRTs; rather, they used a combination of accumulated knowledge and experience, including historical review of previous programmes, and rational interpretation of the expected benefits of the specific components of a programme – based mainly on clinical knowledge and common sense. For example, the now accepted need for access to skilled emergency obstetric care at health facilities, as a prerequisite to averting maternal deaths, draws mostly on the analysis of historical trends in maternal mortality in Western countries, and on clinical knowledge.

Save in exceptional circumstances, evaluation efforts in Safe Motherhood programmes should be descriptive rather than experimental. This is not to say that there is no need for accurate quantitative measurement of indicators – quite the contrary. Descriptive studies should be based on a conceptual framework which includes the existence of feasible programme objectives. As much as possible these studies need to measure whether programme inputs are actually delivered, demonstrate that the inputs are efficacious, and that outputs and outcomes are plausible. Each setting and programme will require many process indicators, many of which will be derived from operations research.

These descriptive efforts should use quantitative and qualitative data to elaborate not only the intervention taking place, but also the wider context, whilst guarding against the trend to seek single technical solutions for complex problems such as maternal health. Indicators should be compared to the conceptual framework to ensure change is going in the expected direction. The presence of change can be interpreted, provided relevant and sufficient data are collected to confirm or refute the role of the intervention. Typically, such relevant data will include:

- information on the timing and coverage of the intervention,
- the potential outside influences such as the presence of other projects in the area,
- the existence of a specific policy environment,
- the coverage/use of existing services on which the intervention relies (e.g. the presence of an obstetrician in a district hospital), and
- the factors which are known to affect maternal health, e.g. levels of fertility, women's attitudes towards the services, etc.

Such descriptive designs, which are usually termed 'before-and-after designs', will not prove that the association between the intervention and the observed change was causal; rather, the different elements will be situated within a conceptual framework to present a plausible argument as to why and how the intervention contributed to change. These can be termed 'before-during-and-after designs', which helps to emphasise that it is not sufficient to measure a single indicator at two points in time.

One or more control areas can help to indicate whether the observed change is part of an existing trend, and is unrelated to the programme. These designs are sometimes called 'quasi-experimental'. However, non-randomly selected control groups or areas may well be systematically different from the intervention area and an apparent effect of the programme may be due to these initial differences. Since it can never be assumed that the comparison groups or areas are similar, it remains necessary to exclude alternative causes for the observed trends. The efforts to document outside influences in the control groups or areas need to be matched by similar efforts in the intervention groups or areas. This limits the use of control groups/areas and suggests that resources put into measuring the control group/area might more profitably be spent on documenting programme inputs and processes better.

For example, the Matlab Maternity Care Project in rural Bangladesh introduced a maternity care programme in which trained, certified midwives assisted women with home births on request, provided prenatal care, carried supplies to stabilise or treat women with obstetrical complications, and had access to transport and referral services for emergency cases. Evaluation of maternal mortality before and after the Matlab

Maternity Care Project in intervention and control areas suggested that the MMRatio was reduced by two-thirds in the intervention area.[43] However, it is unclear how this effect was achieved since very few process indicators were collected. The limitations of the non-randomised design and the difficulties of interpreting mortality data at only two points in time became apparent when subsequent work[44] found a similar decline in a comparison area which had not benefited from the intervention.

Descriptive designs require many indicators, almost all of which will be process indicators, as argued earlier. Numerous groups have derived lists of such indicators for use in monitoring and evaluating Safe Motherhood programmes, including WHO, UNICEF, USAID and UNFPA (see Box 1). Most recently, UNICEF, WHO and UNFPA have published a series of just six indicators to monitor the availability, utilisation and quality of essential obstetric care.[47] Although the relevance of some of these

Box 1. Health outcome and process indicators proposed by various agencies for monitoring maternal health goals

BROAD INDICATORS	USAID[45]	WHO[46]	UNICEF[47]	UNFPA[48]
HEALTH OUTCOME				
Maternal mortality ratio and/or rate	*	*		*
Annual number of maternal deaths		*		
Case fatality rate – all complications	*		*	
Anaemia (prevalence and/or supplementation)		*		*
PROCESS				
Proportion of women with antenatal care	*	*		*
Percentage of pregnant women with tetanus immuniz.	*			*
Proportion of births by trained health personnel	*	*		*
Percentage of adults knowing about maternal complications	*			
Number of EOC facilities per 500,000 population	*	*	*	
Percentage of district hospitals with c-section and blood transfusion				*
Percentage of health facilities with basic obstetric care				*
Percentage of population within 1 hour travel time of EOC/ or geographic distrib.		*	*	
C-sections as a proportion of all births in the population	*	*	*	*
Proportion of expected complications managed at EOC facilities (Met need for EmOC)	*	*	*	*
Admission-to-treatment time interval	*			
SPECIAL TOPICS				
Abortion	*			*
Syphilis screening		*		*
Policy environment	*			*
Client satisfaction with maternal services				*
In-service training for health personnel			*	

Source: (45) based on short list of suggested indicators; (46) based on minimal monitoring list; (48) based on core list of suggested maternal health indicators.

indicators for global monitoring of progress must be acknowledged, it is important to recognise that this form of global monitoring has advocacy as its objective. In contrast, the monitoring of a programme aims to affect programme implementation and functioning. Individual programmes will typically have to collect many more programme-specific input, output and, where possible, outcome indicators to build a convincing case that attributable change has occurred. For example, the national MMRatio is of little use to a programme planner in a district in Indonesia, while the time-from-admission-to-treatment of that district's hospital is unlikely to feature in a UN debate or document arguing for a reduction in maternal deaths.

Conclusions and recommendations

In summary, maternal mortality indicators are intuitive and appealing for measuring progress, but are costly to measure precisely because of the large sample size required. Measures of maternal morbidity are also problematic. Women's perceived obstetric morbidities can be measured, but they agree poorly with biomedical diagnoses. Underlying maternal morbidity, but not direct obstetric morbidity, can be measured via relatively expensive health examination surveys. Facility-based data on maternal complications are a promising alternative to population-based interviews for assessing use of services among women experiencing complications. Some methods for measuring maternal deaths and near-misses, namely audit approaches, are likely to generate many useful process indicators for determining quality of maternal health care.

Experimental study designs are the gold standard for proving causation, but are difficult and costly; descriptive approaches should therefore generally be used for evaluating progress in Safe Motherhood programmes. Such designs require a plausible conceptual framework and many different indicators to build a convincing case. The impracticality of using health outcome indicators leaves process indicators as the main alternative in most settings, possibly supplemented by facility-based data on health outcomes. In many places this means record-keeping systems in facilities will need to be improved and the capacity to analyse and interpret indicators enhanced.

Considerably more work on and documentation of the use of process indicators is needed. Moreover, a venue for publishing and sharing such experience is missing since much of this work is small-scale and not necessarily publishable in peer-reviewed, scientific journals. Furthermore, policymakers and planners need to be educated on the value of piecing together a case study based on process indicators and on the costs associated with measuring maternal mortality.

Evaluation is a valuable tool for improving health programmes and using resources wisely. The obstacles faced in evaluating programmes are not unique to Safe Motherhood programmes; they are common to many other areas of health. Moreover, the difficulties of measuring the MMRatio should not be interpreted to mean that maternal mortality is not a problem. Special studies throughout the 1990s have shown that the burden of maternal ill-health is high, and is amenable to reduction. Such studies of maternal mortality and severe morbidity remain valuable tools for advocacy and for promoting and maintaining political commitment.

Acknowledgements

This paper is based on a presentation to the 1997 Technical Consultation on Safe Motherhood in Colombo, Sri Lanka and on ideas developed in: Campbell O, Filippi V, Koblinsky M et al, 1997. Lessons Learnt – A Decade of Measuring the Impact of Safe Motherhood Programmes. London School of Hygiene & Tropical Medicine, London. Oona Campbell is supported through the Programme on Population and Reproductive Health, funded by the Department for International Development (DFID) UK. Responsibility for the information in this paper and the views expressed belongs to the author alone.

Correspondence

Oona Campbell, Maternal and Child Epidemiology Unit, London School of Hygiene and Tropical Medicine, Keppel Street, London WC1E 7HT, UK. Fax: 44-171-299-4663. E-mail: o.campbell@lshtm.ac.uk

References and Notes

1. Bertrand JT, Magnani RJ, Rutenberg N, 1994. *Handbook of Indicators for Family Planning Program Evaluation*. The Evaluation Project: University of North Carolina.
2. *United Nations Demographic Yearbook 1989*. Department of International and Economic Affairs, Statistical Office. United Nations, New York, 1990.
3. Timaeus IM, 1991. Adult mortality: levels, trends, and data sources. In: *Disease and Mortality in Sub-Saharan Africa*. RG Feachem, DT Jamison (eds). Oxford University Press, World Bank.
4. Lewis G, Drife J, 1998. *Why Mothers Die: Report on Confidential Enquiries into Maternal Death in the UK 1994-1996*. HMSO, Norwich.
5. Bouvier Colle MH, Varnoux N, Costes P et al, 1991. Reasons for the underreporting of maternal mortality in France, as indicated by a survey of all deaths among women of childbearing age. *International Journal of Epidemiology*. 20(3):717-21.
6. Berg CJ, Atrash HK, Koonin LM et al, 1996. Pregnancy-related mortality in the United States, 1987-1990. *Obstetrics & Gynecology*. 88(2):161-67.
7. Campbell OMR, Graham WJ, 1990. *Measuring maternal morbidity and mortality: levels and trends*. Partnership for Safe Motherhood, Population Health and Human Resources Department. World Bank, Washington DC.
8. Campbell OMR, Graham WJ, 1996. Methods for measuring maternal mortality. Paper presented at Seminar on Innovative Approaches to the Assessment of Reproductive Health. International Union for Scientific Study of Population & Population Institute, University of the Philippines. Manila, 24-27 September.
9. Graham WJ, Brass W, Snow RW, 1989. Estimating maternal mortality: the sisterhood method. *Studies in Family Planning*. 20:125-30.
10. Danel I, Graham WJ, Stupp P et al, 1996. Applying the sisterhood method for estimating maternal mortality to a health facility-based sample: a comparison with results from a household-based sample. *International Journal of Epidemiology*. 35(5):1017-22.
11. Rutenberg N, Sullivan J, 1991. Direct and indirect estimates of maternal mortality from the sisterhood method. Paper presented at Demographic and Health Surveys World Conference, Washington DC, August 5-7, 1991.
12. *Revised 1990 Estimates of Maternal Mortality. A new approach by WHO and UNICEF*. WHO/FRH/MSM/96.11. World Health Organization, Geneva, 1996.
13. Graham WJ, Filippi VGA, Ronsmans C, 1996. Demonstrating programme impact on maternal mortality. *Health Policy and Planning*. 11(1):16-20.
14. Stanton C, Abderrahim N, Hill K, 1997. *DHS Maternal Mortality Indicators: An Assessment of Data Quality and Implications for Data Use*. DHS Analytical Reports #4. Macro International Inc, Calverton MD.
15. See, for example: Fortney JA, Susanti I, Gadalla S et al, 1986. Reproductive mortality in two developing countries. *American Journal of Public Health*. 76:134-38.
16. See, for example: Walker GJA, Ashley DEC, McCaw A et al, 1986. Maternal mortality in Jamaica. *Lancet*. 1(8479):486-88.
17. See, for example: Greenwood AM, Greenwood BM, Bradley AK et al, 1987. A prospective survey of the outcome of pregnancy in a rural area of the Gambia. *Bulletin of the World Health Organization*. 65:635-43.
18. Timaeus I, 1991. Measurement of adult mortality in less developed countries: a comparative review. *Population Index*. 57(4):552-68.
19. See, for example: Kwast BE, Rochat RW, Kidane-Mariam W, 1986. Maternal mortality in Addis Ababa, Ethiopia. *Studies in Family Planning*. 17:288-301.
20. *National Maternal Mortality Study: Egypt 1992-1993. Preliminary report of findings and conclusions*. Child Survival Project, Egypt Ministry of Health, Cairo, July 1994.
21. Campbell OMR, Kassas M, Hefni ML, 1995. National Maternal Mortality Study: Egypt 1992-3. Paper presented at Population Association of America Annual Meeting, New Orleans, May 9-11.
22. Campbell OMR, Ronsmans C, 1994. *Verbal Autopsies for Maternal Deaths*. Report of WHO Workshop. WHO/FHE/MSM/95.15. World Health Organization, Geneva
23. Ronsmans C, Vanneste AM, Chakraborty J et al, 1998. A comparison of three verbal autopsy methods to ascertain levels and causes of maternal deaths in Matlab, Bangladesh. *International Journal of Epidemiology*. 27:660 66.
24. Maternal morbidities affect tens of millions. *Network*. 1994; 14(3):8-14.
25. Saftlas AF, Olson DR, Franks AL et al, 1990. Epidemiology of pre-eclampsia and eclampsia in the United States, 1979-1986. *American Journal of Obstetrics and Gynecology*. 163(2):460-65.
26. Statement from a Task Force meeting on validation of women's reporting of obstetric complications in national surveys. *MotherCare Matters*. 1997; 6(2):15-16.
27. Ronsmans C, 1996. Studies

validating women's reports of reproductive ill health: how useful are they? Paper presented at Seminar on Innovative Approaches to the Assessment of Reproductive Health. International Union for Scientific Study of Population, and Population Institute, University of the Philippines. Manila, 24-27 September.

28. Ronsmans C, Achadi E, Cohen S et al, 1997. Women's recall of obstetric complications in South Kalimantan, Indonesia. *Studies in Family Planning*. 28(3):203-14.
29. Barreto TV, Campbell OMR, Davies JL et al, 1992. Investigating induced abortion in developing countries: methods and problems. *Studies in Family Planning*. 23(3):159-70.
30. Llovet JJ, Ramos S, 1998. Induced abortion in Latin America: strategies for future social research. *Reproductive Health Matters*. 6(11):55-65.
31. Bulut A, Yolsal N, Filippi V et al, 1995. In search of truth: comparing alternative sources of information on reproductive tract infection. *Reproductive Health Matters*. 3(6):31-39.
32. See, for example: Goodburn EA, Gaze R, Chowdhury M, 1995. A report: beliefs and practices regarding delivery and postpartum maternal morbidity in rural Bangladesh. *Studies in Family Planning*. 26(1):21-32.
33. See, for example: Filippi V, Marshall T, Bulut A et al, 1997. Asking questions about women's reproductive health: validity and reliability of survey findings from Istanbul. *Tropical Medicine & International Health*. 2(1):47-56.
34. Koblinsky MA, Campbell OMR, Harlow S, 1992. Mother and more: a broader perspective on women's health. In: *The Health of Women: A Global Perspective*. M Koblinsky, J Timyan, J Gay et al (eds). Westview Press, Boulder CO.
35. Graham WJ, Ronsmans CCA, Filippi VGA et al, 1995. *Asking questions about women's reproductive health in community-based surveys: guidelines on scope and content.* Maternal and Child Epidemiology Unit Publication No 6. London School of Hygiene and Tropical Medicine, London.
36. McGinn T, 1997. Monitoring and evaluating the PMM efforts: what have we learned. *International Journal of Gynecology and Obstetrics*. 59(Suppl 2):S245-52.
37. Danquah JB, Appah EK, Djan JO et al, 1997. Improving record keeping for maternal mortality programmes, Kumasi Ghana. *International Journal of Gynecology and Obstetrics*. 59(Suppl 2):S149-55.
38. Abdullah SA, Abdel-Aleem H, Shulman C et al, 1995. *A prospective study to assess patterns of care among pregnant and postpartum women admitted to Assiut University Hospital, Upper Egypt*. Report to the Ford Foundation.
39. Filippi V, Gandaho T, Ronsmans C et al, 1996. The 'near-misses': are life-threatening complications practical indicators for Safe Motherhood programmes? Paper presented at Seminar on Innovative Approaches to the Assessment of Reproductive Health. International Union for Scientific Study of Population and Population Institute, University of the Philippines. Manila, 24-27 September.
40. Belghiti A, DeBrouwere V, Kegels G et al, 1998. Monitoring unmet obstetric need at district level in Morocco. *Tropical Medicine and International Health*. 3(7):584-91.
41. Shulman CE, Dorman EK, Cutts F et al, 1999. Preventing severe anaemia secondary to malaria in pregnancy: a double blind randomised placebo controlled trial of intermittent sulfadoxine-pyrimethamine. *Lancet*. 353:632-636.
42. Hodnett ED, 1997. Alternative versus conventional delivery settings. In: Neilson JP, Crowther CA, Hodnett ED et al (eds). *Pregnancy and Childbirth Module, Cochrane Database of Systematic Reviews*, Cochrane Library. [Updated 4 March 1997]. Database on disk and CDROM. The Cochrane Collaboration, Issue 2. Oxford. (Updated quarterly)
43. Fauveau V, Stewart K, Khan SA et al, 1991. Effect on mortality of community-based maternity care programme in rural Bangladesh. *Lancet*. 338:1183-86.
44. Ronsmans C, Vanneste AM, Chakraborty J et al, 1997. Decline in maternal mortality in Matlab, Bangladesh: a cautionary tale. *Lancet*. 350:1810-14.
45. Koblinsky M, McLaurin K, Russel-Brown P et al, 1995. *Indicators for reproductive health evaluation: final reports of the committee on safe pregnancy*. The Evaluation Project, University of North Carolina. December.
46. *Mother-Baby Package: Implementing Safe Motherhood in Countries*. WHO/FHE/MSM/94.11. World Health Organization, Geneva, 1994.
47. *Guidelines for Monitoring the Availability and Use of Obstetric Services*. UNICEF/WHO/UNFPA. October 1997.
48. *Guidance note on reproductive health programme performance indicators*. United Nations Population Fund, New York, 1996. (Draft)

Measuring Maternal Morbidity

Judith A Fortney, Jason B Smith

Just as the 1980s was the decade of measuring maternal mortality, the 1990s is the decade of measuring maternal morbidity. As the decade ends, the time is right to assess progress. Like maternal mortality, maternal morbidity is not as easy to measure as was originally supposed. Both have multiple causes – clinical, social and administrative; both are time-defined but with antecedents outside the pregnancy and delivery period. Both are characterised, at least in developing countries, by inadequate official records, resulting in a dependence on alternative sources of data. Maternal morbidity has many dimensions: aetiology, severity, duration, time of onset, accumulation and sequelae, each with different causes, consequences and implications for treatment. As with mortality, the understanding of maternal morbidity is enhanced through the use of a variety of data sources. This paper discusses the different sources of data on morbidity, including hospital-based case reviews, hospital discharge surveys, and cross-sectional studies with clinical examination or self-reports or both, and their biases and limitations. It concludes that while there are important reasons to obtain better estimates of the prevalence and incidence of maternal morbidity, there are already sufficient data from existing measures for resource allocation to proceed, and for policies and services to be modified, extended and improved.

MATERNAL mortality is frequently described as 'just the tip of the iceberg', implying that there is a vast base to the iceberg – maternal morbidity – which remains largely undescribed. This is only partly true; the literature is replete with hospital-based studies, case studies and anecdotes describing acute and chronic morbidities associated with pregnancy and delivery. What does remain relatively unknown is the prevalence of morbidity – specific or general – in the population as a whole. The number of such studies is limited, mainly because they are difficult to design, implement and analyse.

Why is maternal morbidity so difficult to measure?

Maternal morbidity, like all morbidity, has several dimensions,[1] including at least the following:

Aetiology

Some disease taxonomies try to classify morbidities by cause (such as infectious agents), but 'cause' is at many levels.[2] What causes a death (such as failure to treat correctly, or to seek treatment) is not necessarily what causes the morbidity in the first place. Maternal morbidity often has many interwoven causes that range from physiology and anatomy (such as pelvic size and shape) to the status of women (e.g. do they need their husbands' permission to seek medical care?) and the political priority (which influences the allocation of resources) given to health care. This view of 'cause' includes both clinical and social causes.

Severity

All morbidities can be measured along a severity continuum which ranges from 'nuisance' to life-threatening. Some become more severe as the condition progresses so that early detection is important (for example, pregnancy-induced hypertension). Some conditions are always life-threatening (such as eclampsia) and others are never so (e.g. backache during pregnancy). Post-partum haemorrhage can be life-threatening immediately or only if it is neglected. In the case of obstetric morbidity, at least in resource-poor countries, severity may often be influenced by lack of appropriate treatment. Several maternal morbidities (for example, haemorrhage or prolapse) have fairly well-defined degrees of severity. While these have been used in clinical studies, they have not, thus far, been used in population-based studies.

Duration
Many obstetric morbidities are short-lived; women either recover with few sequelae, or they die. Still, a few short-lived morbidities do have long-term consequences. Prolonged and obstructed labour is probably the obstetric morbidity with greatest burden of chronic morbidity among survivors. While maternal morbidities are often transient, they are also often recurrent, occurring during each pregnancy. Furthermore, some conditions are inter-generational, either because the same environment persists (such as inadequate nutrition reducing pelvic capacity), or because of conditions of the mother that contribute to relevant ill health in her daughter (such as cretinism in the daughter because of iodine deficiency in the mother).

Time of onset
Obstetric morbidities are concentrated in the reproductive years, especially the early reproductive years, but they may result from conditions which occurred earlier, or the consequences may not be recognised until later. For example, early conditions (such as inadequate nutrition, rheumatic heart disease) can threaten the safety of pregnancy, and the accumulated consequences of repeated pregnancies may not take their toll until middle age.

Accumulation
Some morbidities accumulate over time because of continued exposure to a disease-causing agent (such as pregnancy) or failure to treat. The morbidity may or may not regress when the disease-causing agent is removed. Thus, repeated childbearing may lead to uterine prolapse.

Sequelae
Some morbidities have consequences that are more serious than the original morbidity (for example, choriocarcinoma following a molar pregnancy[3]); the consequences may be curable (such as fistula or choriocarcinoma) or not (such as Sheehan's Syndrome[4] following obstetric haemorrhage). Appropriate treatment of the original morbidity often prevents sequelae.

Each component of maternal morbidity (such as eclampsia or haemorrhage) has different causes, different consequences, and different implications for treatment. They have in common only the fact that they occur in pregnant women during the pregnancy, delivery or post-partum period. Even the post-partum period is somewhat arbitrarily defined and varies from 42 days to three months to one year.

In addition to the six dimensions described above, which apply to all morbidities, there are other reasons why maternal morbidity is difficult to study. Among these is a need for clarity in what is meant by morbidity. Any single morbidity is often a point along a causal pathway with multiple possibilities for intervention.[2] Different researchers may focus on different points in the pathway, but it is not always clear that each point is a distinct morbidity. Take the example of a woman who has a contracted pelvis because of poor diet in childhood and adolescence. The contracted pelvis leads to obstructed – and therefore prolonged – labour, which leads to a vesico-vaginal fistula (VVF) which leads to social ostracism, divorce[5] and suicidal depression. Which morbidity do we wish to measure? For the woman who never becomes pregnant, the contracted pelvis need never create problems – is it then morbidity? The pregnant woman whose condition is recognised will still have an obstructed labour, but it need not be prolonged if properly managed (by caesarean section). Even if she develops a fistula, it can be repaired and she need not suffer the social and psychological morbidities. Hence, this cluster of events may be counted as one morbidity (which would understate it), or six morbidities (which would overstate it).

Research methods
There are several study designs available to the researcher, which are described below. None of these is prospective because prospective designs are prohibitively expensive, and also subject to many of the same biases as cross-sectional ones. In prospective studies, ethical issues emerge in that there is a mandate to treat identified morbidities; while this changes their prevalence, it can be used to confirm their presence. Each of these designs has advantages and disadvantages from a practical (implementation) perspective, and each has its own biases. All, including those involving clinical examination, are subject to diagnostic bias.

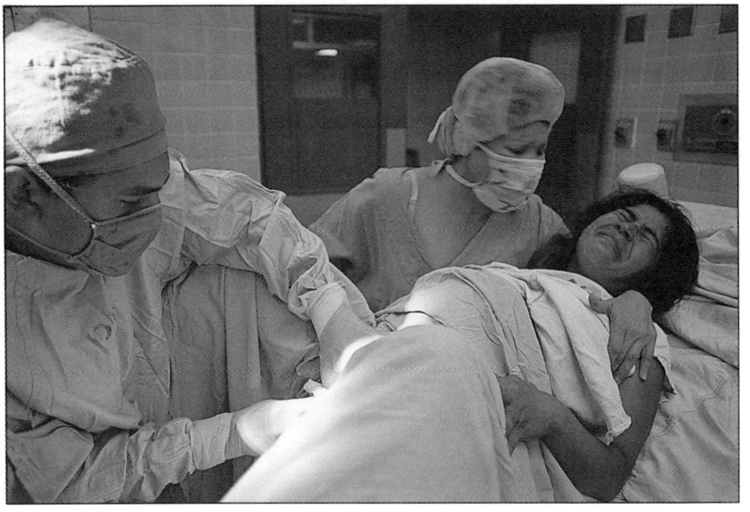

TINA GUE / PANOS PICTURES

Hospital-based case reviews

From these we learn about the nature and cause of the morbidity, and how to treat or cure it. While we can learn something about the burden of the disease, it is impossible to extrapolate from hospital-based studies to the population as a whole. Hospital-based studies include only women who have sought treatment for the condition and do not permit speculation about the nature or magnitude of the untreated segment. In countries with good access to health care, hospital-based reviews are more productive because the untreated segment represents a smaller proportion of the morbid population. There are thousands of studies of this type reported in the literature.

Hospital discharge surveys

In countries with good access to health care, hospital discharge surveys can measure the incidence of conditions serious enough to require hospitalisation. For example, 14.6 per cent of pregnant women in the USA in 1986-87 and 12.3 per cent in 1991-92 were hospitalised during pregnancy for conditions unrelated to miscarriage or delivery.[6,7]

Cross-sectional studies, clinical examination only

This method is ideal for some morbidities. However, it can only be used for chronic conditions that are identifiable upon examination (such as uterine prolapse). It cannot be used retrospectively for acute conditions; it is not possible to determine, for example, if a woman has had a postpartum haemorrhage unless it was very recent. Nor can it be used to detect morbidities with no identifiable signs but with symptoms only, such as dyspareunia or chronic backache.

Cross-sectional studies, self-reports without clinical examination

Table 1 shows studies of maternal morbidity that fall into this category. These studies are based on direct questioning about a recent or current pregnancy; they permit measurement of incidence or prevalence (see Glossary) of morbidity insofar as it is perceived – conditions with no symptoms (such as hypertension) are not perceived and therefore not reported. It should also be noted that this approach can measure only symptoms rather than conditions, and more than one condition (morbidity) may share the same symptoms. For example, loss of consciousness during labour may be because of blood loss, an eclamptic seizure or shock. In studies of past pregnancies, recall becomes an issue. Obviously, studies of this type depend upon women's perceptions of morbidity. A condition that is not perceived, or is not perceived as morbid, is not recorded.

Table 1. Population-based studies of maternal morbidity

Authors	Year of publication	Study site(s)
De Graft-Johnson[8]	1994	Ghana
Stewart & Festin[9]	1995	Philippines
Bhatia & Cleland[10]	1995	South India
CDC & UNFPA[11]	no date	Ecuador
Fortney & Smith[12]	1996	Egypt, India, Bangladesh, Indonesia
Ronsmans[13]	1997	Indonesia
Sloan[14]	unpublished	Ghana

Cross-sectional studies, with self-reports and clinical examination

These combine the above two types of study.[15,16] The incidence or prevalence of specific morbidities varies in these studies. The proportion of women having *any* morbidity during pregnancy or during delivery also varies, but less than might be expected. What no existing research has so far measured is the severity of the condition. The primary difference between countries where most people have access to good medical care and those that do not is that morbidities reach a greater degree of severity in the latter, even when there is little difference in the underlying incidence or prevalence. Though in principle a useful variable, 'severity' is difficult to measure, and no research reports have tried to do so.

The fact that obstetric morbidity is usually acute and for a short time, with the patient either dying or recovering completely, contributes to the difficulty in measuring it. In the absence of medical records – and most births in the world take place at home – only women's or their caregivers' recall and perceptions of events can be measured. It is not possible retrospectively to determine by clinical examination whether a woman experienced a haemorrhage, hypertension, infection or prolonged labour. It is possible to identify clinically conditions that could have been caused by pregnancy or delivery, but also have many other causes – anaemia, hypertension, pelvic inflammatory disease, prolapse.[15]

Some chronic conditions that are usually the result of pregnancy are easily identifiable, and a substantial literature exists on them; vesico-vaginal and recto-vaginal fistulae are the best examples.[16] Research on such conditions is usually limited to women who seek treatment for them; hence, few studies exist which have sought to determine the population-based prevalence of those conditions. While easily identifiable by clinicians when they are asked to treat them, and almost certainly by the women who suffer from them, such conditions are less easily identified by interview techniques. One study,[12] which looked at urinary incontinence including VVF, used questions that were unclear; the women were not familiar with these relatively rare conditions and found the questions difficult to answer.

Reliability and validity

Reliability refers to the ability of a measurement to elicit the same response when repeated. Validity refers to whether a measure is measuring what it purports to measure. Measuring maternal morbidity does not readily lend itself to assessment of reliability, and almost no work has been done in this area. In most developing countries, the only feasible technique for estimating the prevalence or incidence of obstetric morbidity is to interview women about a recent pregnancy (cross-sectional studies without clinical examination). The validity of self-reports, on the other hand, has been under some scrutiny.

Validity is influenced by the fact that questioning elicits symptoms rather than conditions. If a woman says she lost consciousness during delivery, additional questions will be required about hypertension (of which the respondent may be unaware), blood loss (which is notoriously difficult to measure) or shock (which the respondent may not understand). But only if these possibilities can be ruled out will loss of consciousness become a valid measure of eclampsia.

Similarly, even though VVF would appear to be easily identifiable by women suffering from it, efforts to identify VVF in Egypt[16] were less than successful. The questions covered urinary leakage and tried to separate stress incontinence from VVF by the nature of the leakage. In fact, the questions did not distinguish well, perhaps because they were poorly worded, or perhaps because these are quite personal questions. On clinical examination, 17.4 per cent of women reporting urinary leakage were found to have stress incontinence or VVF, and 9.5 per cent of women not reporting leakage were found to have stress incontinence or VVF.

Other conditions for which validity is probably poor include blood loss (it is not well estimated), duration of labour (when does labour start?) and post-partum infection (fever can be caused by other infections).

From an epidemiologic perspective, validity consists of sensitivity and specificity (see Glossary). A few studies have looked at the sensitivity and specificity of questions relating to specific morbidities. There are two ways to do this. The first applies only to chronic conditions and requires a physical examination.[15,16] The two studies referenced showed that, in general, neither sensitivity nor specificity were good.

The second method is more useful for acute conditions of delivery (not pregnancy). Women who delivered in hospital are questioned at some later point about delivery-related morbidity; both women with morbidities and those without are interviewed. Interview responses are compared with hospital records.[13,14,17,18] Table 2 shows the sensitivity and specificity of individual morbidities from the five studies that have measured them. Comparisons are difficult because each study examined slightly different questions. In addition, as with validation studies of chronic morbidity, studies vary in what is included in the numerator and the denominator because of case definitions and study design.

Two difficulties exist with this approach. First, hospital records are often less than complete, and are not always reliable, especially for less severe conditions.[19] Second, women who deliver in hospital are different from those who deliver at home. Uncomplicated hospital deliveries are more likely to be better educated women who may also be better able to report their condition. Women who experienced a complicated delivery in hospital are probably more likely to report their condition correctly (because they may have been told its name) than women who delivered at home. (Danel et al, however, reported quite small differences.[19]) Thus validation through the use of hospital records may over-estimate the accuracy of self-reports.

Table 2 shows that self-reports can be a valuable tool in determining the gross burden of obstetric morbidity. However, it is not yet possible to use self-reported information to diagnose conditions, and self-reports cannot provide accurate estimates of prevalence or incidence.

Ronsmans[20] provides elegant mathematical

Table 2. Sensitivity and specificity of individual maternal morbidities as recalled and reported to interviewers*

Morbidity	Philippines 1995[17]	Bolivia 1998[18] **	Ghana 1996[14]	Indonesia 1997[13]
Post-partum haemorrhage	Sensitivity: 0.53 (0.39-0.66) Specificity: 0.90 (0.84-0.94) ('lost a lot of blood around delivery')	Sensitivity: 86.7 (59.5- 98.3) (thought she would die) Specificity: 88.9 (82.7- 95.1) (fainted)	Sensitivity: 0.70 (0.35-0.93) Specificity: 0.91 (0.87-0.94)	Sensitivity: 0.51 Specificity: 0.90 (0.91) (excessive bleeding during labour or delivery)
Prolonged labour	Sensitivity: 0.41 (0.26-0.57) Specificity: 0.88 (0.79-0.94) ('more than 12 hours')	Sensitivity: 21.2 (11.3- 31.1) (extended pushing) Specificity: 98.7 (96.9-100) (extended labour)	Sensitivity: 0.74 (0.6-0.85) Specificity: 0.83 (0.78-0.87) (dysfunctional labour)	Sensitivity: 0.31 Specificity: 76.7 (89.1) ('more than 24 hrs' response in hours)
Eclampsia	Sensitivity: 0.44 (0.21-0.69) Specificity: 0.96 (0.92-0.98) (convulsions during pregnancy or delivery)	Sensitivity: 50.0 (28.2-71.8) Specificity: 98.6 (97.5-99.7) (any seizures)	Sensitivity: NA Specificity: 0.99 (0.99-1.0)	Sensitivity: 0.75 Specificity: 0.99 (0.96) (convulsions during pregnancy)
Post-partum infection	Sensitivity: 0.56 (0.23-0.84) Specificity: 0.93 (0.88-0.96) ('very high fever' post-partum)	Sensitivity: not calculated (too few cases) Specificity: 99.3 (98.5-100) (presence of infection)	Sensitivity: 0.25 (0.01-0.81) Specificity: 0.99 (0.97-1.0)	Sensitivity: NA Specificity: 0.86 (0.92) (high fever post-partum)

**The denominator used in the calculation of the specificity given in parentheses includes women who reported a complication other than the one specified and women who had the condition. The denominator used in the calculation of the specificity outside the parentheses refers to women who had uncomplicated deliveries and women who had the condition.*

*** Several different questions used. The one cited is the one with the highest sensitivity or specificity.*

Table 3. How sensitivity and specificity influence the estimates of prevalence (adapted from Ronsmans[20])

Sensitivity	Specificity	Estimated prevalence where: Actual prevalence = 1%	Actual prevalence = 5%
50%	80	20	21
	90	10	12
	95	5	7
	98	2	4
	99	1	3
	100	1	3
70%	80	20	22
	90	11	13
	95	6	8
	98	3	5
	99	2	4
	100	1	4
90%	80	21	23
	90	11	14
	95	6	9
	98	3	6
	99	2	5
	100	1	5
95%	80	21	24
	90	11	14
	95	6	10
	98	3	7
	99	2	6
	100	1	5

arguments to suggest that self-reports tend to over-estimate morbidity, especially if the underlying true prevalence of morbidity is low. Assuming the sensitivities exceed 50 per cent, specificities must be very high to produce accurate estimates of morbidity, and small variations in specificity can result in large over-estimates of prevalence. Because high specificity may be easier to achieve for some morbidities than for others, the accuracy of self-reports may vary by condition. Table 3, which is adapted (and abbreviated) from Ronsmans, shows that specificity has a greater influence on the accuracy of estimates than sensitivity – in other words, it is more important to identify correctly women who did not have a condition than it is to identify correctly those who did.

Where the true prevalence of disease is around 5 per cent, high specificity (0.98 or greater) in conjunction with low sensitivity (0.80 or less) can lead to under-estimates of prevalence; but where specificity is less than 0.98 – as is often the case – even sensitivities as high as 0.99 lead to over-estimates. Lower prevalence of disease is even harder to estimate correctly. Higher prevalences are somewhat easier; for example, where actual incidence is 20 per cent, a sensitivity as low as 0.60 in conjunction with a specificity as low as 0.90 will lead to an accurate estimate (data not shown in Table 3). With high prevalences, of course, the possibility of an under-estimate is greater. Table 3 emphasises just how high the specificities need to be; many of those shown in Table 2 are high, but not sufficiently high.

In countries where most births take place outside of institutions, and in spite of their limitations, self-reports in response to well-designed and well-worded interviews may be the only way to collect information about some maternal morbidities. Furthermore, health-seeking behaviour is based on the perception of morbidity (and options for care) regardless of clinical reality. Thus self-reports are critical for understanding how women interact with their health services.

Short of all births taking place in institutions and comprehensive data collection on all deliveries, there is little choice but to continue to use self-reports. Hence, we should seek to refine the means by which we ask women about their experience of obstetric morbidity. This means improving questionnaires (through use of formative research), and interview techniques. All available sources of data should be used, including hospital-based studies, national-scale surveys (such as Demographic and Health Surveys) and case-series. In addition, designing questions to improve specificity would be valuable.

In the meantime, activities to improve measurement of maternal morbidity need not delay sensible and reasonable decisions on health resource allocations and programme priorities. Data presently available, while statistically unsatisfying, are adequate to begin to address the problems of inadequate health services that cause so much suffering to mothers worldwide.

Program implications: why do we need to know?

Why study maternal morbidity – is it to inform policy? to plan programmes? to know the burden of maternal ill health? Different reasons suggest different definitions of morbidity, and will influence which dimensions are important. Knowing the true (i.e. population-based) incidence or prevalence of disease is potentially important for three main reasons.

First, we need the information in order to plan to address morbidity. This means allocating money, and having the necessary skills and supplies in health facilities. High (rather than low) incidence or prevalence is more likely to catch the attention of those who allocate resources. However, it is not clear that precise, population-based estimates of morbidity are required for this – especially where medical services are known to be poor. We know that maternal morbidity is high and that current resources are insufficient to address it; the less-than-robust combination of measurements already available is adequate for making policy and programme decisions.

Glossary

Sensitivity is the proportion of persons with the condition who are correctly identified. For example: it is the proportion of women who suffered a post-partum haemorrhage who were correctly identified by an interview to have had a post-partum haemorrhage.

Specificity is the proportion of persons without the condition who are correctly identified. For example: it is the proportion of women who did NOT suffer a post-partum haemorrhage who were correctly identified by an interview as having been free of this condition.

Incidence is the proportion of the population who experience a condition for the first time during a given time period. For example: the proportion of women who have a post-partum haemorrhage after their delivery.

Prevalence is the proportion of the population who have a condition at any one time. This measure is better used for chronic conditions, such as uterine prolapse or fistula, than it is for acute conditions, such as post-partum haemorrhage or eclampsia.

It is true that if we knew the proportion of women who can be expected to need medical care during delivery, the number of hospital beds, doctors, nurses, drugs and other supplies to treat them could be provided. No developing country or donor has the resources to do this all at once. Furthermore, in many areas, hospital beds stay empty because the skills and supplies are lacking, or patients are poorly treated. Upgrading medical facilities so that women seek care is the first step; expanding services (more hospitals, clinics, beds, staff, etc) when current services are overloaded is the next step. Neither of these require better statistics than are available now.

Second, we need to be able to measure maternal morbidity so that we can learn whether interventions have been successful. There are pitfalls here, which better measurement of incidence or prevalence does not necessarily avoid. Moreover, because most maternal morbidities cannot be prevented, the incidence of the morbidity is not the outcome of interest; the number treated and case-fatality rates are more useful to know. But there are important exceptions. For example, interventions to prevent infection should be evaluated by their impact on the incidence of infection, and for that we need to be able to measure infection better.

Finally, we need to be able to measure maternal morbidity in order to learn more about its causes. It was the high incidence of puerperal infection in the 19th century that led Semmelweiss to investigate its causes and identify an intervention.[21] Today, a change in the incidence of infection in a particular location would also lead to an investigation of its causes.

In summary, while there are scientific reasons for wanting to know the true incidence or prevalence of specific obstetric morbidities, there are already sufficient data from existing, imperfect measures from the perspective of policy and programmes. Thus, resource reallocation can proceed, services can be modified, extended and improved, and policies can be put in place simultaneously with innovation and improvements on the research front.

Acknowledgements

The authors are grateful to Patricia Bailey and Emelita Wong for their many helpful suggestions.

Correspondence

Judith Fortney, Family Health International, PO Box 13950, Research Triangle Park, NC 27709, USA. Fax: 1-919-544-7261. E-mail: Jfortney@fhi.org

References and Notes

1. Fortney JA, 1995. *Reproductive Morbidity: A Conceptual Framework*. Family Health International, Research Triangle Park NC, September. Also presented at the IUSSP seminar Innovative Approaches to the Assessment of Reproductive Health. Manila, Philippines, September 1996. (To be published in the seminar proceedings.)
2. Fathalla M, 1987. Why did Mrs. X Die? *People*. 14:8-9.
3. A molar pregnancy is one in which a part of the placenta (the chorion) develops abnormally. Left untreated, this tissue may become cancerous and spread to other parts of the body.
4. Sheehan's Syndrome is a condition of the pituitary gland resulting from circulatory collapse caused by severe blood loss during or after delivery.
5. Divorce and social ostracism are social, rather than clinical, morbidities.
6. Franks AL, Kendrick JS, Olson DR et al, 1992. Hospitalization for pregnancy complications, United States, 1986 and 1987. *American Journal of Obstetrics and Gynecology*. 166:1339-44.
7. Bennett TA, Kotelchuck M, Cox CE et al, 1998. Pregnancy-associated hospitalizations in the United States in 1991 and 1992: a comprehensive view of maternal morbidity. *American Journal of Obstetrics and Gynecology*. 178:346-54.
8. De Graft-Johnson JE, 1994. Determinants of maternal morbidity in Bosomtwe-Atwima-Kwanwoma District (of Ghana). Dissertation, University of North Carolina, Chapel Hill.
9. Stewart MK, Stanton CK, Festin M et al, 1996. Issues in measuring maternal morbidity: lessons from the Philippines safe motherhood survey project. *Studies in Family Planning*. 27:29-35.
10. Bhatia J, Cleland J, 1996. Obstetric morbidity in south India: results from a community survey. *Social Science and Medicine*. 43:1507-16.
11. *Ecuador: Encuesta Demografica y de Salud Materna e Infantil. Informe General*. Centers for Disease Control and Prevention, United Nations Population Fund. Atlanta & New York, 1995.
12. Fortney JA, Smith JB, 1996. *The Base of the Iceberg: Prevalence and Perceptions of Maternal Morbidity in Four Developing Countries*. Family Health International, Research Triangle Park NC, December.
13. Ronsmans C, Achadi E, Cohen S et al, 1997. Women's recall of obstetric complications in south Kalimantan, Indonesia. *Studies in Family Planning*. 28:203-14.
14. Sloan NL, Arthur P, Amoaful E et al. Validity of self-reports to identify major obstetric complications. (Submitted for publication)
15. Younis N, Khalil K, Zurayk H et al, 1994. *Learning About the Gynecological Health of Women*. Number 2, Policy Series in Reproductive Health, Population Council, New York.
16. Ezzeldin HO, El-Nahal N. Saleh S et al, 1995. Study of the prevalence and perception of maternal morbidity in Menoufeya Governorate, Egypt; Final report to the Ford Foundation. Egypt Fertility Care Society, Cairo, 1995. (The study reported here was part of the study reported in reference [9].)
17. Stewart MK, Festin M,1995. Validation study of women's reporting and recall of major obstetric complications treated at the Philippine General Hospital. *International Journal of Gynecology and Obstetrics*. 48:S53-S66.
18. Seoane G, Castrillo M, O'Rourke K, 1998. A validation study of maternal self reports of obstetrical complications: implications for health surveys. *International Journal of Gynecology and Obstetrics*. 62:229-36.
19. Danel I, Ponce de Leon R, Lozado P, 1996. Validation study of responses to maternal morbidity modules of the 1994 Ecuadoran Reproductive Health Survey. Presented at IUSSP seminar Innovative Approaches to the Assessment of Reproductive Health. Manila, Philippines, September. (To be published in the seminar proceedings.)
20. Ronsmans C, 1996. Studies validating women's reports of reproductive ill health; how useful are they? Presented at IUSSP seminar Innovative Approaches to the Assessment of Reproductive Health. Manila, Philippines, September. (To be published in the seminar proceedings.)
21. Loudon I, 1992. *Death in Childbirth: An International Study of Maternal Care and Maternal Mortality 1800-1950*. Clarendon Press, Oxford. Chapter 3.

National policies and programmes

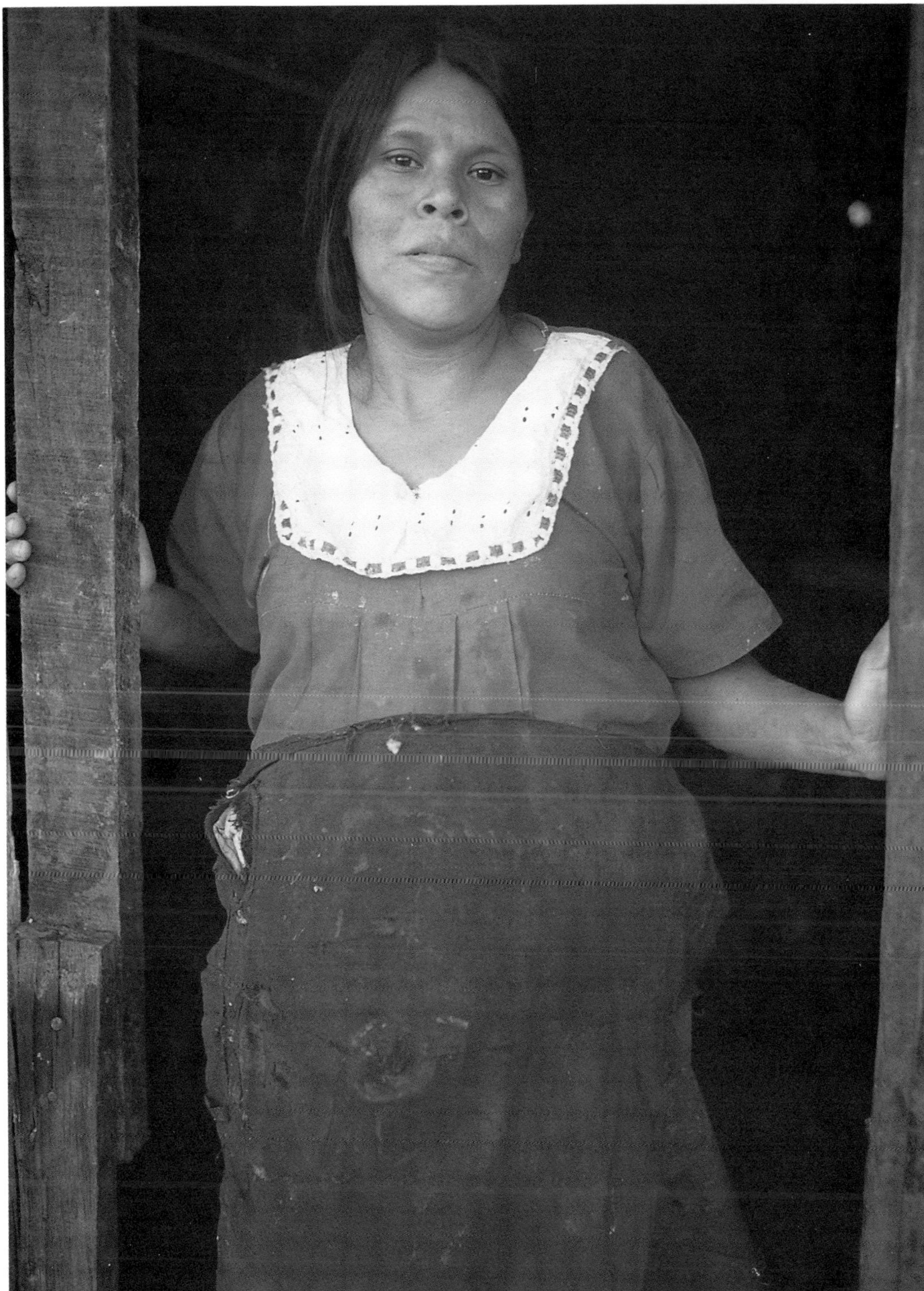

JENNY MATTHEWS / NETWORK

Safe Motherhood Programmes in Bangladesh

Zahidul A Huque, Margaret Leppard, Dileep Mavalankar, Halida Hanum Akhter, TA Chowdhury

Despite substantial decline in infant and child mortality in Bangladesh during the last decade, and a number of activities to reduce maternal mortality, a decline in maternal mortality is yet to be observed. For this reason, an assessment of the maternal health programme was commissioned by the government in 1997. The assessment found that despite an impressive health infrastructure, home birth is almost universal, still mostly carried out by untrained TBAs. Women's poor health and low status in society, the poor quality of maternity care services, lack of trained providers, low uptake of services by women, and infrastructural and interdepartmental difficulties are all contributing to the high rate of deaths. Many non-governmental organisations have undertaken innovative pilot projects to reduce maternal deaths, with impressive results in some project areas, which may be valuable in informing the direction of the national programme. A consensus has been reached among relevant government agencies and donors on an Essential Service Package for Bangladesh, which includes reproductive health care. Improvements in maternity care are an important part of this package. Major policy strategies include a focus on patients, improvement in the quality of services, cost recovery, and reorganisation of Health and Family Planning Directorates to improve integration of planning and programmes.

DESPITE efforts on the part of the government and many non-governmental organisations to improve the health of the women and children for more than a decade, Bangladesh, one of the poorest and most densely populated countries in the world, continues to experience high maternal mortality. The maternal mortality ratio (MMR) is estimated to be 420-850 per 100,000 live births,[1,2] and has not fallen significantly since data were first reported in the 1970s. The three leading causes of deaths are post-partum haemorrhage, complications of abortion, and eclampsia, though the distribution of these may vary by region and study. This mortality is associated with reports by women of a high level of perceived morbidities: 57 per cent antenatal morbidities, 26 per cent intra-partum, 62 per cent post-partum, and 29 per cent chronic or residual morbidities.[3] About 70 per cent of mothers suffer from nutritional deficiency anaemia and 50 per cent of babies are born with low birth weight.[4,5]

For more than a decade, the Government of Bangladesh (GOB) has recognised safe delivery as a key component of its maternal and child health strategy. The GOB responded to the 1987 global Safe Motherhood Initiative by conducting its first assessment of delivery services for maternal health care in 1988.[6] The findings influenced the maternal health components of the Fourth Health and Population Project (1991-1998), and several maternal health pilot projects were implemented both in the government and NGO sectors. Safer delivery for women was one of the six objectives of the Fourth Population Project. Interventions to support this objective included:

- training of TBAs;
- screening and referral of high risk pregnancies;
- strengthening of antenatal, delivery, and post-partum care;
- funding of a special maternal and neonatal care project; and
- strengthening of obstetric and gynaecological services at sub-district health complexes and district hospitals.[6]

While the MMR has remained at high levels, Bangladesh witnessed a 37 per cent decline in the infant mortality rate between 1985 and 1995.[7] This decline is attributable to the child health programmes implemented in this same period, such as immunisation, outreach clinics, and diarrhoeal disease control programmes. To find out why government efforts to bring about a reduction in maternal deaths were not being achieved, the Government of Bangladesh commissioned an assessment of the Maternal Health Programme in 1997.

This paper is based largely on the findings of that assessment, which was conducted by a team of experts from the Indian Institute of Management in Ahamedabad, India; London School of Hygiene and Tropical Medicine, UK; Canadian International Development Agency, Dhaka; World Bank, Washington DC; Bangladesh Institute of Research for Promotion of Essential and Reproductive Health and Technologies (BIRPERHT), Dhaka; and an independent consultant. Technical, management and financial support for this assessment were provided by MotherCare, a global project on maternal and neonatal health, based in Washington DC.

The assessment team spent three weeks in October 1997 in the field visiting health facilities at all levels and holding discussions with policymakers, programme managers, hospital staff and field level workers. The team also met with the directors of special projects to discuss the lessons learned from their projects. The information gathered from these visits was supplemented by a review of published and unpublished literature on maternal health status and programmes in Bangladesh, and health information records provided by national and local level officials. The study findings and recommendations were presented to the Government of Bangladesh at a workshop in Dhaka.[8]

The assessment found that women's low status in society, the poor quality of maternity care services, a lack of trained providers, low uptake of services by women, and infrastructural and interdepartmental difficulties all contribute to the high rate of deaths.

Women's status in Bangladesh

Social and cultural conditions in Bangladesh can to some extent explain the plateauing of the MMR. Women's choices are restricted with regard to childbearing and fertility preference, and their educational attainment and economic participation are also limited. Nor have women achieved equal rights and freedoms in the society. The onset of menstruation and puberty are viewed as a potential threat to the honour of a girl's family,[9,10] which is mitigated only at marriage. Within marriage, pregnancy and birth are welcomed, especially in the case of newly married couples, and a woman's ability to carry and bear a child is regarded as something to be celebrated and the source of status for her family.[11]

Pregnancy is kept hidden from the public eye as long as possible. A woman is not supposed to complain about her suffering during pregnancy to her husband or mother-in-law unless it becomes unbearable. She is also expected to continue her household tasks for as long as possible. There is a strong sense of pride if a woman can do her household work throughout pregnancy, and give birth with the help of a relative or traditional birth attendant (TBA) without troubling her husband or other male members in the family to arrange a hospital delivery.

Some rituals surrounding childbirth may negatively affect the health of women and newborns. In many situations, immediately after delivery the woman takes a cleansing bath to remove the gross ritual pollution associated with birth and blood. However, she then remains, to a greater or lesser extent, secluded from the rest of her family and from outsiders, i.e. she may be kept in a separate room or have a separate mat on the floor. Often, fire smokes are lighted to remove the evil spirit from the room where she sleeps. The period of post-partum seclusion ranges from 7-40 days[12] and serves to limit women's access to health services and trained service providers.

Service delivery infrastructure

Bangladesh has developed an impressive primary health care infrastructure over the years. Maternal health services are provided at community and facility levels through a network of domiciliary field workers, 'satellite' clinics,[13] health clinics and hospitals. Health service workers are employed by one of two separate directorates in the Ministry, either the Directorate of Health Services or the Directorate of Family Planning. The Ministry's bifurcation into these two wings dates back to the

1970s. Although the organisational structure of the Ministry has gone through many changes since then, these Directorates and the services they are responsible for have not been integrated at all levels. The present structure does not adequately address identified needs, especially for maternity services, which require co-ordination between primary, secondary and tertiary levels of care. Furthermore, across the divide between the two directorates, health workers who are employed by the Directorate of Family Planning do not co-ordinate with those employed by the Directorate of Health Services, and this is also true at all levels of care.

At community level, female family welfare assistants (FWAs) provide domiciliary family planning primarily and some maternal health services to households in the villages. These workers are recruited locally and must have ten years' education. Male health assistants (HAs) also provide domiciliary services, including distribution of vitamin A capsules, immunisation, detection of malaria, and prevention and treatment of diarrhoeal diseases, among others. The population served by each FWA and HA is approximately 5,000-6,000. By 1992, 23,000 FWAs had been trained and 95 per cent of communities now have FWAs.[7] Health and family planning supervisors are posted at union level to oversee the work of the FWAs and HAs in the villages.

At union level,[14] there are 3,000 Union Health and Family Welfare Centres (UHFWCs) and 30,000 satellite clinics throughout the country, which provide primary level care to a rural population of about 20,000-30,000 people. UHFWCs are staffed by paramedical staff, family welfare visitors (FWVs) and medical assistants, who provide promotive and simple curative services. In some unions, qualified medical doctors (MBBS) are posted, but obstetric first aid is virtually absent at union level.[15] Twice a week satellite clinics are held by FWVs to provide antenatal care, immunisation and family planning services to a cluster of villages. Ninety-one per cent of women live in communities where a satellite clinic is available.[7]

At thana (sub-district) level, there are 349 Thana Health Complexes (THCs) which provide preventive and curative services to a population of 200,000-400,000 each. The THC provides the first level of indoor care, with 31 beds and a professional staff of eight doctors, one dentist, five staff nurses, and some basic medicines and equipment. Outpatient antenatal services are primarily provided by family welfare visitors (FWVs), who are female paramedical staff under the Directorate of Family Planning. FWVs do not receive adequate technical and management support from the doctors at thana level, who are under the Directorate of Health Services. Anyone requiring admission is seen by a medical officer.

THCs have a post for a gynaecologist, but this position is usually filled by a medical officer with no special training in obstetrics/gynaecology. Nor are trained anaesthetists normally available or posted at THCs, unless they are part of special projects. Basic Essential Obstetric Care (Basic EOC) services, including administration of parenteral antibiotics, oxytocic and sedative drugs, assisted vaginal delivery, and manual removal of placenta, are available in about 56 per cent of THCs, according to a national survey in 1995.[16] Only a few THCs with special projects offer Comprehensive EOC (Basic EOC plus caesarean section, anaesthesia and blood transfusion).

At the district level, there are 64 Maternal and Child Welfare Centres (MCWCs), each serving a population of 1 to 2 million. A 1995 survey found that only 69 per cent of the MCWCs were found to be offering Comprehensive EOC,[16] so the rest are currently being upgraded to do so. Comprehensive EOC services are also supposed to be provided at the 64 district hospitals; however, the same 1995 survey revealed that only 39 per cent of district hospitals were delivering Comprehensive EOC.

Tertiary-level care is provided in 13 medical college hospitals. There are also 12 private medical colleges, but many of them do not have hospitals of their own. The Institute of Post-Graduate Medicine and Research (Bangabandhu Post-Graduate Medical College), the premier graduate medical faculty with a large hospital, is located in the capital city of Dhaka and is supported by the government. Other specialised hospitals are administered both by private organisations and by the government.

Antenatal, delivery and post-partum coverage and quality

Despite the existing health services infrastructure, the majority of pregnant women do not receive antenatal care in Bangladesh – only 29 per cent of women giving birth between 1992 and 1996 had received some antenatal care. Yet a strikingly high number (75 per cent) of women received a tetanus toxoid injection.[7] Of those who did receive antenatal care, 20 per cent received it from a doctor, and 7 per cent from a nurse, a midwife, or a family welfare visitor. Less than 1 per cent were visited by a TBA. Use of antenatal care has not increased over the last few years. Although awareness of the benefits of antenatal care is high among pregnant women (85 per cent), this knowledge has not been translated into care-seeking behaviour.[7]

About 6 per cent of deliveries in rural areas are attended by trained medical personnel and 95 per cent take place at home, mostly at the husband's residence.[3,7] In most cases, the decision about who should deliver the baby is taken before labour pains start. In only 20 per cent of cases do women themselves take the decision about who will deliver their baby. In 30 per cent of cases, the decision is made by the husband and in 27 per cent by the family as a whole; outside family members are involved in the remaining cases.[17]

Deliveries at health facilities and by trained providers take place more often in urban settings (35 per cent), more often among women with secondary level education and those who have received at least four antenatal visits. There are not many differences in the use of delivery services among women by age, birth order or geographic region.

Institutional deliveries can be risky due to the lack of emergency drugs, sterilised equipment and poor hygiene practices of providers. One member of the Maternal Health Assessment Team noted that institutional delivery is, in many respects, very similar to that performed by an untrained TBA. In higher referral centres, obstetricians spend substantial time with normal cases that could well have been handled by trained midwives.

TBAs remain more accessible to women than professional providers. The majority of deliveries continue to be assisted by TBAs, with 25 per cent assisted by relatives and 8 per cent by medically trained personnel.[7] The government had trained more than 45,000 TBAs as of October 1997, to provide delivery care for women in their homes; however, 65 per cent of deliveries were conducted by untrained TBAs. Even trained TBAs, however, like many professionals providing delivery care in Bangladesh, continue to ask women to bear down during the first stage of labour and perform multiple vaginal exams. Correspondingly, post-partum care is also primarily provided by TBAs and is not well organised.

Village doctors are often called upon when labour is not progressing normally, yet they are mostly not trained in clinical skills and they too have been observed to provide incorrect treatments (such as intra-muscular syntocinon to increase painful contractions). This wastes critical time that could have been used by clinically-skilled providers to manage complications. Co-ordination among the various levels of care is lacking, and even where referral systems are in place in project areas, they rarely function well.

Dysfunctional staffing configurations, unclear job descriptions, under-skilled staff and staff who lack confidence in their skills, are some of the problems facing the provision of Comprehensive EOC on a daily, 24-hour basis. To compound these problems, supplies are often lacking, and equipment is frequently not working or is inappropriate. Many of the facilities are poorly designed in terms of patient flow, lighting and ventilation, hand-washing facilities and consideration for traditional practices. Furthermore, there are frequent delays in the provision of treatment because the family who accompany the woman have to purchase drugs and blood. Thus, most facilities are not in a position to provide quality EOC services. The challenges are systemic, requiring change on a variety of levels to overcome the barriers to improving quality of care.

Response of the government: proposed strategies

Bangladesh recently published a new strategy for the health sector, the Health and Population Sector Strategy (HPSS), which lays the foundation for the Fifth Five-Year Plan (1998-2003).[4] The strategy paper defines an 'Essential Service Package' (ESP), which includes:

- reproductive health care,
- child health care,
- communicable disease control,
- limited curative care, and
- behaviour change communication (BCC).

The content of the reproductive health component of the ESP is defined as:

- care and counselling of women during pregnancy, delivery and the post-partum period, including neonatal care,
- menstrual regulation and post-abortion services,
- adolescent health care, and
- family planning services.

The HPSS also recognises a need for organisational and managerial reform and increased integration of health services at grassroots, union and thana levels. The ESP will provide increasingly sophisticated services at each of these levels. Public sector hospitals will be improved, including caesarean section capability at specified thana and district hospitals, through greater autonomy of management, local level accountability, cost recovery and a revolving drug fund.

To expand and improve overall hospital care, partnerships or commissions for services with NGOs and private, not-for profit hospitals will be explored along with a larger and better regulated private sector. Strengthening the referral system is part of the strategy, along with setting up a specialised, self-sustaining, autonomous agency to provide blood bank services. Upward referral of serious and complicated cases and periodic downward visits of specialists will be arranged. Cost-recovery procedures, based on pilot-testing, will be introduced for out-patient registration, drugs, inpatient care, surgical operations and diagnostic services, while protecting the poor.

Service delivery of the ESP at the community level will be provided as one-stop services through community clinics run by a team of an FWA and an HA. The FWV based in the union-level UHFWC will provide technical backup and supportive supervision. Each union will have four community clinics, each covering a population of 6,000. Community clinic services will include:

- registration of pregnant women,
- information given to pregnant women, in advance, about attending for clinical services,
- maintenance of records for women's expected delivery date,
- referral of problem pregnancies and deliveries to a higher health centre,
- provision of family planning methods, particularly the pill and condoms,
- provision of information, education and communication activities on hygiene, diet, immunisation, intestinal parasites and breast-feeding,
- information given to families in advance about outreach clinics and ensuring that children are immunised at the right time,
- provision of Oral Rehydration Solution and vitamin A, and
- treatment for worms, malaria, acute respiratory diseases and tuberculosis.

These community clinics and the FWA/HA team will offer these services at a clinic to the same number of people as were previously covered by them through visits to households. However, family planning and maternal health services will no longer be provided routinely at the doorstep. Any household visits made will focus on women who are the most neglected and who are at highest risk, or who drop out of family planning or have an infectious disease. They will be carried out in most cases one day per week by one of the team members of the community clinic.

The infrastructure within which family planning services are provided, and existing channels of communication and service provision, can be used and expanded for maternity care. One of the major strengths of the Bangladeshi health system is the political commitment and support which has characterised the family planning programme. Through a strong outreach programme, Bangladesh managed to raise the contraceptive prevalence rate from 11 per cent in 1978 to almost 50 per cent in 1996. A similar level of commitment is required to provide 24-hour emergency obstetric care in hospitals 365 days of the year, to complement community-level services. Policymakers and programme managers will need to allocate additional resources in order to implement these services successfully.

Information for women and their families

Until recent years, the major effort of the Bangladesh maternal health programme has been aimed at improving health service facilities. With almost all women delivering at home with relatives or briefly trained TBAs, it will take time to change this pattern of birthing. Hence, under the Fifth Five-Year Plan for 1998-2003, policy-makers and health service managers are committed to promoting behaviour change communication (BCC) with regard to maternal and neonatal health care, and other aspects of health care as well.

The current BCC strategies were lacking both in quantity and quality in 1997 for maternal and neonatal health care. Few materials explained clearly the signs of complications in pregnancy and exactly how the woman and her family should prepare for action if a complication develops. The Maternal Health Assessment Team found that printed materials were available for health workers, but there were few available for women to take home. Where take-home materials existed, rural people did not always seem to understand the messages. These problems indicated a need for more rigorous pre-testing of messages and materials with the intended audiences.

Improving quality of care: innovative schemes by NGOs

Several pilot projects initiated by non-governmental organisations (NGOs) have tested innovative ways to improve the quality of care in maternal health services. In one area of the Chandpur district, for example, the Bangladesh Association for Voluntary Sterilisation (BAVS) initiated a training programme for village nurses (*palli* nurses) to perform normal deliveries and to recognise and refer complications. These women, with a prerequisite of eight years of basic schooling, are selected by their communities to receive six months of training to become community nurses. The training includes one month of theoretical class with demonstration sessions of ten antenatal and ten counselling clients, followed by a month-long, clinical, hands-on training at Azimpur Maternity Hospital in Dhaka, and four months of practical training at the district headquarters under the supervision of nurses and doctors. Each *palli* nurse conducts 10 to 15 supervised, normal deliveries during the training period.

In the BAVS pilot study area, with a population of 145,000, 28 palli nurses provided services to 64 per cent of deliveries in 1995.[18] However, the coverage declined to 52 per cent in 1997, the phase-out year of the project. Each *palli* nurse conducted on average seven deliveries per month. They referred nine per cent of the women they attended to a higher facility, and almost all of the women complied with the referral. With the training programme in place, 90 per cent of pregnant/post-partum women in the project area received antenatal care and post-partum visits from a *palli* nurse. Among the deliveries conducted by the *palli* nurses, the stillbirth rate was 25 per 1000 deliveries and the neonatal mortality rate 29 per 1000, which are lower than national rates (41 and 53 respectively). Unlike many trained senior providers, *palli* nurses are eager to provide 'hands-on' delivery services. Moreover, *palli* nurses work out of their homes in the villages and are empowered by performing valued work in their communities.

In another pilot project, carried out by the Bangladesh Red Crescent Society, community midwives with four years of training and junior midwives with 18 months of training, following at least eight years of basic education, provided delivery services. Under the aegis of this project, 22 MCH centres were operational in 1994-96 in Barisal and Khulna district pilot areas, each staffed by a community midwife, a junior midwife and a guard. These midwives charge Tk.25 (US $0.50) for a normal delivery. The project has also introduced a cost-recovery programme for medicines, currently recovering about 60 per cent of the cost. A number of voluntary health workers, who have received eight weeks of training, are also working with the midwives. In this pilot project population, the MMR fell from 410 to 230 per 100,000 live births. However, although the initial trend is encouraging, the numbers may be too small to be statistically significant.

Another NGO, the Bangladesh Rural Advancement Committee (BRAC) has mini-health centres in numerous sites throughout Bangladesh,[19] each staffed by a nurse and a doctor. These centres have established linkages with the community through the placement of TBAs on a 12-hour rotation in these centres. The TBAs gain on-the-job clinical training from the nurse and doctor, and become efficient in referring patients with complications to district hospitals, using referral slips and escorting the patients if necessary. The TBAs maintain good rapport with the referral facilities to facilitate a better reception for the referred cases.[19]

The International Centre for Diarrhoeal Diseases Research, Bangladesh (ICDDR,B) in Matlab developed a scheme for the placement of trained midwives in the villages to provide

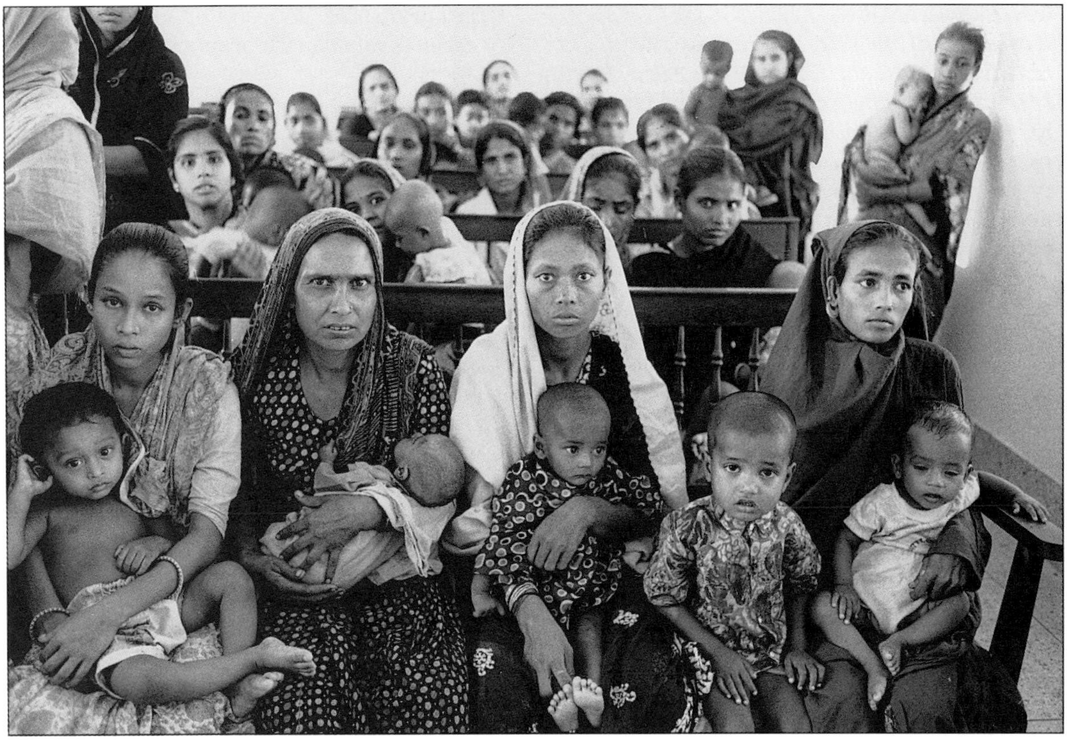

JENNY MATTHEWS

services for pregnancy and delivery and referrals as required. The midwives were linked to community-level health workers, who referred pregnancy and delivery cases to these midwives. The midwives saw two-thirds of the cases with complications; they managed 40 per cent of them and referred the rest to the Matlab Clinic. An important aspect of this pilot project was the availability of a boatman for referral services. The intervention was reported to be successful in reducing maternal mortality rates in the project areas.[20] Interestingly, however, recent analysis of Matlab data indicated that a similar decline in maternal deaths also took place in the 'control' areas of the project.[21]

Conclusions

The situation for maternity care in Bangladesh is an example of the fact that construction of clinics and recruitment of health workers are necessary but not sufficient conditions for improving maternal health status. Substantial investment in midwifery training, the improvement of referral facilities and the establishment of a timely referral system are also necessary. Quality of services from the perspective of both women and providers is also a pre condition for convincing women to deliver in a health-care facility when they face complications. Community-based programmes to generate greater demand for utilisation of maternal health services have not received much attention in the past and must be addressed on a priority basis. Behaviour change communication interventions must address the harmful effects of traditional practices and mobilise social support that will allow women to seek care from health facilities.

As exemplified by the deployment of boatmen for the midwifery programme in Matlab, the NGO-initiated pilot projects have contributed many ideas and strategies for the next Bangladesh Health and Population Sector Strategy. The sustainability of the maternal health programme depends on community participation in programme design and evaluation, and the introduction of innovative finance mechanisms, such as cost recovery for services and drugs.

Recommendations

A number of detailed recommendations were drawn up in the light of the 1997 Maternal Health Assessment and the experience of the innovative NGO projects described here, which are summarised below. These recommendations are preliminary and remain under review in Bangladesh, but they also provide useful strategies for other large-scale programmes.

- ***Create awareness of healthy behaviours during pregnancy, delivery and the post-partum period. Encourage health service providers to be responsive and respectful to clients.***

Informational materials and their use need to be evaluated to determine their effectiveness. A patient-centred approach should also be encouraged among providers. Implemented together as part of the Essential Services Package, these efforts will help create an awareness of services and quality standards in such services, thus increasing demand to improve services.

- ***Expand and improve the quality of normal delivery at home by trained providers and introduce post-partum visits.***

Selected FWAs should receive basic midwifery training. TBAs must continue to receive training in the detection of complications, referral, post-partum care and avoidance of harmful practices. Programme planners should take advantage of programmes where service utilisation is high (e.g. tetanus toxoid immunisation) to screen for pregnancy complications and advise women about danger signs and contingency plans in case they suffer a complication.

- ***Expand and improve the quality of Essential Obstetric Care (EOC).***

These efforts should focus on selected Thana Health Complexes (THCs), which should be upgraded to provide Basic EOC services, and a few THCs to provide Comprehensive EOC. Blood transfusion capacity must also be available in all Basic and Comprehensive EOC facilities. Standards for quality of care must be established, and training provided accordingly.

- ***Integrate the delivery of maternal health services at all levels of service.***

Structural barriers separating the Health and Family Planning Directorates must be eliminated. Private practitioners, NGO clinics, and community health workers need to be involved in the promotion of Essential Obstetric Care services.

- ***Establish effective links between community-level facilities and referral facilities.***

For example, linkages among midwives, FWVs, nurses, TBAs and FWAs must be improved.

- ***Develop an effective data collection and monitoring system.***

Instruments for data collection and monitoring must be integrated so that family planning and other reproductive health data and reporting systems are linked. Data should be easy to understand, analyse and use by staff at THC, district and national levels.

- ***Develop technical expertise to provide guidance for the design, implementation, monitoring and evaluation of maternal health programmes from the national level.***

This effort will help to ensure that programmes are relevant to national objectives and meet national standards. National guidance will also help to promote leadership for maternal health interventions and research.

Acknowledgements

The authors are grateful to the Government of Bangladesh for facilitating the Bangladesh Maternal Health Assessment, and to USAID, the World Bank and the Canadian International Development Agency for funding the assessment. Many thanks are also due to Ms Carla Chladek and Dr Marge Koblinsky of MotherCare for editorial and technical support.

Correspondence

Zahidul A Huque, UNFPA Representative for Sudan, GCPO Box 1608, New York, NY 10163, USA. E-mail: Huque.Zahid@undp.org

References and Notes

1. Rahman F, Whittaker M, Hossain MB, 1991. Maternal mortality in rural Bangladesh, 1982-1990: Data from Verbal Autopsies. Presentation at ICDDR,B (unpublished).
2. UNICEF, WHO, 1996. *Revised 1990 Estimates of Maternal Mortality: A New Approach by WHO and UNICEF*. Geneva.
3. Akhter HH, Chowdhury MI, Sen A, 1996. *A Cross-Sectional Study on Maternal Morbidity in Bangladesh*. Dhaka: BIRPERHT.
4. Government of Bangladesh. 1997. *Bangladesh Health and Population Sector Strategy*.
5. Nahar N, 1997. Recent trends in perinatal health in South Asia: Bangladesh. Paper presented at International Conference on Improving Health of Newborn Infants in Developing Countries, Nepal.
6. MOHFW, 19[illegible]. *Maternal Health Sub-Committee Assessment of Health Services for Maternal Health*. Dhaka: National MCH Co-ordination Committee.
7. The infant mortality rate was estimated at 71 per 1000 live births in 1995. *Bangladesh Demographic and Health Survey 1996-97*. National Institute of Population Research and Training (NIPORT), Mitra and Associates and Macro International Inc.
8. The full report of the assessment is available from MotherCare/ JSI, 1616 N. Fort Myer Drive, Arlington, VA 22209, USA.
9. Blanchet T, 1984. *Women Pollution and Marginality: Meanings and Rituals of Birth in Bangladesh*. Dhaka: University Press.
10. Maloney C, Aziz KMA, Sarker P, 1981. *Beliefs and Fertility in Bangladesh*. Dhaka: ICDDR,B.
11. Hartmann B, Boyce JK, 1983. *A Quiet Violence: View From a Bangladeshi Village*. Dhaka: University Press.
12. Gazi R, Goodburn E, Chowdhury AMR et al, 1995. *Case Studies on Practices during Post-Partum Period in Rural Bangladesh*. Dhaka: BRAC.
13. Satellite clinics are temporary facilities to provide family planning and maternal health services by FWVs, FWAs and HAs. Typically the clinics are organised at the houses of prominent village leaders or teachers where women can visit without reservation.
14. This is the lowest administrative geographical unit.
15. World Health Organization, 1996. *Reproductive Health Care in Bangladesh. A Review of Recent Data and Some Proposals for Future Strategies and Activities*. WHO, Dhaka.
16. Ahmed YH, Rahman MH, Chowdhury FK et al, 1995. *A Report on Baseline Survey for Assessment of Emergency Obstetric Care Services in Bangladesh*. Bangladesh Institute of Research for Promotion of Essential and Reproductive Health and Technologies (BIRPERHT), Dhaka.
17. Akhter HH, Rahman H , Mannan I et al, 1995. *Review of Performance of Trained TBAs*. Dhaka: BIRPERHT.
18. Barkat A, Rahman A, Majid M, 1998. *Evaluation of Palli Nurse (Community Midwife) Project of BAVS*. University Research Corporation (Bangladesh).
19. Margaret Leppard, London School of Hygiene and Tropical Medicine, personal communication, 1997, 1999.
20. Fauveau V, Stewart K, Khan SA, Chakraborty J, 1991. Effects on mortality of community based maternity care programme in rural Bangladesh. *Lancet*. 339(Nov 9): 1183-86.
21. Ronsmans C, Vanneste AM, Chakraborty J, Ginneken JV, 1997. Decline in maternal mortality in Matlab, Bangladesh: a cautionary tale. *Lancet*. 350(Dec 20/27):1810-14.

Safe Motherhood in Indonesia: A Task for the Next Century

Coeli J Geefhuysen

The Indonesian Ministry of Health has addressed the problem of Safe Motherhood with great energy and many activities, in line with World Health Organization recommendations, but the maternal mortality rate has not yet dropped. Modern midwifery is the mainstay of the programme, but traditional birth attendants are still preferred by the community. Midwives need more skills for the tasks expected of them. Referral is confounded by poverty, geography and climate, and health centres and district hospitals often have inadequate resources for supervision or emergency care. Central policy decisions and action are still required to develop an integrated approach, give senior midwives more responsibility at health centre level, improve record keeping, provide community education about pregnancy and its complications, make a concerted effort to contain costs of maternal and child health, and reduce poverty and illiteracy. Projects in overlapping departments could be integrated and decentralisation made more effective. Initiatives to improve training of midwives will eventually bear fruit, but maternal mortality cannot be made to disappear through midwifery training alone. Even with the substantial efforts being made, Safe Motherhood will remain a task for the next century.

SAFE Motherhood is the culmination of services for women from the beginning of life and the ability to choose when to become pregnant. Indonesia has all the problems which lead to high levels of maternal mortality and morbidity,[1,2] made worse by the recent monetary crisis. In 1989, Indonesia embraced the recommendations of the 1987 WHO Safe Motherhood Initiative, including the recommendation to provide skilled attendance at birth, mainly by trained midwives, as the most likely way to reduce pregnancy-related mortality and morbidity.[1,3-8]

This reversed a previous policy decision of the mid-1970s. Following the trend in industrialised countries and recommendations in publications in the 1960s,[7] it had generally been thought best that all deliveries take place in hospital, conducted by medical staff. Indonesian specialists had embraced this concept, and in 1975 midwifery courses were phased out nationally. Existing midwives went on providing services in private practices in towns and in hospitals and aimed to maintain standards through the IBI, the national midwives' professional organisation,[9,10] but no new midwives were trained.

The Indonesian Safe Motherhood Initiative was launched in 1989 with the aim of reducing the maternal mortality ratio (MMR) and the infant mortality rate (IMR). This is a vertical programme,[3-5] directed by the Ministry of Health and assisted by international loans and donor funding. Midwifery training has been reinstated as a central pillar of the Initiative. The President of Indonesia decreed in 1989, on the recommendation of the Ministry of Health, that a sufficient number of village midwives be trained to place one midwife in every village within five years. The population of Indonesia is over 200 million, with an annual national birth rate reported at 2.4 per cent.[9,11] To place a midwife in every village, 54,000 midwives had to be trained by 1996,[3,5,6] an enormous undertaking.

The direct causes of the high MMR in the country are similar to those found elsewhere in the tropics.[2,5,6,12-14] Perinatal mortality has also remained high, estimated at 30 to 60 per 1000 live births. Efforts to reduce the MMR have been carried out with great energy and many activities. It was therefore an unpleasant surprise for everyone concerned to discover in 1997 that these activities had not yet achieved the hoped-for results nationally.[6,9] However, although the MMR has remained at between 420 and 450 per 100 000 live births,[5,9] studies based on accurate records have shown higher maternal mortality at the beginning of interventions and improvements later on.[10] During the 1990s, projects in different regions have created a patchwork of improvements; much still remains to be done.

In this paper, Indonesian maternity and midwifery services are described in the context of health service organisation, including family planning and outreach services for child health which include limited antenatal care; the hierarchy of medical responsibility for midwifery and obstetric services; the management and training of village midwives and permanent midwives; and what still needs to be done at community, service delivery and central levels to reduce maternal and perinatal deaths.

Maternity and midwifery services within health service organisation

Health services are organised and health policy determined at Health Ministry level. Though there have been moves toward decentralisation, budgeting and major policy decisions, as well as the direction of all vertical programmes, remain centralised.

District health offices are responsible for subdistrict health centres and the adequate functioning of district hospitals. Health centres are placed in subdistricts, with volunteer and outreach services (*posyandu*) to the villages. The national aim is to hold an outreach clinic within five km of each home once a month. Though policy is in place, however, few health centres are equipped with adequately trained staff, tools and drugs for obstetric emergencies, or even running water. Many do not have a telephone or radio and in remote areas it is difficult to get staff.[6,15] Some health centres in remote areas have been rebuilt to accommodate a few in-patients, mainly for obstetric care.

Immediately after graduation from medical school, doctors are placed by the central authority in health centres on contract, and are in charge of the clinic. Most stay less than a year, especially in the most remote areas. Only a few health centres have permanent posts for doctors, some of whom have achieved excellent services. National prizes are given yearly for the best health centres,[9,15] as examples of what can be achieved.

Health centre staff size varies with the size of the population and the number of villages. At a minimum, this includes one permanent (i.e. tenured) midwife. These permanent midwives, though often more skilled than village midwives, cannot act without the doctor's permission in emergencies. Contract placements of new village midwives to each village are done from a central office, though the village midwives come under the health centre administratively.

Some villages have special 'birth houses', paid for in part by the community, which the midwife should use for her practice and sometimes live in. These are also meant to be used for other community activities. Quality and number vary from excellent to very poor across the country. To date, there are more village midwives than birth houses. One birth house I saw was tiny, built on a hill away from the village, without a well and poorly equipped. The midwife had to carry water up the hill; there was no toilet and she could not have lived there. Another, on a small island, was an ample house with a verandah, well equipped, in the village itself. The midwife did live there and the village was proud of the house and their midwife. Nevertheless, the midwife did not want to stay on. She had no connections in the village, it was too lonely, not a 'complete' life.

As village midwives do not have tenure, their salaries are relatively high, higher than those of the permanent midwives in the health centres. In addition, they are allowed to charge a fee per delivery, the amount of which is decided in discussion with health centre staff; this varies regionally. In some regions it is higher than the fee for the lowest class of hospital patient; in others it is about the same as the local honorarium for traditional birth attendants (TBAs).

Between 1991 and 1997, some 56,000 young midwives were placed on three-year contracts, but some villages are still without village midwives. Every three years village midwives are supposed to be replaced by new graduates. Recently, they have been allowed to elect to stay on for a second term. Those who are replaced are encouraged to go into private practice, preferably near their village post. However, because villages are too poor to support a private midwife, many former village midwives try to set up practice in the smaller towns.

Permanent midwives are responsible for the supervision of the village midwives in their area; they do few deliveries themselves. They are also responsible for meeting with trained TBAs and in the past were responsible for TBA training. Many of these senior midwives were trained many years ago, but their junior staff come from the ranks of the newly trained.

Each subdistrict has a population of 50,000-100,000 people, depending on population density, and the number of villages varies according to the cultural patterns in each region. Some are very small, resulting in numerous villages per health centre, while in other areas 'villages' can be 7,000 people spread over a fairly wide area. This may determine the proximity of the village midwife to potential patients in her area.[15]

District hospitals are supposed to maintain readiness for emergencies and play a role in continuing education through clinical meetings, perinatal audit, visits to the periphery and in-service training. However, district hospitals often do not have the necessary staff, equipment or blood available to respond adequately to many emergencies.[6,12,13,15] At night, drivers may have to be fetched, and the ambulance may have to be used to bring the doctor, midwife and laboratory/blood technician. Blood donors may also have to be found.

Each province is responsible for the proper functioning of provincial and district health services and for equipment. Decentralisation is intended to put the main focus on the district level, yet it is at provincial level that training facilities exist and where most medical specialists reside. Problems of vertical to horizontal integration persist.[6]

Tertiary hospitals are linked to universities (often in provincial capitals). Other hospitals are the provincial and district public hospitals and an extensive network of private hospitals in urban centres. There is a move towards privatising parts of the public hospital system to raise income for better services, the effects of which need careful monitoring.

Internal reports and needs assessments have found that service providers at all levels spend much of their time in meetings and on administration,[9] and comparatively little time on community or clinical activities at health centres or on outreach by specialists. Further, there is hardly any reference material in most health centres.[15]

Pre-placement training for village midwives

Before the Safe Motherhood Initiative there were no trained midwives in the villages. To fulfil the large quota of entrants required under the Presidential decree, admission after nine years of schooling (± age 17) into training was permitted; this may soon be raised to 12 years of schooling. The midwifery curriculum is centrally co-ordinated. There are three different training programmes based in nursing schools, with different intake criteria. Courses include a variable length of general nursing training, followed by one year of midwifery training. National examiners attend final examinations. The first new midwives graduated in 1993 and began to be placed in the villages.[9,16] Initial support came from international loans and grants.

The difficulties of absorbing so many trainees at one time appear to have been underestimated. To cope with this, the more highly qualified, top graduates were promoted immediately to trainer status to assist the few senior midwives still in place who had been trained before 1975. Even so, many young midwives have graduated with little experience in conducting a delivery and even less experience of handling complications.[15,16] Student loads have often exceeded patient availability near the schools. Failure rates in examinations have deliberately been kept low, with those who fail being allowed to sit examinations again, most of whom pass the second time around.[9]

Assessments have shown deficiencies in overall course design, overlap between nursing and midwifery training, and a particular lack of training in communication skills, problem-solving and hands-on experience. There are insufficient numbers of training models (phantoms) in schools as well, but the greatest need is for more hands-on training in actual delivery settings, which continues to be confounded by student numbers.

Evaluations in practice have consistently shown that the skills of the new midwives are insufficient for the tasks they face, particularly with regard to decision-making.[2,16,17] Revision of teaching materials and methods, based on recommendations in evaluation reports, was begun in 1997.[2,9] Midwives trained under the revised curricula are due to graduate in 2000 and 2001. With less pressure on the training programme when initial placements are complete, schools will have a better chance of giving students hands-on experience.

Replacing traditional birth attendants with trained midwives

In the past, those TBAs interested in being trained were invited to present themselves at health centres and, until recently, permanent midwives provided this training along with free delivery kits. Then the Ministry decided that TBAs should be phased out and that support for TBA training should be stopped wherever village midwives had been placed. Some district staff believe that TBA training should be continued; they think it is unrealistic to expect the population suddenly to patronise only the new midwives.

Health centre staff have expressed fears that the number of untrained TBAs, and therefore the number of unsafe deliveries and complications, would increase. In some areas training has been continued as 'meetings', though free delivery kits for TBAs are no longer available. In most areas, however, trained TBAs can obtain sterile cord-cutting sets at cost from village midwives or the health centre, as required.[15]

The Indonesia Demographic and Health Survey (1997) showed that the majority of births (68 per cent) still take place in women's homes, 11 per cent in the homes of midwives or others, 9 per cent in government facilities and 12 per cent in private facilities.[18]

Midwives do most of the hospital delivery care, and hospital midwives take a major role in the practical training of undergraduates and in-service training. In towns, private midwifery services have been popular for many years. However, most people live in villages.

Apart from doing as many deliveries as possible herself, the village midwife is expected to supervise deliveries done by TBAs and deal with emergencies as they arise, thereby improving her own reputation and attracting more deliveries to her own practice. The WHO stipulates that a midwife should attend at least 30 deliveries per year to maintain practice standards;[19] however, this number is reached by very few of Indonesia's midwives.

Based on calculations of estimated deliveries per village population, district crude birth rates, reported antenatal contacts, new marriages as recorded at subdistrict level (which must be reported by law) and the statistics of the family planning programme (which are considered reliable), I found that far more deliveries than reported were still being attended by TBAs and others rather than by midwives.[9,15]

TBAs are independent and their fees are generally lower than those of the village midwives, and they can be paidin kind and with deferment. TBAs have usually completed their own families by the timethey become birth attendants, and there is no age or time limit on when they stop practising. In contrast, it is hard for a young midwifeto win the trust of village women, and hard for a much older TBA to accept her 'supervision'. The following is a compilation of the kinds of remarks about and attitudes towards the village midwives that I have personally encountered:

Just imagine being 'that young girl", aged 20, unmarried, fresh from academic training,having seen and dealt with only a few deliveries and usually no complications, placed alone in a village amongst people you don't know, who may have a different language and culture. You know older people will not have respect for you – 'not even married'! You are not even supposed to 'know about these things'. There has been minimal training in how to 'invade' such a closed environment. Moreover, you are often no more able to deal with the emergency than the TBA and have less skill to persuade families to fund expensive hospital transfers by borrowing money or selling land or an animal.

This is the situation encountered by the majority of village midwives. Of course, some are better at gaining trust and confidence than others, some may know the community they are placed in, but these are exceptions. By the time they have gained some trust and experience, and made a place for themselves in the community, their contracts are finished and they are replaced by new, inexperienced village midwives. Many elect to leave at the end of their first terms and return to less remote environments in order to go into private practice, or have to follow their husbands elsewhere.

In-service training for village midwives

In-service training at health centre level or below became urgent when the problems faced by village midwives working alone were realised. This is a responsibility of the Ministry of Health.[15,16] There are well-developed training facilities at provincial level, but improvisation had been the norm at district level. An abundance of short courses was developed centrally, to be offered at district level. Both participants and independent evaluators complained, however, that there were too many participants and too little hands-on care.[9,15,16] Travel time could be as long as course time for those attending from distant areas or islands, and staff could find themselves away from their villages for a week or more every month. Distance-education modules were well received, but access to practical training has remained difficult.[17]

Training in life-saving skills for emergency obstetric care, developed from a US model for which excellent technical manuals are available,[20] also has to include exposure of each trainee to actual emergencies and case management.[16] Indonesian obstetricians, particularly those in tertiary hospitals, have been critical of the modules because they do not include the underlying principles on which actions are based. In response, specialists in different regional centres of the country developed protocols for decision-making for different emergencies, as adjuncts to the modules.

In-service training for permanent midwives and midwifery trainers

Permanent midwives, including those in hospitals, are not familiar with all the materials that village midwives are taught to use, such as the partograph,[21] and do not always feel confident about supervising them. They are sometimes also unsure they have the respect of young graduates and can find it hard to be a sympathetic and knowledgeable supervisor. Because of the pressure to train village midwives who are in-service, permanent midwives have not yet had their training updated through refresher courses. Although a new course has been developed to train permanent midwives in the area of supervision,[9] the material still relies heavily on checklists and adherence to administrative routine. While this is important, it minimises training in case management, and improving communication between permanent and village midwives and between village midwives and the community.[9,15]

The two national training centres for the training of trainers provide in-service training, for medical specialists, but these centres are also overwhelmed by the numbers of trainers required. Courses address teaching methods as well as technical matters, but only a few in each group are able to practise the new interactive techniques under supervision.[9,15,20,22] Indonesian obstetricians running some of the courses are not always aware of global activities and literature. However, they do consider nationally accepted protocols essential for the training of trainers.[9,15] This requires reviews, based on international standards,[23] of protocols from several regions and coordination of the results.[15]

Barriers at community level

Perceptions on the part of families of the risks of pregnancy and of recurring problems are limited,[2,15,24] and it is hard for most village women to perceive that one mother's death in 200 deliveries is far too many. An infant death is also often accepted as unavoidable. Decisions about funding and transport are not always made before labour starts, money may not be to hand during delivery, and family decisions to raise money in the event of an emergency may be time-consuming, as has been found elsewhere.[12,15]

A small percentage of families are entitled to the health card for the 'poor', on application, which provides free health care in hospitals, but it is not given to everyone classified as 'poor'. 'Poor' is defined by the Indonesian government as not having enough income to eat more than once a day; the percentage of people below this level, which was reported at 10-13 per cent in 1996, more than tripled after the financial crisis began in mid-1997, and many people are only just above this level.

The literacy rate for women overall is over 80 per cent, but lower in remote areas,[6,10,15] and the national language taught in schools is not understood by all women. Nor do all local leaders accept that girls too need education.

Costs of transport and medical care are also barriers to the use of modern health services. Village savings schemes have been used in some places, administered by women's clubs or health volunteers, for example, but these have often failed in the past as more people tend to require help than can contribute.[11] Public health services are not free in Indonesia, and although fees are considered low by staff, large numbers of people have a problem with the expenses involved in hospitals and emergencies, resulting in underutilisation.[9] Despite the current drive to self-funding of hospitals, for maternal health care to improve it will remain necessary to support peripheral services and protect essential services for women and children.

Problems with referral in cases of obstetric emergency

Guidelines for obstetric referral[6] specify that the attendant at a delivery should refer problems arising to the next level of care. This means that TBAs should call the village midwife, then the woman should be referred to the health centre, and finally to the hospital. An ambulance resides at the health centre. If a woman requires transfer, someone may have to go to the health centre first, request the ambulance, raise the driver, and finally transport the patient. If other means of transport nearer than the health centre can be found, the woman is usually taken directly to the hospital.

Analysis[5,6] has identified problems in all aspects of implementation of the Safe Motherhood Initiative, but particularly in the referral system. Many deliveries are conducted more than two hours' travel away from any emergency care.[6,12] People live scattered over numerous islands, and on the larger islands many areas are remote due to forest or mountains. During wet weather, roads are often closed, and transport may not be available for emergencies or is expensive.

Limited antenatal care through outreach services

Child Survival programmes for under-fives have been running in Indonesia since the early 1980s, mainly with health volunteers (*kader*), who are involved in child health monitoring and curative outreach clinics (*posyandu*). Health volunteers are appointed by the village women's organisation;[25,26] they are frequently busy women with many social responsibilities. Health centres are responsible for a brief training of all health volunteers. Monthly village-based outreach sessions have been successfully implemented, though they tend to be directive and co-operation usually means obeying instructions.[25]

Initially, the only activity included for pregnant women was tetanus toxoid injections. Preventive activities have increasingly been combined with integrated curative services, provided by staff from sub-district health centres. More recently, antenatal care, including the provision of iron and folate tablets, has been added in areas where there are village midwives, and where the clinic can be held in a building providing some privacy. In populous areas, approximately 60 per cent of pregnant women (based on 1996 census data) were receiving at least a tetanus toxoid injection and one antenatal examination.

Most outreach clinics are very busy and the amount of time per consultation is limited. The team arrives mid-morning and departs by midday; I have myself seen clinics deal with 50-70 mothers, some with several children, in one morning. Pregnant women are often seen with their other children and referred to the midwife by the health volunteers; some primiparae are brought by other women attending the outreach clinic. However, in one district I visited, district reports revealed that less than half of the deliveries of those seen at least once antenatally were later attended by trained staff. Those living far away, or with large families or embarrassed by poverty – i.e. high-risk groups – often attend outreach services only occasionally. Non-attenders are rarely followed up.[9,15]

Separate family planning services

Family planning services, which started in the 1960s, are run through a separate organisation (BKKBN), which is corporatised. BKKBN works together with the Health Department at district and subdistrict level. They have their own training teams and statistics department,[7] and they do their own yearly census, which is not integrated with national health statistics. BKKBN is financially and managerially strong, with links to the pharmaceutical industry, and has been strongly supported by government and by donor agencies.[15]

Community family planning workers, recruited on recommendation of the sub-district head and usually younger than health volunteers, are paid a retainer; they are specially trained by BKKBN in different methods of contraception, health promotion and communication with the community. They are affiliated to the health centres and usually take part in outreach clinics.[15]

The national family planning policy of two children per couple is aimed at married couples; the services also cover prostitutes living in designated areas but not unmarried young people. Indirectly, this was the first programme in Indonesia to address maternal health; however, education on the possible complications of pregnancy and delivery is not included in consultations.

Into the 21st century: what more is needed?

The Safe Motherhood Initiative has been instrumental in moving the Ministry of Health to understand and address the problem of maternal mortality. This is an important achievement, and a necessary pre-condition for improvements to be made as and when conditions allow.

It was an unpleasant surprise for everyone concerned to discover that initial activities had not yet achieved the hoped-for results nationally.[6,9] However, an integrated approach, using community education, increasing the competence of village midwives, improving supervision and follow-up, and proper record-keeping have all contributed to improved statistics in some project areas.[10]

To make programmes effective down the line to community level is a Herculean task, expensive in manpower and resources. The strong, centralised reins and budget control are often felt as constraints at more local levels. Decentralisation might help in allowing more peripheral decision-making in those provinces which have stronger management.

Village level interventions are important to create appropriate demand for the services of the village midwives who are already in place, who are under-utilised because village people do not see that they know more than TBAs and have more hygienic practices. But planning of services at district level or below would not achieve coherent practice or training across referral levels. Basic principles could be laid down in an overall plan, including the content of training, with the possibility of different approaches for the different cultural settings across the country, and developed through detailed planning at provincial level with district input.

Community education

Health volunteers have received health education materials about pregnancy in many areas, but there is no community education programme.[10,15] Village-based education is needed, as many in the population do not yet see the need for women to be able to choose whether to become pregnant, that there is an unpredictable risk of complications with any pregnancy and at any age, or that antenatal care, trained care during delivery and readiness for referral in case of emergencies are all important.

Midwives: professional and training needs

There is widespread awareness of midwifery training problems, and new ideas are continually being tried out to improve quality of service.[16,19,22,27] If efforts are continued at the rate of the last few years, both in pre-placement and in-service training, the results will begin to show in statistics in the first decade of the 21st century, when a sufficient number of midwives in villages may be working more effectively than at present. Provincial planners would like longer and more effective courses at all levels, more hands-on training and smaller numbers being trained at one time. Some provinces have submitted training plans; but these may not be implemented rapidly because of budgetary constraints.[15]

As a profession, midwifery requires separate recognition in order to guarantee a sufficient level of staffing and experience in training centres, schools and university departments. Schools have insight into what is required, but it will take more time to change teaching methods and improve curriculum content. Managers of training programmes consider it necessary for those members of the nursing profession training nursing and midwifery trainers to get further university education overseas, though this may be delayed by the financial crisis. Fellowship holders would not return to their teaching posts for several years, but would then be more competent to train others and stimulate change.[15]

In the end, attention to midwifery training is only part of the solution however. It will not reduce maternal mortality unless midwives actually deliver the babies and can refer women adequately.

Provincial and district level responsibilities

As attempts to date have failed to increase the coverage by village midwives in many areas, incentives have been suggested to improve their profile, e.g. that they are offered lower salaries plus incentive payments to follow up antenatal cases and for each delivery they attend. TBAs could be encouraged to call village midwives to all deliveries through a small incentive as well. However, incentives are generally a double-edged sword.

A village midwife at a well-organised health centre should have the means to start an infusion on any emergency transfer even now. However, problems with referral and lack of resources and staff at district level remain serious problems, which need to be given greater priority.

It requires policy decisions to transfer the supervision of midwifery at the health centre primarily to the senior permanent midwife, and to allow midwives to carry out all life-saving procedures necessary in their particular situation.[8] Everyone practising midwifery needs to be trained to a level of proficiency for the work required. Senior midwives also need to be trained in how best to support the village midwife in gaining access to the community. Permanent midwives' salaries could be boosted to include active case-management supervision.

Health centre doctors with tenure, especially those in remote areas, should have special training in general and obstetric emergency care. Experiments with this are in progress. Some specialists are involved in training health centre doctors with tenure to meet the needs of patients in remote areas.[15]

It should also be required for hospitals to become 'women- and baby-friendly'[3,28] though few are at the moment. With the help of donors, the equipment in many hospitals and clinics is being improved, but many are not yet up to the standard required for the conditions they have to deal with.[11,28,29]

Neonates in many cultures, including in Indonesia, are kept indoors for the first 40 days after birth. Home visits by the midwife to treat neonatal illness and to do a post-partum check on the mother would be a practical proposal; this is not done in current practice.[28-30]

Maternal-perinatal audit of difficult cases has recently been introduced as a learning tool at district level. The guidance material mentions that audit should be for training and not used primarily as a corrective activity. However, sessions are also supposed to take place in a formal meeting at district level, where 'the person involved' presents 'the case' with all the stakeholders present. The presenter in one session, a young health centre doctor, told me that the specialists present criticised her for taking life-saving actions that are 'only allowed for specialists', even in the absence of transport to bring the woman to hospital. Experiences like this have in some cases resulted in resistance to reporting cases for audit.[9,15] The suggested format could be altered, however, in ways that create a more acceptable learning situation.

Record-keeping

Poor record-keeping is not unique to Indonesia.[10] Although vital statistics are essential tools for monitoring IMR and MMR,[31] registration of births and deaths is not compulsory and certificates from local authorities are relatively expensive in Indonesia.[15]

Provincial and district annual reports are separate for hospital and clinic services. Based on recapitulation of monthly tables, they frequently differ from ward records and attendance registers. Errors in copying and arithmetic are multiplied inconsistently so that provincial and national figures merely give a rough guideline as to the occurrence of events.[9,15] This also affects maternal morbidity statistics, which reflect morbidity only for the small percentage of pregnant women in public hospitals.

Maternal record cards, which record some routine information, and a follow-up record designed by the Ministry and held by the mother, were seldom available peripherally. The village midwife uses a summary form for all antenatal cases under her care at the monthly clinic and a personal notebook for deliveries. Only these are used for monthly tables.[15]

Individual patient records are indispensable for case-management supervision and peer review, and for appropriate record-keeping to determine the impact of programmes. Recently proposed designs[15] use an individual record for reporting vital information, and incorporate the features of existing models and principles of the WHO home-based maternal record[32] in a form that can be used to aid decision-making and supervision, and to make the importance of the data clear to the provider.[31] If these were distributed and used for every pregnancy, data would become more reliable. There are moves to concentrate data processing in the district and provincial authorities, but this would require radical changes in the current system of data collection and compilation. A decision on the new record design was pending at the end of 1997.[15]

Central level responsibilities

Responsibilities for health, health services, and midwifery training and education are split between three different departments in the Ministry of Health. This contributes to delays in implementing changes, even when these are considered essential. Ministerial departments benefit from the project funds they attract, making them less likely to share project responsibilities, even when a combined effort might lead to a better result. This is not a purely Indonesian problem and can be exacerbated by donors.

The independence of the BKKBN from other health services for women results in much duplication of efforts. Vertical structures in the Safe Motherhood and Child Survival programmes also continue to dominate activities, and budgeting remains centrally organised. This hampers integration of services, as well as the funding of provincially planned initiatives such as new training programmes.[15] Integration of village midwifery care, family planning services and maternal and child health services (and statistics) would require radical decisions at Ministerial level, and safeguards would be needed to maintain efficiency. More broadly, however, services for women and children need protecting in the general push towards privatisation of health services, and funds will be needed to keep essential services free.

Maternal mortality cannot be made to disappear through equipment and midwifery training alone. Safe motherhood cannot be achieved without a coherent health policy at all levels and 'best practice' at the village level. Many dedicated people are working towards this goal. Initiatives in health will have slowed down due to the economic crisis at a time when anti-poverty programmes and health promotion need new impetus. It will be an achievement if Ministerial departments in Indonesia continue to work towards defining the steps necessary, and to set priorities to achieve improvements. Donors need to rethink project funding, given the economic crisis and the political upheavals that followed, with continuing effects of increased poverty among ordinary people.

Safe motherhood is difficult to achieve. When motherhood becomes safe in Indonesia, many other goals will have been reached as well.

Acknowledgements

As an international consultant for Education and Training, Rural Health and Population Project (Asian Development Bank III loan), Ministry of Health, Republic of Indonesia, in 1997, I visited four provinces in Sumatra, and Surabaya, Bandung and Yogyakarta to carry out an assessment of training for the Safe Motherhood programme. Much of the information reported in this paper comes from my own observations on these visits. My final report Ref [15] used many of the references described in Ref [9]. These are unpublished and confidential reports but workers on projects in Indonesia can ask to see this material at the Ministry of Health. I wish to acknowledge with gratitude my co-consultant Dr Kartini Binol, whose enthusiasm, personal support, knowledge of related projects and the literature available locally, facilitated my work in Sumatra and formed a background for my own observations and this paper. I thank the Indonesian Ministry of Health for access to internal reports; the Asian Development Bank III for the opportunity to stay in Indonesia through SAGRIC in 1997; Pascale Allotey for comments on an earlier draft; and the ACITHN/Tropical Health Program for use of facilities.

Correspondence

Coeli J Geefhuysen
E-mail: j.geefhuysen@mailbox. uq.edu.au

References and Notes

(NOTE: * = Starred references are not available through public libraries)

1. *World Health Day: Safe Motherhood*. WHD 98 1-11, Division of Reproductive Health (Technical Support), World Health Organization, Geneva , 1998.
2. Sibley L, Armbruster D, 1997. Obstetric first aid in the community – partners in safe motherhood. A strategy for reducing maternal mortality. *Journal of Nurse Midwifery*. 42(2):117-21.
3. *Human Resource Development for Maternal Health and Safe Motherhood: Report of a Taskforce*. Meeting 2-4 April, MCH/HRD/90.1. World Health Organization, Geneva, 1990.

*4. *Executive Summary of Assessment and Recommended National Strategies. Safe Motherhood*. Volume 4 of Assessment of Maternal Health Situation and Health Services, Usha Shah, Sunarti Sudomo; Ministry of Health, Indonesia/UN Development Programme/World Health Organization, 1991.

*5. Stokoe P, 1995. *The Indonesian Safe Motherhood Initiative with special emphasis on the contribution of the Rural Health and Population Project, Briefing Document*, Asian Development Bank. The Asian Development Bank has provided several loans for health service strengthening to improve service delivery and record keeping for maternal health, and was also involved with midwifery training.

*6. *Proceedings of the First World Congress on Maternal Mortality (Marrakesh), Workshop on Managing the Referral System – An Agenda for Improvement*. Country Case History: Reducing the Maternal Mortality in Indonesia. Ministry of Health, Indonesia, 1997. (Draft) This includes summaries of the following document: Assessment of Maternal Health Situation and Health Services, Safe Motherhood, Usha Shah, Sunarti Sudomo; Volume 1; Volume 2, Assessment of Socio- Cultural Aspects; Volume 3, Assessment of Midwifery Services and Education Practices; Volume 4, Executive Summary of Assessments and Recommended National Strategies; Volume 5, Recommended Plan of Action, Ministry of Health Indonesia, UNDP/WHO,1991.

7. Butler NR, Alberman ED (eds), 1969. *Perinatal Problems*. E&S Livingstone, Edinburgh.
8. Kwast BE, 1992. Midwives: key rural health workers in maternity care. *International Journal of Gynecology and Obstetrics*. 38(Suppl):S9-S15.
9. In Indonesia, as elsewhere, the Safe Motherhood Initiative has led to national needs assessments, internal reports, evaluations and data collection that are used for internal purposes and reports to donors and never reach publication. Much of the information in this paper is based on such reports, a list of which is available from me. As a consultant, I saw these in confidence and have not referenced them here to protect that confidence. Other unpublished documents, of a less sensitive nature and possibly available from organisations outside Indonesia, are marked with a star.

*10. Rochjati P, 1997. Conducting research on community based improvements in MMR in two provinces. Personal communication at Airlangga University, Medical Research Department.

11. *World Population Data Sheet*, Haub C, Cornelius D (eds). Population Reference Bureau, Washington DC, 1998.
12. Feuerstein M, 1993. *Turning the Tide. Safe Motherhood*. Macmillan/Save the Children, London.
13. Tarimo E, 1996. Safe motherhood and district health systems. *European Journal of Obstetrics & Gynaecology, and Reproductive Biology*. 69(1):5-10.
14. Sweet B, Tickner V, Maclean G, 1995. Midwifery in Indonesia: a professional snapshot. *Modern Midwife*. 5(6):8-13.

*15. Geefhuysen J, 1997. Rural Health and Population Project (ADB III), Department of Health, Ministry of Health RI Final report on Medical Education and Training.

*16. With support from the World Bank, midwifery training evaluations of midwifery pre-placement programme A and C, the life-saving skills and distance in-service training were carried out under the Population V project with the assistance of the British Council. (a) Population V Evaluation of Programme A Midwifery Training, Report and Executive Summary, British Council, 1996; (b) MacClean GD, Sweet BR, 1995. Evaluation of Programme C midwifery training. Population V Project, Consultants's report, British Council. (c) Maclean G, Sweet BR, Tickner VJ, 1995. Evaluation of Effectiveness of the Life Saving Skills Programme for Bidan di Desa in Indonesia, British Council, Population V Project Part B Report and Executive Summary.

*17. Fordham J, 1996. *Midwifery*

Training – Executive Summary Report on Long Distance Learning. British Council, Development and Training Services for World Bank Population V Project.
18. *Indonesia Demographic and Health Survey 1997*. Indonesian Central Bureau of Statistics and Macro International Ltd. Jakarta and Calverton MD, 1998.
19. Tinker A, Daly P, Saxenian H, Lakshminarayanan R, Gill K, *Women's Health and Nutrition: Making a Difference*. World Bank Discussion Paper, 1994.
*20. DepKes/BinKes 1996/1997 Modules on Delivery: on Life Saving Skills; based on: Marshall MA, Buffington ST, *Life-Saving Skills Manual for Midwives*. American College of Midwives. Adapted and translated by UPK-UnPad, 2nd edition.
21. *The Partograph. A Managerial Tool for the Prevention of Prolonged Labour*, Section I; World Health Organisation 1988 WHO/FHE/MSM; Geneva.
*22. (a) Sullivan R, Magarick R, Bergthold G et al, 1995. *Clinical Training Skills for Reproductive Health Professionals*; (b) Johnson R, Lewison D (eds), 1996. *Overview: Issues in Training for Essential Maternal Health Care*. Workshop Report 24-26 April; (c) *Clinical Training Skills Course Handbook – Guide for Participants*; (d) *Clinical Training Skills Course Notebook for Trainers*, 1997. JHPIEGO (Johns Hopkins University Program for Reproductive Health and Education), Baltimore.
23. Standards of midwifery practice for safe motherhood. Field testing version. World Health Organization SEARO, New Delhi, 1997.
24. Geefhuysen CJ, Rahman Isa A, Hashim M et al, 1998. Malaysian antenatal risk coding and the outcome of pregnancy. *Journal of Obstetric and Gynaecological Research*. 24(1):13-20.
25. Grace J, 1996. Healers and modern health services: antenatal, birthing and post-partum care in rural East Lombok, Indonesia. In: *Maternity and Reproductive Health in Asian Societies*. Rice PL, Manderson L (eds). Harwood Academic Publishers/OPA, Amsterdam.
26. Hunter C, 1996. Women as good citizens: maternal and child health in a Sasak village (Lombok). In: *Maternity and Reproductive Health in Asian Societies*.(as [13]).
27. *Evaluation of Midwifery Training, Draft Field Manual and Guidelines*. Safe Motherhood Initiative, World Health Organization SEARO, New Delhi, 1997.
28 (a) *Mother-Baby Package – Implementing Safe Motherhood in Countries*; and (b) *A Safe Motherhood Planning Guide*. WHO/FHE/MSM 94.11. Division of Family Health, World Health Organization, Geneva, 1994.
29. *Integrated Management of Childhood Illness: Global Status of Implementation*. World Health Organization, Division of Child Health, Geneva, 1997.
*30. (a) MotherCare Indonesia Project – Overview and Update, 1997; (b) Beck D, Buffington ST, McDermott J, (no date). *Healthy Mother and Healthy Newborn Care*, American College of Nurse Midwives: (i) *A Reference for Caregivers*; (ii) *A Guide for Caregivers*. MotherCare, John Snow Inc, Washington DC, 1997.
31. (a) *Indicators to Monitor Maternal Health Goals, Report of a Technical Working Group*, Geneva 8-12 November 1993; and (b) *Painting the Big Picture: Assessment of maternal and peri/neonatal health at country level, including methodologies for assessing maternal and peri/neonatal health at community level*. WHO Maternal Health and Safe Motherhood Programme, Division of Family Health, Geneva 1994.
32. *Home Based Maternal Record – a training module for trainers and a training module for health providers*. Division of Family Health, WHO, Geneva, 1997.

Safe Motherhood, Unsafe Abortion: A Reflection on the Impact of Discourse

Susanna Rance

Ten years ago, in 1987, the International Conference on Safe Motherhood was held in Nairobi. As a result of this event, greater attention has been given to the previously 'unseen tragedy' of maternal mortality and its significance as a development indicator. A goal was set to halve the number of maternal deaths in developing countries by the year 2000. In Bolivia, the past decade has seen considerable developments in reproductive health policies and services, including a number of programmes designed to reduce maternal mortality, at least one third of which result from the complications of unsafe abortions. However, due to opposition from conservative forces within the Bolivian government influenced by the Catholic hierarchy, efforts to reduce deaths from unsafe abortion took a step backwards in 1996. This paper shows that discourses which condemn abortion have material effects on women's bodies and lives. It argues that the advances brought about by Safe Motherhood initiatives should be recognised and consolidated, and calls for these inititiatives to be revitalised with new concepts and fresh objectives, which construct women's diverse identities and needs as women and not only as mothers.

IN the decade since 1987, Safe Motherhood initiatives have raised global awareness of the causes, consequences and extent of maternal morbidity and deaths, stimulating action through partnership between governments, private agencies, local, national and international organisations, health professionals, donors and the media.[1]

These initiatives have led to a number of highly positive experiences in the Latin American region. The Andean Safe Motherhood Conference, held in Santa Cruz, Bolivia in 1993, was attended by key participants from state and non-governmental organisations. This event marked a watershed in opening public discussion on maternal mortality, including issues pertaining to induced abortion. The recommendations of the Andean Declaration are still pertinent today and many of them are currently being taken up by national and regional Safe Motherhood Committees.

The Mexican Safe Motherhood Conference, also in 1993, stimulated inter-institutional action at national, regional and local levels. To date this has included lobbying for changes in relevant legislation; state conferences; roundtable discussions on topics such as quality of care, and post-partum and post-abortion contraception; workshops with journalists; activities on gender relations within reproductive health services; operational research on health posts for pregnant women, and research on maternal mortality and its associated factors, using methods such as verbal autopsies.[2,3]

Public recognition of maternal deaths and the resources invested in preventative action brought valuable support to the international women's health movement, which had long campaigned on these issues with varying levels of success. In 1987 the time was perhaps not ripe for questioning the ideological foundation of the widespread support which was made available for promoting Safe Motherhood initiatives. Now, however, it seems an opportune moment to evaluate this discourse critically and examine the impact it has on health policies and services for women.

As Barbara Bradby has said, international programmes have been drawn towards women's issues yet they have been taking no chances. The name 'Safe Motherhood' sums it up: women are repeatedly defined with reference to their role as mothers. The name attempts to reassure that even in the face of so much conflicting evidence, motherhood must still be the safest place for women.[4]

In 1987, deaths associated with pregnancy and childbirth were constructed as a human tragedy whose moral dimension was closely associated with the social value assigned to motherhood. 1996 newspaper headlines in Bolivia continued to represent those who die not as women, but as actual or potential mothers and nurturers:

'Mothers are dying'

'Bolivia loses mothers'

'Mothers leave abandoned orphan children'

Children need a healthy, living mother. In their reproductive role, mothers are essentially good, needy and deserving of protection from the patriarchal state and church. 'Mothers must be helped in all circumstances, above all unfavourable ones', reads a recent editorial from a Bolivian Catholic daily newspaper. But further on, the article expresses the deeper significance of this 'help', in a warning aimed at the woman who is tempted to abdicate her maternal duty: 'All her life she will hear the voice of her own conscience, challenging her: "Where is your child?"'[5]

Following this moral logic, Safe Motherhood is the reward promised to mothers who accept a destiny fundamentally oriented towards their children's welfare. These apparently benevolent discourses construct female bodies and lives as vulnerable. The naming of a programme such as Safe Motherhood is more than a matter of political convenience. Rather, it is an ideological statement which constructs women as mothers, who deserve protection and safety only as such.

The power of discourse

Discourses – our own and those of others – have tangible effects on our identities, bodies and lives. These discourses are not fixed, but changing and susceptible to negotiation. Diverse social groups – including feminists – seek power and influence through contesting the discourses of others, creating and recreating their own and disseminating representations of the world in accordance with their particular and varied interests.

Discourse theories reject the notion of an objective, universally valid and scientifically provable reality. Instead, these theories postulate the construction of multiple representations of contrasting realities. Their application implies a willingness to recognise – but also to contest – discourses which construct the world on the basis of identities and interests which enter into conflict with one's own.

Far from assuming a relativism aloof from political commitment, some post-modernist philosophers such as Lyotard have claimed the discursive arena as a battlefield: 'To speak is to fight.'[6] As Rita Felski points out, the struggle for change need not be limited to defensive postures: 'While feminism certainly contains a negative moment which exposes the illusory or repressive nature of patriarchal discourses, it also develops alternative cultural and political positions.'[7] In this process, language acquires crucial importance as a tool for feminist action. In negotiating discourses, feminists assert their own identities, voices, bodies and right to exist in the world.

Two steps forward...

In Bolivia, the past decade has seen considerable developments in reproductive health policies and services. In 1989, the heritage of pro-natalism was relegated to the past with the introduction of a national reproductive health programme and campaigns to promote its use. Since 1991, state health services have offered increased access to contraceptive information and methods.

In 1994, the Bolivian government's 'Plan for Life' was launched, with the goal of rapidly reducing maternal mortality rates. In the same year, the Bolivian delegation to the Cairo conference proclaimed 'respect for women's decisions concerning sexuality and fertility and democratisation of women's roles in the family and in society.' The official Bolivian country statement for Cairo, subsequently published as the Declaration of Principles on Population and Sustainable Development,[8] was the first explicit formulation of a national population policy. This document is markedly progressive, given a regional context dominated historically by the Roman Catholic hierarchy.

Official figures attribute 27 to 35 per cent of all maternal deaths to abortion complications,[9] an estimate that is recognised as conservative due to under-reporting.[10] Feminists have contributed to discussions on abortion through a public debate increasingly centred on women's health and experiences. In 1994, the Working Group on Unwanted Pregnancy and Abortion was set up as a forum for linking and reinforcing the efforts of some 35 institutions and individuals to increase public awareness about these issues. The Working Group has contributed to a process of humanisation and feminisation of the abortion debate in Bolivia, producing and disseminating up-to-date research findings, and lobbying for change.

At both the Cairo and Beijing conferences in 1994 and 1995, the Bolivian government explicitly recognised abortion as a public health issue. In its Declaration of Principles, the Ministry for Human Development stressed that 'women who have resorted to abortion must be humanely treated and offered appropriate counselling'.[8] The National Health Secretariat had already begun supporting research on abortion as a basis for the production of educational materials, awareness-raising and training courses for health service staff on gender-sensitive post-abortion care.

In a climate of growing openness, in May 1996 the Health Secretary, Dr Oscar Sandóval Morón, pointed out Bolivia's sovereign right and obligation to publicly discuss the legalisation of abortion and to reach some conclusion on the matter: 'Not to do this is simply to devalue human life as less important than certain concepts and prejudices, and to ignore what is staring us in the face.'[11]

In the weeks and months that followed, a flood of contrasting positions on abortion made daily headlines and monopolised the media. On 28 May, the International Day of Action for Women's Health, in a press conference in the National Congress, a committee of feminist activists belonging to the Working Group declared the need to recognise and address the reality of abortion, and to develop a debate free from hypocrisy, focusing on gender equity and sexual and reproductive rights.

The founding in February 1996 of the National Safe Motherhood Committee in Bolivia augured new advances in the prevention of maternal deaths. However, in Bolivia today, 'safe motherhood' represents a conservative discourse when contrasted with the post-1994 emphasis on gender and sexual and reproductive health. An instrument which, in its time, served to call international attention to the needless deaths of women, has become a two-edged sword, which is being used to cut back the assertion of women's autonomous identities.

...One step back

Despite the ground gained, the power of discourses focused on motherhood began to undermine Bolivia's progressive policies. In 1996, government politicians offered maternal health as a Mother's Day gift to the female population, while moralists continued to label abortion as criminal and anti-life. These discourses hindered the efforts of feminist activists to build on past gains and resist a forced return to the restrictive language and practices of mother-child unity.

Clear evidence of this tendency was exposed through the National Insurance Programme for Mothers and Children, which was launched on 1 July 1996. This new initiative put the government to the test concerning its political willingness to address women's reproductive health needs in an integrated fashion.

From July 1996, the government began to publish reports on the coverage of the new Insurance Programme, including the numbers of women served with free antenatal and post-partum care, and the numbers of vaginal births and caesareans. Statistics were also provided on the numbers of infants and children receiving perinatal care, vaccinations and treatment for diarrhoea and respiratory infections.

From the start, the Insurance Programme achieved a considerable impact: official figures indicate that in its first five months, overall use of maternal and infant health services rose by over 30 per cent. While cultural and geographical obstacles to coverage remained, the removal of economic barriers was shown to significantly increase rates of use.[12]

Ambiguity on abortion reasserted

However, there was a singular gap in the figures published. No mention was made of Insurance Programme coverage of treatment for abortion complications, although official intentions to include such care had been suggested in the months preceding the Programme's inauguration. Given governmental declarations that rapid reduction of maternal mortality was a priority, the inclusion of free post-abortion care seemed a logical as well as necessary step.

In mid-July 1996, the Departmental Health Chief for Cochabamba, Rigoberto Siles, stated that in its first week of operation, the Insurance Programme had provided medical coverage for a total of 185 women and children, including three women with abortion complications.[13] Given regional reports of 200 cases of abortion complications monthly in some maternity hospitals, three in a week seemed very few. However, the Cochabamba data were of key importance as the first public evidence that free post-abortion care was actually being provided under the Mother-Child Insurance Programme.

Two days later, the Undersecretary for Medical Insurance, Guillermo Aponte, also presented a public report on the Programme's national achievements. Once again, any mention of treatment for incomplete abortion had disappeared from view. Aponte gave the figures for three types of services provided for women: antenatal care, vaginal births and caesareans.[14] Where were the three cases of abortion complications treated in Cochabamba? Apparently, these women had been erased from the national figures.

Thus, the matter of free treatment for abortion complications appeared to be ambiguous. It seems that the three Cochabamba women – and an unknown number of other women in Bolivia's other eight Departments – did manage to infiltrate the programme of free care meant for women marching firmly towards the goal of maternity. Theoretically, having had abortions, they should have been excluded. But lack of clarity in official declarations, and the habitual practice of rule-bending under oppressive systems, led to an unspecified degree of institutional and statistical slippage. While some women who were treated for abortion complications may well have been covered – others almost certainly were not.

This scenario of denial and confusion in reporting occurred within the context of official efforts to mask the reality of clandestine abortion and deny the need for non-discriminatory hospital treatment of abortion complications. Requests for clarification from feminists active on the issue met with silence and evasion from official quarters. No clear answers were given, but a revealing statement was made (off the record) by a lowland provincial health authority: 'Best not talk about it. It might get in the way of providing free care for these women on the quiet.'[15]

In response to press articles and letters to the authorities, an official explanation was made public on 26 July by the Undersecretary for Health, Dr Javier Torres-Goitia: 'The Insurance Programme covers all obstetric emergencies, such as haemorrhage in the first trimester of pregnancy, which are spontaneous and carry the risk of loss of the pregnancy, but it in no way contemplates curettage or incomplete abortion.' Torres-Goitia insisted that the Programme covered treatment for bleeding which occurs spontaneously, since 'such treatment is urgent, because otherwise the woman's life is put in danger'. He also said: 'The National Insurance Programme for Mothers and Children in no way seeks to cover induced abortion, so it must remain clear that the practice of abortion is not being promoted, although women who arrive with bleeding are indeed treated, whatever the cause.'[16]

The then Director of the Women's Hospital in La Paz, Dr Fernando Alvarez, clarified that 'induced abortion is not covered, so the woman has to pay for her own care'.[16] Reporters investigating this statement for a feminist news network asked Alvarez how the hospital determined whether a complicated abortion had been spontaneous or induced. He replied: 'That's a difficult question to answer, because right from the start, we mistrust the woman.'[17] Such mistrust, far from being restricted to women's statements about how they came to lose their pregnancies, reflects a more widespread misogyny which remains rife in medical circles.

Differing views among the medical profession

A discourse of control and moral protection of women from their own acts is also used by members of the medical profession. In the early stages of the debate, the Bolivian Society of Gynaecology and Obstetrics stated in a paid announcement: 'Induced abortion is an intervention which, because of its complexity, involves a high level of risk for women's health; facile comments on its supposedly innocuous nature lack veracity and scientific rigour.'[18] One prominent leader of the Society, when questioned about this claim, replied (off the record) that danger to the woman is 'not just physical but emotional and spiritual'.

The first woman president of the La Paz Medical College, Dra Ana María Aguilar, expressed a contrary position: 'From the technical/scientific point of view, an abortion does not have fatal consequences for a woman when it is carried out in hygienic conditions and in an appropriate way.'[19] She also referred to the Code of Professional Ethics which states: 'The interruption of a pregnancy will only proceed by therapeutic indication agreed by the medical committee and with due authorisation from the patient or her immediate relatives.'[20] These differences reveal the ideological discrepancies among the medical sector.

Within both state and private health services, however, medical control of abortion practice remains intact. This control, exercised by a patriarchal and predominantly male profession, is highly discretionary. Doctors' decisions, far from being based only on therapeutic indications, as established by current law and medical ethics, are also influenced by social stereotypes and moral prejudice,[21] not to mention financial considerations.

The government backs down

Opposition from the Catholic hierarchy had a considerable impact, and not only on the abortion debate. The church also attacked the national reproductive health strategy and the social marketing of condoms by the private sector to the adolescent population. Church pressure was a key element in the premature silencing of the debate, and influenced the government in June 1996 to cut short an official mass media information campaign on contraceptive methods.

In August 1996, the Santa Cruz Junior Chamber of Commerce launched a campaign 'In defence of the most defenceless' and distributed posters warning women 'Abortion can make you a mother with empty hands'. Activities were organised to raise the awareness of close to 30,000 young people regarding the 'physical, psychological, spiritual and moral damage' caused by abortion.[22]

In the same month, the Health Secretary drew back from his progressive stance on abortion by declining an invitation from the same committee of feminist activists from the Working Group to participate in a public forum entitled 'Abortion: A Public Health Issue', planned as part of its campaign for the 28 September International Day of Action on Abortion. Sandóval stated:

'The National Government, through the Ministries of Justice and Human Development and the Health Secretariat itself, has decided that its official position on this matter is that it cannot be considered as a subject of modification within the framework of current governmental plans.'[23]

Unsafe abortion: a self-fulfilling prophecy

Maternal mortality is defined by the World Health Organization as 'the death of a women while pregnant or within 42 days of termination of pregnancy, irrespective of the duration and the site of pregnancy, from any cause related to or aggravated by the pregnancy or its management.'[24] Deaths from abortion complications are therefore included under maternal mortality. When an abortion has been induced, there is a need to look critically at the categorisation as 'maternal' of an event which is generally (although not always) characterised by the woman's decision against becoming a mother, at least with this specific pregnancy.

In Bolivia today, deaths from badly practised abortions are still labelled 'maternal deaths'. Yet the unsafe nature of such abortions is the price women are expected to pay for having transgressed by refusing maternity. This punishment is socially selective, however, and those women who can least afford to pay for qualified care are triply sanctioned. As well as being the ones most at risk from unsafe interventions, they are also the ones who are publicly accused of reckless self-exposure, and if they die, their deaths are cited as evidence that abortion is physically and morally dangerous. Conservative discourse, in attempting to block attention to abortion issues, uses pseudo-scientific arguments to represent the procedure as inherently dangerous.

In opening the public debate on the legalisation of abortion, the Health Secretary had based his argument on the need to prevent the deaths of young and healthy women from badly practised interventions.[25] If the prevention of unsafe abortion were merely a technical matter, however, the solution would be relatively simple. It is the interference of moral prejudice that blocks solutions to health problems like this. This same type of interference falsifies statistical data on the causes of maternal mortality. Deaths from haemorrhage and sepsis associated with abortion are whitewashed and grouped under these same causes of deaths in pregnancies reaching full term.

Abortion is constructed as socially dangerous for reasons far removed from any concern for public health. Rather, it is represented as risky because it puts at risk patriarchal control of women's sexuality and fertility, a system of belief which fears rejection of maternity by a woman-mother. Abortion must remain unsafe according to the unwritten law of patriarchal power, the law of the father: 'Not the flesh and blood father, nor the father in a purely symbolic sense, but a certain type of society and of organisation of power.'[26]

Mother-womb, embryo-subject

This discussion leads to the analysis of discourses which construct the embryo or fetus as the main actor on the reproductive stage. The impact of these discourses can be observed in recent reports, reprinted in the Bolivian press, concerning the destruction of 'orphan' frozen embryos in the UK.[27] Should these embryos, in storage for five years and not wanted by their progenitors, be destroyed or transferred to other women? The issue has stimulated intense debate among the Catholic hierarchy. From the Vatican's 'profound perplexity', a proposal emerged:

'Once the embryos have been conceived in vitro, they must be transferred to the mother, and only if immediate transfer is impossible they may be frozen, but with the intention of taking them, immediately the conditions present themselves, to the maternal breast, which is the only "place" worthy of the person.'

The Vatican newspaper *L'Osservatore Romano* also raised the possibility of 'antenatal adoption':

'If the mother is unreachable or rejects the "transfer", some authors – including Catholics – have considered the possibility of transferring the embryos to another woman.... This solution, suggested as extrema ratio *to save the embryos from being abandoned to certain death, has the merit of taking seriously the value of the embryos' life, and courageously taking up the challenge of cryopreservation.'*[28]

In Argentina, where *in vitro* fertilisation is also posing dilemmas, Edgardo Youn, professor of human reproduction at the University of Buenos Aires stated similarly: 'Frozen embryos have a destiny and there are no cases of abandonment.' Argentinian experts like him have also declared themselves in favour of the 'antenatal adoption' of the few embryos which might remain frozen in the country.[29]

These discourses, with their complicity between scientific and moral agendas, construct an interchangeable mother-uterus whose individuality is invisible if not ultimately disposable. The embryo-subject, on the other hand, is given a unique human value which must be defended at all costs. These are representations which support the protection of the maternal function primarily for the good of the child. The Roman Catholic columnist quoted previously maintains, for example, that: 'It is erroneous to defend the woman's right to abortion on the grounds that the fetus is her property, a part of her being; the conceived is a being independent of its mother, a complete person.'[5]

Such discourses are latent in the approach of certain antenatal programmes, whose primary aim is to promote fetal development rather than women's well-being. Antenatal classes can be highly beneficial for a woman with a wanted pregnancy. However, from a sexual and reproductive rights perspective, it is possible to assert that she herself, through her decision to procreate, infuses life into her pregnancy and constructs the human quality of the embryo/fetus. The unborn child, as such, is a creation of the woman. The viability of a given pregnancy is not merely a biological matter.

Jorge Villarreal maintains that from the point of view of the obstetrician-gynaecologist, 'Pre-viable fetuses are only patients as a function of the woman's decision.'[30] Far from constructing the woman as a uterine receptacle for the embryo, this ethical proposition situates the woman as subject at the centre of the reproductive stage, recognising and respecting her decisions regarding her pregnancy, as a crucial element in its viability.

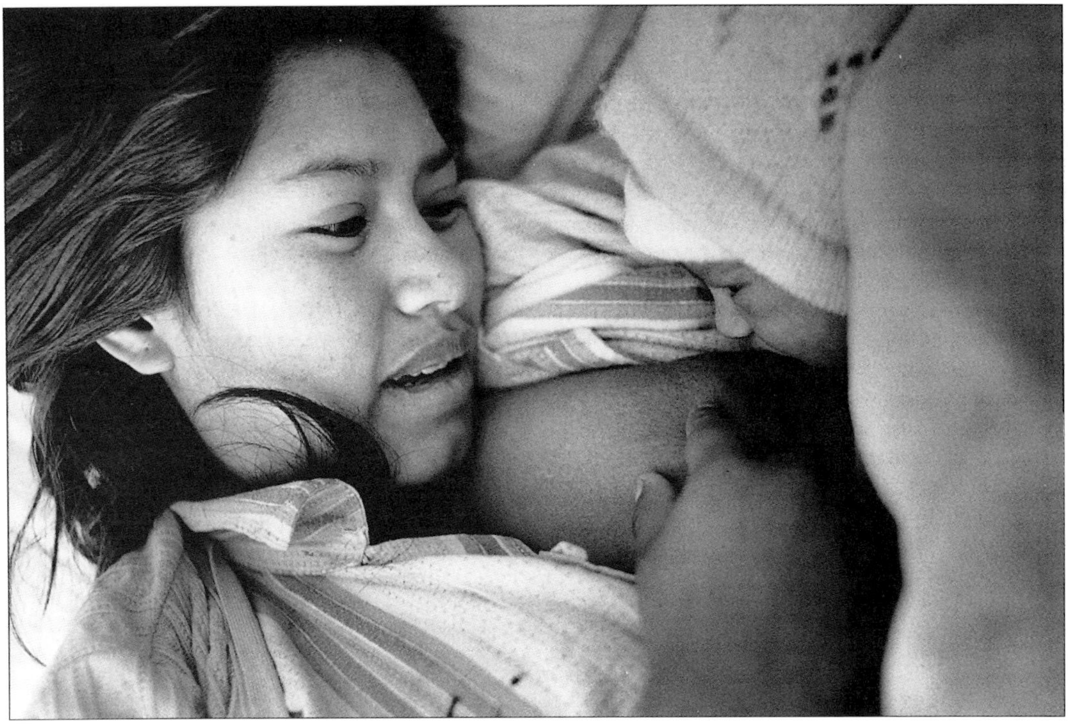

JENNY MATTHEWS

Maternal mortality: a political question

Maternal mortality is above all a political question. At the National Seminar on Maternal Morbidity and Mortality in Brazil in August 1989, Brazilian feminists debated the best way to campaign against maternal mortality. In past debates concerning the Integrated Programme for Women's Health in Brazil (PAISM), they reached conclusions which remain valid and important today: First, we must address women's needs as these are defined by women themselves. These needs include access to birth control. Second, pro-natalist or anti-natalist population policies which have any coercive elements violate the basic right of women to decide whether or not they want to have children, how many children they want, and when to have them. Hence, coercive policies deserve to be repudiated by progressive groups.[31]

As Carmen Barroso said in a paper presented at that seminar, there are three crucial areas for feminist action in health: 'redefinition of the issues, demands for increased decision-making power for women, and support for the right to abortion.' She concluded that:

'...it is up to the feminist movement to give priority to campaigning for the right to abortion, not only because clandestine abortion is one of the leading causes of maternal mortality, but also because decriminalisation of abortion is an important step towards making women full members of the community. In the campaign for legalisation of abortion, statistics are vital in the defence of women's lives and health. But we must not lose sight of the most important issue at stake: the autonomy of women to become aware, responsible and capable of making decisions about our own bodies, sexuality and lives. Our aim is to affirm the morality of women and refuse the protection of church and state.'[31]

After a decade of Safe Motherhood programmes, her three challenges are still valid and can be applied in the following ways: redefining the problem of deaths associated with pregnancy, childbirth and abortion; consolidating women's decision-making power within health systems; and giving priority to campaigns for the right to abortion which resist a focus that is restricted exclusively to women's maternal role.

It was in this spirit that despite the lack of official approval, the Bolivian feminist activists' committee went ahead with its 28 September 1996 campaign, with support from the Latin American and Caribbean Women's Health Network and the International Women's Health Coalition. A variety of media and cultural activities were carried out to raise public awareness on the following issues:

- the importance of continuing a broad public debate on the question of abortion;
- support for humane and appropriate care for women with abortion complications;
- free treatment for such complications within the National Insurance Programme for Mothers and Children;
- provision of services for abortion that are permitted under current Bolivian law, that is, in cases of rape, incest or risk to the woman's life. Abortions for these 'non-punishable' reasons continue to be practised clandestinely, without official recognition or support.[32]

Ten years on: time for change

'Maternal health is not an isolated problem: the [Safe Motherhood] Initiative has encouraged decision-makers to deal openly with many women's issues – such as unwanted fertility, women's low status, legal rights, sexually transmitted diseases, violence against women and unsafe abortion – and to take action, despite potential controversy, in the interest of public health.'[1]

Feminists in the Bolivian women's health movement have been key actors in a process of evolution of concepts that had an important influence on and were further developed during the Nairobi, Cairo and Beijing conferences. They have contributed to changing use of language, which has moved from the unity of 'mother-child' to 'maternal and child health', to a distinct 'maternal health' and more recently into the wider arena of women's sexual and reproductive health and rights.

The term Safe Motherhood, and the discourses which sustain it are not written in stone. They can be replaced by others which explicitly promote sexual and reproductive rights. Over the past years, feminists and health activists have challenged and changed a series of terms which carry ideologies contrary to their interests. For example, those who wanted to talk about voluntary fertility regulation stopped referring to birth spacing, responsible parenthood or family planning. What used to be called venereal diseases are now known as sexually transmitted diseases. The stigmatising notion of 'risk groups' with relation to HIV transmission has been contested through the identification of risk behaviours. In 1973, homosexuality was removed from the WHO Diagnostic and Statistical Manual of Mental Disorders, and there are now moves to get 'gender dysphoria' off the list as well.[33] Referring to 'battered women' diverts attention away from those who batter them.[34] Denouncing 'domestic violence' as such can also backfire against women as a discourse, by implying that the home or the domestic environment are themselves intrinsically violent, thus turning a blind eye to (mostly male) gendered aggression.

To this end, some new terminology can be suggested as a substitute for currently used terms:

- women's health (instead of maternal health),
- women's sexual and reproductive health (instead of safe motherhood),
- reproductive mortality (instead of maternal mortality),
- fertile age (instead of reproductive age).

The term 'reproductive mortality' was first suggested by Valerie Beral[35] in 1979 as a more appropriate index:

'Reproductive mortality includes deaths due to complications of pregnancy, induced abortion, and contraception among women of reproductive age.'[36]

The interests of groups active in the women's health movement lie not only in issues of public health nor of maternity. Their framework is, rather, one of gender equity and sexual and reproductive rights. Within their particular and local situations, the controversy which faces these groups is precisely the public re-definition of women's diverse identities and needs. Any controversy generated by the re-negotiation of discourses will ultimately be beneficial in terms of putting these issues firmly on the table for discussion.

Safe Motherhood programmes in Bolivia and in many other countries worldwide have made significant contributions to women's health over the past decade. But during this period, the discourse of Safe Motherhood has reinforced drives to protect and control women as mothers. This focus, in the hands of conservative forces, has begun to create conflict with feminist advocacy of women's empowerment and the exercise of sexual and reproductive rights within an integrated framework.

The ten-year anniversary of Safe Motherhood provides an opportune moment for reflection. Its advances to date should be recognised and consolidated, but the discourse of Safe Motherhood has fulfilled its historic purpose. The initiative should now be revitalised with a new name and fresh objectives, which construct women's diverse identities and needs as women and not only as mothers.

De-maternalising safety, in-suring abortion

Women do not need the credential of maternity to deserve and demand safety in their sexual and reproductive lives. Neither should women have to accept the punishment of unsafe abortion if they opt at some moment – in a particular pregnancy and a given situation, determined by them individually – not to become mothers.

The strategy proposed by the Safe Motherhood Initiative can be applied to the reality of abortion, without moral condemnation, just as to other aspects of pregnancy and childbirth. This includes recognition of the problem, identification of barriers women experience in making and carrying out decisions to seek care, and improving access to and quality of care, with training for health workers to provide humane and appropriate treatment.[37]

Rather than assigning blame for women's deaths to health workers, communities or family members, it may be more productive to challenge the material impact of discourses which construct women as uterine environments destined primarily for reproduction. Discourses too can kill, through the power of their exponents to control health policies and services. Unsafe abortion is a clear example of the impact of discursive power, in which danger is a self-fulfilling prophecy and promises of safety are reserved for an idealised and socially approved motherhood.

Feminists have already succeeded in transforming and creating many discourses which support women's rights and autonomy. There is no need to lose the opportunities gained through the Safe Motherhood Initiative. In many spheres, women are already recognised as women. The deaths of women from causes associated with pregnancy, childbirth and abortion have been identified as a problem and unsafe abortion has been identified as a public health issue. Feminists and health activists have voices, votes and a degree of power and can take responsibility for the construction and dissemination of new discourses. Without relinquishing the spaces and resources we have already gained, let us take a fresh look at our own use of the Safe Motherhood discourse. It is an ideological trap, from which we should now take action to extricate ourselves.

POSTSCRIPT

Since 1997 when this article was written, what has changed in Bolivia? Treatment for women with complications of induced abortion is still not covered by the National Insurance Programme for Mothers and Children. The current government has announced its inclusion from the year 2000, but under another scheme – and another name.

Treatment of haemorrhage...

A new Basic Health Insurance, which will offer a more comprehensive package of services to wider sectors of the population, was approved by supreme decree in December 1998 and officially launched in May 1999. Public affiliation will continue throughout 1999 and services are due to be offered from the year 2000. These are to include 'treatment for haemorrhage of the first trimester of pregnancy'.

This terminology has evolved through various stages of discussion in two successive government administrations. Language negotiated between health authorities and international donor agencies has gone full circle from 'haemorrhage in the first trimester of pregnancy' to 'haemorrhage in the first semester', to 'the first half of pregnancy' and back again to 'the first trimester'.[38] At certain moments, each of these definitions has been included within – or replaced by – the wider bracket of 'obstetric emergencies'. Representatives of the Health Ministry continue to insist that 'abortion complications' should not be openly mentioned in the promotion of Basic Health Insurance services.

...or post-abortion care?

Less publicly, a discursive and technological innovation was officially approved in a ministerial resolution of 31 March 1999.[39] This establishes a measure to improve the quality of obstetric emergency services, reducing the cost and length of interventions – the introduction of manual vacuum aspiration (MVA) within post-abortion care, at last explicitly named. Use of MVA had been officially vetoed over the past decade on the grounds that in the 'wrong hands' it could be used to induce illegal abortions. The US-based agency Ipas is currently assisting the Ministry of Health with a pilot MVA staff-training project in two regional hospitals. At the same time, the national interagency Post-abortion Care Committee is drawing up norms for this area of treatment in preparation for its inclusion next year within Basic Health Insurance services.

The Ministry of Health is simultaneously drawing on conservative and progressive approaches to addressing the problem of unsafe abortion. Alternations in official discourse and practice can be explained by the government's need to steer a course between two key pressure points. One of these is political: national and international 'sensitivity' concerning abortion among decision-makers, influenced by Catholic Church hierarchies. The other is economic: sectoral reforms and structural adjustment measures make MVA a cost-cutting necessity if the new services are to be made widely available.

A recent Ipas publication states that 'a visit by high-level Bolivian Ministry of Health officials to neighbouring Peru convinced them to implement a comprehensive post-abortion care programme using MVA to address the needs of women throughout Bolivia'.[40] Internationally, the economic rationale has spoken the loudest in favour of such innovations. These require monitoring in specific contexts to ensure quality of care .

Implementing the Cairo agenda

Over the past two years, Bolivian women's health advocates have continued to campaign for decriminalisation of abortion, with slogans such as 'Let's talk about abortion' and 'Abortion: for the right to choose'.[41] Both of these demands conflict with current government policy.

However, Bolivia does remain at the forefront of a minority of Catholic Latin American countries which explicitly defend the Cairo and Beijing agendas on sexual and reproductive health and rights, and recognise unsafe abortion as a major public health problem. Bolivian official delegations have maintained this position at the Cairo+5 conferences in the face of moves from some delegations to fracture the 1994 consensus. Feminist organisations and health sector NGOs active within the Ministry of Health-led National Forum for Sexual and Reproductive Health are insisting on going forward, not back, from the 1994 and 1995 agendas.

The reality of unsafe abortion: from pillar to post

In the gap between discourse and practice, women's lives continue to be threatened:

At 9:30am on 3 February 1999, following three visits to negotiate an advance payment of 350 Bolivianos,[42] M, aged 22, had an abortion by curettage in a doctor's surgery in La Paz. At midday she was woken by the nurse who told her to leave immediately: 'She practically threw me out.'

M bled profusely for the three hours it took her – on foot, by minibus and taxi – to reach her home in a suburb of the neighbouring city of El Alto. She said nothing to her family. At 5pm, finding her unconscious and haemorrhaging, they took her to XX Octubre Hospital, the main tertiary care centre in the city of half a million inhabitants. After waiting two and a half hours, she was told she could not receive emergency care because there was no anaesthetist and the hospital did not have the necessary drugs.

Still bleeding copiously, M was taken by relatives to the Women's Hospital in La Paz. She was examined by interns but could not be treated until the duty resident returned. After a long wait, M was taken for a scan which showed her uterus was perforated. While awaiting treatment she went into hypovolemic shock. Obtaining blood from the hospital blood bank presented further difficulties and delays.

At 2am, M's family decided to take her to a private clinic. Following the operation she suffered a cardiac arrest and almost died. After three weeks of intensive treatment, during which her operation wound became infected, M is steadily recovering. She continues to meet with a researcher who works with the clinic.[43] Together they are reconstructing the details of M's 'case', an odyssey in search of care.

First legal abortion in Bolivia

The Bolivian Penal Code permits 'non-punishable abortion' in cases of rape, incest, abduction not followed by marriage, and danger to the woman's life or health.[44] After 26 years of this legislation, the first legal abortion in Bolivia's judicial history was performed. On 10 August 1998, a judge authorised the termination of pregnancy of a 14-year-old girl who had been raped by her father.

A feminist institution in the city of Sucre, Centro Juana Azurduy, supported the demand for a legal abortion which was presented by the girl's mother. Medical tests confirmed a ten-week pregnancy. For the first time, the judicial authorities responded promptly, authorising the abortion three days later.

When the girl was referred to the Women's Hospital in Sucre, five doctors in succession refused to admit her, citing 'ethical reasons' for not complying with the judicial order. For three days the girl was denied admission and subjected to verbal aggression from doctors, who accused her of 'committing a crime'. The hospital director intervened and the girl was finally admitted. However, the treatment administered – induction via intravenous drip – was not effective as it was systematically interrupted by the doctors on duty. In response to a further judicial demand by Centro Juana Azurduy, medical resistance was finally overcome. After six days in hospital, the pregnancy was terminated surgically.[45]

Both M in La Paz and the 14-year-old girl in Sucre finally obtained the post-abortion and abortion care to which they were entitled under Bolivian health policy and legislation. Both were subjected to traumatic and potentially damaging experiences. They both survived. Many women do not. Despite gradual changes in discourse, policy and practice, unsafe abortion in Bolivia remains an all too common reality.

Acknowledgements

This paper is reprinted in full from ***Reproductive Health Matters*** *Vol 5, Number 9, May 1997. The Postscript was written in 1999 to update the paper for inclusion in this book. The original paper was adapted in English from a paper presented in Spanish to the Seminar 'Saude Reprodutiva na América Latina e no Caribe: Temas e Problemas' in Caxambu MG, Brazil, 5-7 October 1996. The Seminar was organised by PROLAP (Programa Latinoamericano de Actividades en Población), ABEP (Asociación Brasilera de Estudios en Población) and NEPO/UNICAMP, Brazil. Quotations from texts originally in Spanish have been translated into English by the author.*

Correspondence

Susanna Rance, Casilla 10640, La Paz, Bolivia. E mail: srance@latinwide.com

References and Notes

1. *Safe motherhood, steps ahead.* Family Care International, New York 1994. (Leaflet)
2. Elu M del C. La experiencia de maternidad sin riesgos. México DF. (Unpublished, undated draft)
3. Verbal autopsy uses a participatory methodology to analyse specific maternal deaths with community organisations and identify points at which life-saving interventions could have been made.
4. Bradby B, 1996. Community-level research within a reproductive health programme: from participation to dialogue. Paper presented to EC Reproductive Health Research Meeting. Ghent, Belgium, 23-25 June.
5. de Anasagasti P, 1996. Contra la vida. *Presencia* (La Paz). 19 Sept.
6. Lyotard JF, 1984. *The Postmodern Condition: A Report on Knowledge.* Manchester University Press, Manchester.
7. Felski R, 1989. Feminist theory and social change. *Theory, Culture and Society.* 6(2):219-40.
8. *Declaración de Principios sobre Población y Desarrollo Sostenible.* Ministerio de Desarrollo Humano/PROSEPO/ UNFPA, La Paz, 1994.
9. *Plan Vida: Plan Nacional para la Reducción Acelerada de la Mortalidad Materna, Perinatal y del Niño, Bolivia, 1994-1997.*

Ministerio de Desarrollo Humano/Secretaría Nacional de Salud/UNFPA/USAID/UNICEF La Paz, 1994.
10. *La Niñez y la Mujer en Bolivia, Análisis de Situación*. UNICEF Bolivia. La Paz, 1994.
11. *Hoy* (La Paz). 14 May 1996.
12. *Correo de los Comités*. 1(December):2. Comité Nacional por una Maternidad Segura, La Paz.
13. *El Diario* (La Paz). 17 July 1996.
14. *La Razón* (La Paz). 20 July 1996.
15. Alexia Escóbar, Personal communication, 17 August 1996.
16. *Ultima Hora* (La Paz). 26 July 1996.
17. Goyzueta J and Orellana O, 1996. *Los abortos inducidos tienen un costo*. RED-ADA, Red Nacional de Trabajadoras de la Información y Comunicación - ERBOL. No 11. La Paz, 15 August.
18. *El Diario* (La Paz). 23 May 1996.
19. *El Diario* (La Paz). 16 August 1996.
20. Código de Etica Médica, Artículo 15. *Estatutos y Reglamentos 1993*. Colegio Médico de Bolivia, La Paz, 1993.
21. Rance S, 1997. Discursos médicos en torno al aborto: Estudios de caso en contextos hospitalarios de los sistemas de salud pública y seguridad social. Ipas/National Health Secretariat/DFID, La Paz. (Unpublished report)
22. *El Mundo* (Santa Cruz). 15 August 1996.
23. Letter from the National Health Secretary to members of the 28 September Campaign Committee, La Paz, 16 August 1996.
24. *International Classification of Diseases, Injuries and Death*, 9th Edition. World Health Organisation, Geneva 1979.
25. *Hoy* (La Paz). 14 May 1996.
26. Muraro L, 1994. *El Orden Simbólico de la Madre*. Horas y Horas, Madrid.
27. *Ultima Hora* (La Paz). 15 August 1996.
28. *Presencia* (La Paz). 23 July 1996.
29. *Los Tiempos*. 4 August 1996.
30. Villarreal J, 1996. Presentation to the Annual Meeting of Trainees, Fundación Educación para la Salud Reproductiva (ESAR), Pachacamac, Peru. 31 August.
31. Barroso C, 1990. Maternal mortality: a political question. Maternal mortality and morbidity; a call to women for action. Paper presented to National Seminar on Maternal Morbidity and Mortality, Itapecerica da Serra, Brazil. 28 May.
32. Aliaga S, 1994. Qué dice la ley Sr. Juez? Equidad, *Hoy* (La Paz). 18 May. In 1993, an application for legal abortion was made in court on behalf of two teenage sisters who had been raped and made pregnant by their father. The judge, who holds evangelical religious beliefs, systematically caused delays in consideration of the case, which was finally abandoned when the girls' pregnancies were in the second and third trimesters.
33. Taylor J, 1995. The third sex. *Esquire*. April:102-12.
34. Stark E, Flitcraft A and Frazier W, 1979. Medicine and patriarchal violence: the social construction of a 'private' event. *International Journal of Health Services*. 9(3):461-93. Cited in De Lauretis T, 1987. *Technologies of Gender*. Indiana University Press, Bloomington.
35. Beral V, 1979. Reproductive mortality. *British Medical Journal*. 2:632-34.
36. Rosenberg MJ and Rosenthal SM, 1987. Reproductive mortality in the United States: recent trends and methodologic considerations. *American Journal of Public Health*. 77(7):833-36.
37. Koblinsky M, 1996. *Para salvar la vida*. MotherCare-Bolivia/JSI/USAID, La Paz.
38. *Por una Maternidad Segura en Bolivia*. Ministerio de Salud y Previsión Social/Comité por una Maternidad Segura/UNFPA/Family Care International. La Paz, May 1999, p3.
39. Resolución Ministerial No. 0133, Ministerio de Salud y Provisión Social, 31 March 1999.
40. Hord CE, 1999. ICPD Paragraph 8.25: A Global Review of Progress. Issues in Abortion Care 5. Chapel Hill, NC: Ipas.
41. Bolivian slogans of the 1996-97 and 1997-98 September 28 campaigns for decriminalisation of abortion in Latin America and the Caribbean.
42. Equivalent to US$ 60.
43. Sociologist Silvia Benítez provided this information with M's consent.
44. *Codigo Penal 1972*, Art.266. Republica de Bolivia. Editorial Serrano, Cochabamba, 1997.
45. Caso de interrupción judicial de embarazo. Centro Juana Azurduy, Sucre. August 1998. (Unpublished report)

Costing Safe Motherhood in Uganda

Eva Weissman, Olive Sentumbwe-Mugisa, A K Mbonye, Craig Lissner

The Ugandan government is implementing a comprehensive safe motherhood programme in an effort to reduce high levels of maternal and neonatal morbidity and mortality in the country. The 'Mother-Baby Package' of the World Health Organization is used to set standards regarding the scope and quality of the health care provided to pregnant women and newborn babies. To provide programme planners with a better appreciation of the costs entailed in implementing the Mother-Baby Package, a costing study was done using a standard WHO methodology. It was found that the Ugandan government presently spends about US$0.50 per capita on maternal and newborn health care. To upgrade this care to conform with the standards and guidelines set forth in the Mother-Baby Package would cost approximately US$1.40 per capita, representing an incremental cost of US$0.90. The inclusion of capital and overhead costs would raise the cost to approximately US$1.80 per capita, bringing the incremental cost up to US$1.30. This study assisted national authorities, donor governments, and other partners at the national level in considering the substantial recurrent cost implications of providing higher-quality maternal and newborn care, and in doing so it has facilitated an important dialogue on maternal and newborn health care financing and sustainability issues.

THE Mother-Baby Package,[1] which defines an essential cluster of health interventions for the reduction of maternal and neonatal mortality in developing countries, was developed by the World Health Organization (WHO) in 1994. The interventions in the package include antenatal and delivery care, basic newborn care, the management of obstetric complications and post-partum care, including family planning services. One of the tenets of the Mother-Baby Package is that the management and provision of services must be integrated into a country's existing district health system. The development of a 'vertical' programme for maternal health, as has proven successful for immunisation, diarrhoeal diseases and some other health issues, is deemed not practicable for as broad and complex an area as maternal and neonatal health. This has important implications for the financing of any maternal and neonatal health programme, since it makes it difficult to distinguish the specific cost elements of the interventions in the programme from other, unrelated health interventions.

A large number of maternal health costing studies have been carried out in recent years, most of which are limited to specific services or components of maternal care. In the area of family planning, for example, costs have been well-researched.[2] In integrated maternal care, one of the few published estimates for a comprehensive maternal health programme was made by the *World Development Report 1993*,[3] in which an investment of about US$4 per capita was found to be among the most cost-effective investments in health, in terms of disability-adjusted life years (DALYs) saved. Another estimate is found in *Making Motherhood Safe*,[4] in which the estimated cost of reducing maternal mortality ranged from US$2 in a weak health system to just above US$6 in a more developed health system. A more recent study on the cost of safe motherhood estimated that an integrated package would cost US$2.60 in a low-income setting, and up to US$5.60 in a middle-income scenario.[5] However, these estimates are all based on hypothetical models; in 1998 a comprehensive review of the literature on the cost of reproductive health identified only one country-specific study of maternal health cost.[6] Furthermore, many researchers have lamented the lack of country-specific cost data for integrated packages of maternal health interventions.[7]

The paucity of relevant global, let alone local,

information on cost poses a challenge to maternal health planners and managers in developing countries, for in the development of health financing schemes, programme costs are critical. Without a firm grasp of these, as well as of the cost structure, the development of a realistic and sustainable financing scheme is problematic.

Whilst Uganda has actively embraced the concept of Safe Motherhood, there has been little discernible improvement in maternal and neonatal health indicators over the past decade. High fertility rates and restricted access to quality maternity care continue to expose Ugandan women to a high risk of dying from pregnancy- and delivery-related complications. The maternal mortality ratio has been estimated to be as high as 1,200 per 100,000 live births,[8] and the neonatal death rate is 41 per 1,000 live births.

In its recently issued National Poverty Eradication Action Plan, the government of Uganda has reaffirmed its commitment to improving the health and welfare of all Ugandans, with special emphasis on the health of women and young children. The National Safe Motherhood Programme[9,10] is the foundation of Uganda's strategy to achieve a significant reduction in maternal and infant morbidity and mortality.

The major objectives of the Ugandan National Strategic Plan for Safe Motherhood are to:

- reduce maternal mortality by 30 per cent by the year 2001 by providing a comprehensive range of high quality reproductive health services.
- contribute towards the reduction of the infant mortality rate (IMR) by 30 per cent by the year 2001 through an accelerated reduction in the neonatal component of the IMR.

Improving the quality of maternal and newborn health care is seen as one of the major means of achieving the above objectives. In this context, the Uganda Ministry of Health implemented WHO's Mother-Baby Package.

The WHO Mother-Baby Package

The WHO Safe Motherhood programme developed the Mother-Baby Package in 1994. It contains treatment guidelines and standards for the 12 essential health interventions identified in Table 1.

Table 1. Mother-Baby Package interventions

Antenatal care	Basic antenatal care
	Management of syphilis, gonorrhoea and chlamydia
	Management of severe anaemia
	Treatment of malaria
Normal delivery care	Clean and safe delivery
	Basic newborn care
	Post-partum care
Essential obstetric care	Management of eclampsia, sepsis, haemorrhage and abortion complications, plus provision of emergency caesarean sections
Family planning	Family planning information and services

WHO, working with the World Bank, also developed a companion costing methodology[11] which enables programme planners to estimate the local cost of implementing the package. Besides calculating the costs directly associated with the provision of the 12 interventions, the model contains the option of calculating capital and overhead costs. Since Uganda already had a detailed budget plan detailing the latter costs, this study concentrated on generating estimates of treatment cost.

Methodology

Two cost estimates were generated. The current practice model was used to estimate current expenditure on maternal and newborn health services at the district level. The standard practice model was used to estimate expenditure required to upgrade this care, according to the standards of the Mother-Baby Package. The difference between the two estimates represents the incremental cost, or additional investment, required to provide this higher level of care.

Information about current treatment practices was collected at approximately 20 randomly selected government health facilities in two of Uganda's 21 districts – Iganga and Mbarara. Treatment was assessed at health centre as well as hospital level. Using questionnaires developed specifically for this purpose, medical personnel in charge of maternal care at the facilities (doctors, nurses and midwives) were interviewed about the treatment provided at the facility for each of the 12 interventions contained in the Mother-Baby Package. Information was collected regarding the drugs administered, the amount of time clinical staff spent with the client, and any other supplies (surgical, laboratory, etc) used. The survey also assessed other items, such as the number of staff, the total number of clients and major equipment.

The 'standard' for treatment practice was based on the treatment guidelines and standards outlined in the Mother-Baby Package, with changes and modifications based on national guidelines.[12,13] The cost of providing this standard of treatment was calculated using population projections for the year 2001.[14]

Cost data for drugs and other supplies were collected from national sources, including the essential drugs programme and the Ministry of Health. When local unit cost data were not available, international and indicative costs were used as proxies.[15]

Results and discussion[16]

Two factors determine the total cost of maternal health care services. The first is the average treatment cost per client, which for almost all interventions will increase when care is provided according to the new standards. The second is the number of women who will require these services.

The Ugandan government has also set ambitious goals relating to the number of women that it is trying to reach. By the year 2001, it aims to:

- provide 90 per cent of all pregnant women in Uganda with quality antenatal care, based on a four-visit protocol;
- increase the percentage of women who deliver at health facilities/under supervision of skilled personnel from the current 38 per cent to 50 per cent; and
- increase the contraceptive prevalence rate from 15 per cent to 30 per cent.

These initiatives will have a major impact on the demand for maternal health services, as illustrated in Figures 1-3.[17]

Figure 1. Current and Projected Number of Antenatal Care Visits

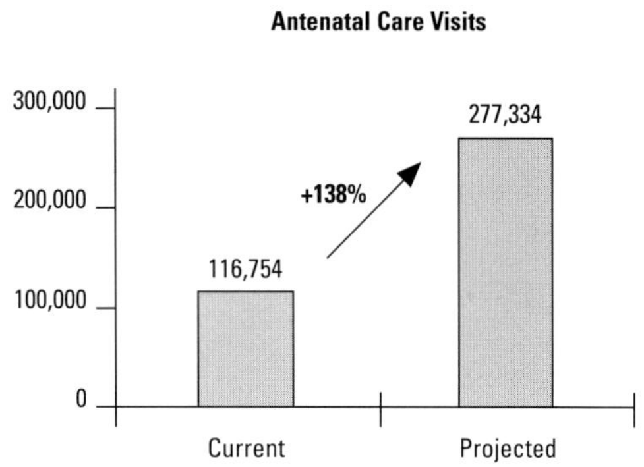

Figure 2. Current and Projected Number of Attended Deliveries

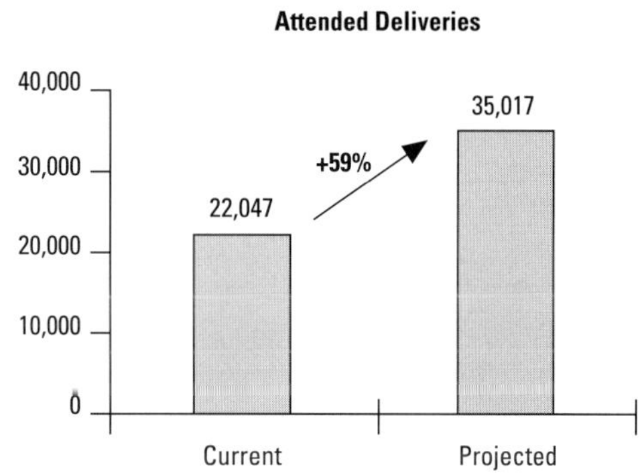

Figure 3. Current and Projected Number of Family Planning Clients

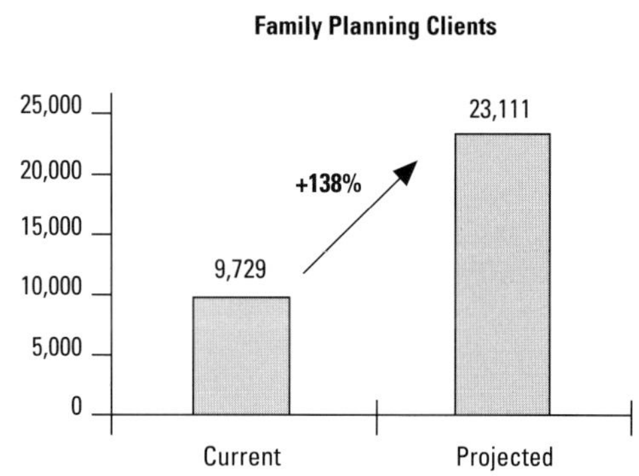

Demographic and Health Survey data for Uganda indicate that 90 per cent of all pregnant women already receive some type of antenatal care. Under the new policy, however, every woman is expected to have at least four antenatal care visits. This will effectively double the current number of antenatal care visits. Combined with the expected growth in population, this will mean a 138 per cent increase in antenatal care visits by the year 2001. The projected increase in facility-based deliveries and in the number of women using family planning will further increase the demand for health services, by 59 per cent and 138 per cent respectively.

Similar increases are projected for the other interventions provided in the package. The more antenatal care women receive, based on the Mother-Baby Package interventions, the more likely it is that underlying conditions such as anaemia, malaria and sexually transmitted diseases will be treated during pregnancy. Currently, these conditions often go undetected and untreated. As regards delivery-related complications, if those attending birth have more skills and training in handling normal deliveries and managing and making timely referrals when necessary, the more likely it is that women will receive proper care should complications arise.

Average treatment cost per case

Figure 4 compares the current and standard treatment cost per client for each of the 12 interventions at the hospital level.

As the graph shows, the per-case treatment cost will increase for almost all interventions. The cost differential is attributed to the fact that current treatment is well below the standards of the Mother-Baby Package. For example, at present, for the treatment of syphilis and gonorrhoea, in many cases treatment of the woman's partner is not provided. Another reason for the increase in per-case treatment cost is the simple fact that at present the necessary drugs and supplies are often unavailable.

Total treatment cost by intervention

Figures 5 and 6 provide a breakdown of the total treatment costs,[18] which are the product of the average treatment cost per case and the number

Figure 4. Average Treatment Cost per Client at Hospital Level (in US dollars)[7]

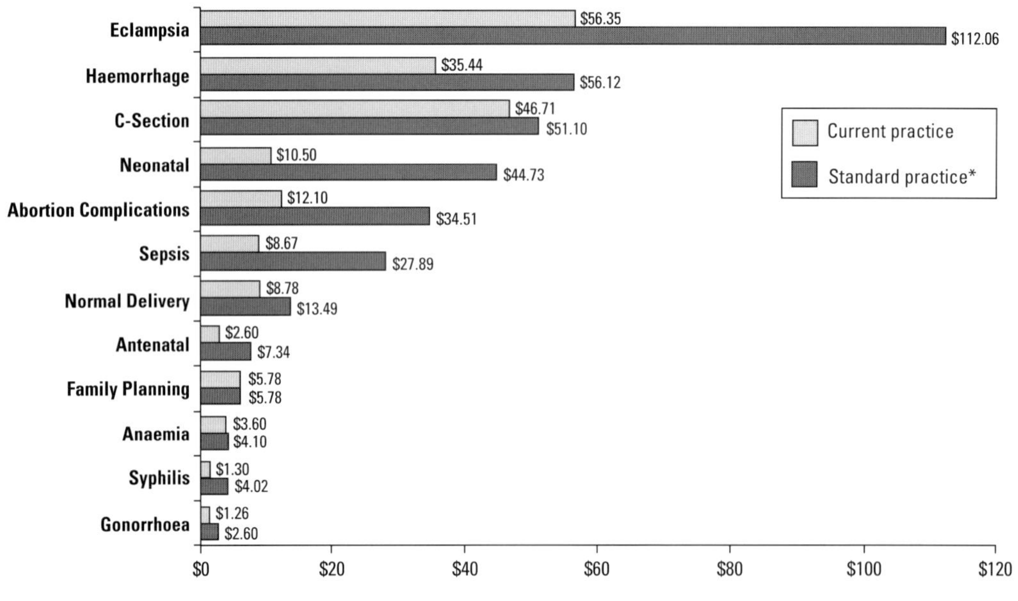

** Standard = based on the Mother-Baby Package*

Figure 5. Current and Standard Treatment Cost by Intervention (in US dollars)

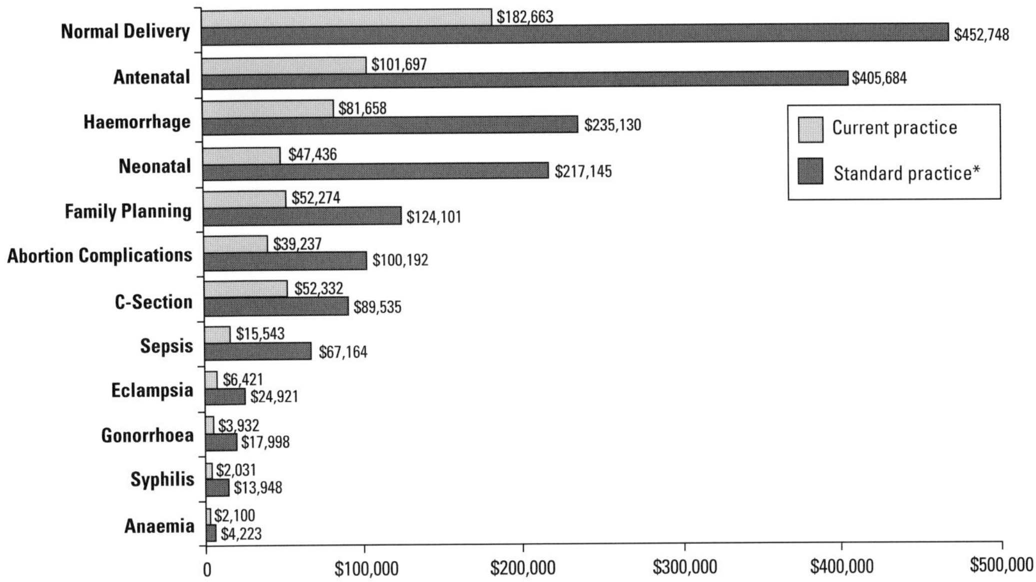

** Standard = based on the Mother-Baby Package*

of women who require the intervention. Antenatal and delivery care, even though relatively inexpensive on a per-case basis, represent major costs because of the large number of women who require these interventions. Treatment for eclampsia, which, on a per-case basis, is the most costly intervention (US$112 for the average case), makes up only a small share of total costs due to the low incidence of this complication (0.5 per cent of all pregnancies). The total costs of treatment for haemorrhage and neonatal complications are high, because they both have a relatively high incidence and a high per-case cost (US$56 and US$45, respectively, under the new guidelines at the hospital level).

Figure 6. Incremental Treatment Cost by Intervention

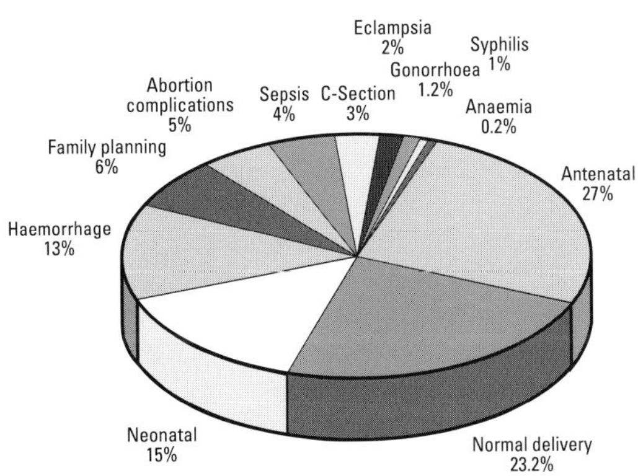

Total treatment cost by input

Figures 7 and 8 show the total treatment cost broken down by input, or cost category. Figure 7 compares the total cost for the six input categories under the current and the Mother-Baby Package standard scenarios. Clinical staff time, currently the single largest cost item at approximately US$324,000, will account for almost US$1 million in the year 2001. A large part of this increase can be attributed to the increase in the number of women treated by the health system. Average treatment time per woman, however, will also increase once the new treatment standards are adopted. Currently, the

Figure 7. Current and Standard Treatment Cost by Input (in US dollars)

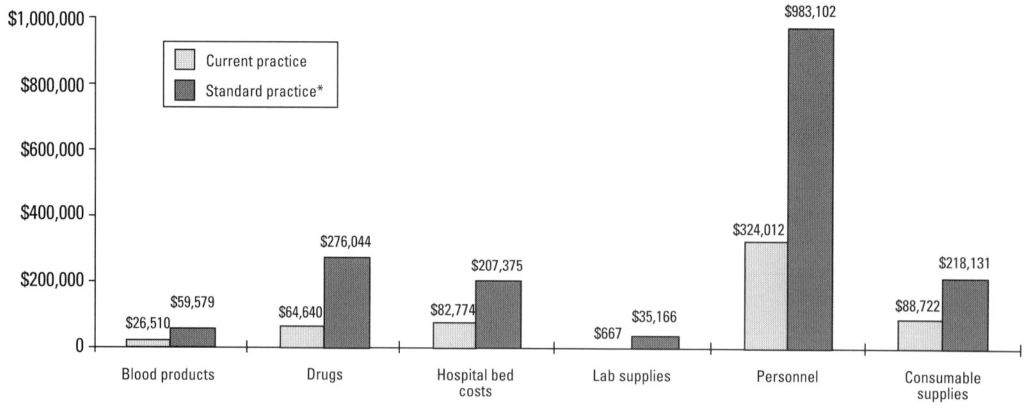

** Standard = based on the Mother-Baby Package*

average woman receives a total of 10 minutes of antenatal care over the course of her pregnancy. Under the new standard she is expected to be seen by a nurse or midwife four times, with each visit lasting at least 20 minutes. Deliveries will be attended by better qualified, and thus more expensive, staff.

The largest percentage increase is projected in laboratory supplies (US$700 to US$35,000 a year, due mainly to the introduction of routine lab tests in antenatal care) and in drug costs (US$65,000 to US$275,000).

Figure 8. Incremental Treatment Cost by Input

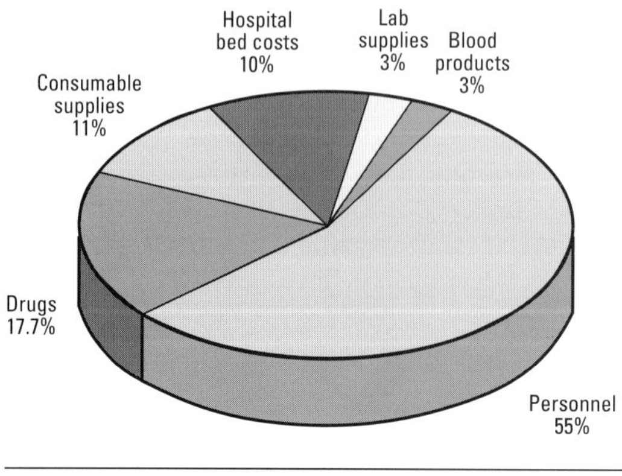

Capital costs

The increase in medical treatment costs constitutes only a fraction of the total cost of a Safe Motherhood programme. Substantial investments will be required in the country's physical and human infrastructure. Existing facilities have to be renovated and equipped. New facilities might have to be built, equipped and staffed. Service providers at all levels have to be trained to provide care according to the new treatment guidelines. Numerous other measures, including the strengthening of supervision, referral, monitoring and evaluation systems, will have to be taken to ensure quality and accessibility of care. Because the Ministry of Health had already prepared a comprehensive budget covering the capital costs associated with the upgrading of infrastructure; for the costing study new estimates of capital cost requirements were not made; the analysis relied on the existing budget. Figure 9 shows the distribution of total capital costs.

Almost half of the total capital cost of US$45 million is to be spent on the renovation and upgrading of Uganda's ageing health facilities. Another 22 per cent is to be spent to improve the referral system (setting up a communication system between facilities and purchasing ambulances and other forms of emergency transport). Clean delivery kits for traditional birth attendants and the basic obstetric and

Figure 9. Capital Cost Components

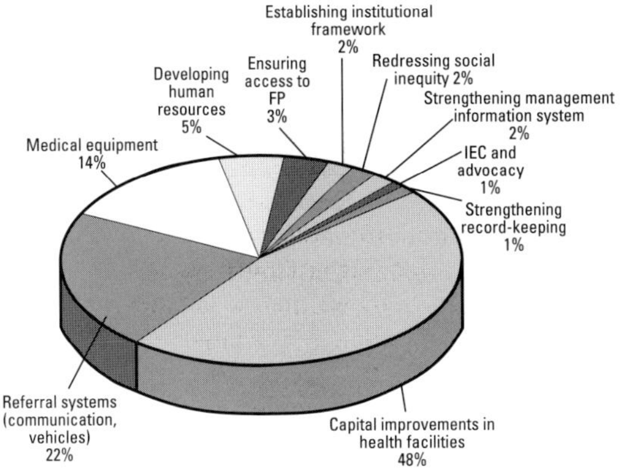

surgical equipment necessary to provide maternity care according to the Mother-Baby Package standards, will account for another 15 per cent of total capital expenditure. While expenditure for the development of human resources accounted for only five per cent of capital costs planned for 1999-2001, it is recognised that this figure will need to rise in the coming years in order to meet the need for more skilled attendants at birth.

Table 2. Annual Treatment Cost

	Total cost per District	Cost per capita
Current treatment practice	$600,000	$0.50
Treatment according to Mother-Baby Package guidelines and standards	$1,800,000	$1.40
Difference/incremental cost	$1,200,000	$0.90

Table 3. Total Annual Costs, including Capital Costs

	Total cost per District	Cost per capita
Treatment cost	$1,800,000	$1.40
Capital costs (annualised over 5 years)	$450,000	$0.40
Total annual costs	$2,250,000	$1.80

Conclusion

The summary cost findings are displayed in Tables 2 and 3. It was found that the Ugandan government presently spends about US$0.50 per capita on maternal and newborn health care. To upgrade this care to conform with the standards and guidelines set forth in the Mother-Baby Package would cost approximately US$1.40 per capita, representing an incremental cost of US$0.90. The inclusion of capital and overhead costs would raise the cost to approximately US$1.80 per capita, bringing the incremental cost up to US$1.30.

The spreadsheet proved very useful to national authorities, donor governments and other partners at the national level in considering and addressing the substantial cost implications of providing higher-quality maternal and newborn care. For example, the results proved invaluable in discussions in the planning group of the Ministry of Health, in advocating for an increased budget allocation for safe motherhood interventions. In addition, in the context of the development of a new national budget, the estimates were used to validate, and in some cases increase the budget allocations for certain lines relating to maternal health. Finally, when the decentralised district-level budgets are developed, the estimates will be used again to advocate an increased allocation for maternal health. In summary, the results of the spreadsheet have proved invaluable in Uganda in facilitating an important dialogue on maternal and newborn health care financing and sustainability issues.

Acknowledgements

This study was funded by the UK Department for International Development and the World Health Organization.

Correspondence

Craig Lissner, Department of Reproductive Health and Research, World Health Organization, 1211 Geneva, Switzerland. Fax: 41-22-791-4189. E-mail: lissnerc@who.ch

References and Notes

1. World Health Organization, 1996. *Mother-Baby Package: Implementing Safe Motherhood in Countries*. World Health Organization, Geneva. WHO/FHE/MSM/96.11.
2. Janowitz B, Bratt JH, 1992. Costs of family planning services: a critique of the literature. *International Family Planning Perspectives*. 18:137.
3. World Bank, 1993. *World Development Report: Investing in Health*. World Bank, Washington, DC.
4. Tinker A, Koblinsky M (eds), 1993. *Making Motherhood Safe*. World Bank Discussion Paper No. 202, World Bank, Washington, DC.
5. Lissner C, Weissman E, 1998. How much does Safe Motherhood cost? *World Health*. 51(1):10-11.
6. Mumford EA, Dayaratna V, Winfrey W et al, 1998. *Reproductive Health Cost: Literature Review*. Working Paper Series No. 3. Futures Group International, Washington DC, July.
7. Tinker A, Koblinsky M, Daly P, 1994. Programming for Safe Motherhood: a guide to action. *Health Policy and Planning*; 9(3):252-66.
8. World Health Organization, Maternal and Neonatal Health/Safe Motherhood Unit,1996. Revised 1990 estimates of maternal mortality: a new approach by WHO and UNICEF. WHO/UNICEF, April. WHO/FRH/MSM/96.11 and UNICEF/PLN/96.1.
9. Uganda Ministry of Health, 1997. *Uganda Safe Motherhood Strategic Plan (1997-1999)*. Uganda Ministry of Health, Kampala.
10. Uganda Ministry of Health, 1997. *Maternal Child Health and Family Planning 5-Year Strategic Plan (1997-2001)*. Uganda Ministry of Health, Kampala.
11. World Health Organization, 1999. *Mother-Baby Package Costing Spreadsheet User Guide*. WHO, Geneva. WHO/RHR/99.17. (In press)
12. Uganda Ministry of Health, 1995. *Uganda Family Health Manual*. Uganda Ministry of Health, Kampala.
13. Uganda Ministry of Health, 1993. *National Treatment Guidelines*. Uganda Ministry of Health, Kampala.
14. Uganda Ministry of Health, 1995. *Uganda Demographic and Health Survey*. Uganda Ministry of Health, Kampala.
15. UNICEF, 1997. Essential Drugs Price List. UNICEF Supply Division, Copenhagen, January 1997.
16. A more detailed analysis, prepared for planners at the national and district level, is available from the authors. Weissman E, Sentumbwe O, Mbonye AK et al, 1999. *Uganda Safe Motherhood Programme – Costing Study*. World Health Organization, Kampala/Geneva. WHO/RHR/99.9.
17. All graphs in this paper depict results for the Iganga district.
18. Total treatment cost combined the cost data from the health centre and the hospital level, weighting the respective average treatment costs by the number of women treated at those levels.

The Impact of Free Maternal Health Care in South Africa

Helen Schneider, Lucy Gilson

In a global context of a return to user fees for health services, one of the first policies announced by the new South African government in 1994 was free maternal and child health (MCH) care, part of a series of social policies aimed at reducing inequalities in health status and access to health care. Most pregnant women in South Africa receive some form of antenatal care during pregnancy, but a significant proportion deliver without the assistance of a health professional, and access to safe abortion and emergency referral are still low for many women. The impact of free MCH has been to increase utilisation of existing antenatal and paediatric services, but does not appear to have influenced the numbers of deliveries within facilities. Furthermore, strong reactions against these policies have come from front-line providers, e.g. beliefs that the new policies are encouraging women to become pregnant and that pregnant women do not deserve free care. Although definitive conclusions will only be possible in the longer term, early evidence suggests that free maternal health care, on its own, is not a sufficient condition for reducing the large burden of avoidable maternal and perinatal mortality in the country. However, free care should be seen as one of several measures which may help to increase access to and quality of maternal care services . In addition, it has signalled that the state is sensitive to the needs of the poor and disadvantaged, contributing to a sense of entitlement to services, which may have longer-term, beneficial effects.

SOUTH Africa is an upper middle-income country[1] with a population of 40 million people, 55 per cent of whom live in urban areas.[2] Years of apartheid governance have made South Africa one of the most unequal societies in the world – the poorest 40 per cent of households account for only 11 per cent of total income, while the richest 10 per cent of households account for 40 per cent of total income.[3] Income inequalities in South Africa are primarily determined by race (reflecting a long history of intense racial discrimination), but also by gender and rural location. Thus 95 per cent and 75 per cent of people falling below the poverty line are African[4] and live in rural areas, respectively.[5] Female-headed households have a poverty rate of 60 per cent compared to 30 per cent for male-headed households.[3]

The new post-apartheid government, elected in 1994, has committed itself to reducing these and other inequities inherited from the past. This is reflected in several social policies, including those within the health sector. In a global context of a return to user fees (i.e. payment by users for health care received), one of the first policies announced by the new South African government was free maternal and child health (MCH) care, which was later extended to all public sector, primary health care services.

This article reviews the South African experience of free maternal health care and its possible impact on maternal health. After summarising the status of maternal health and health care in South Africa, it describes the user fee systems in operation prior to 1994, and the content and process of policies adopted post-1994. The evidence on the impact of free care on utilisation of maternal care services is then presented. The research conducted to date has assessed the early impacts of free care and measured output (utilisation) rather than outcome (mortality and morbidity) variables. The conclusions should be seen in the light of these limitations.

The introduction of user fees for health care services in many countries has had as its primary objective to raise revenue and therefore increase the financial sustainability of health services.[6] Subsidiary benefits are seen to include a gain in efficiency by discouraging inappropriate or 'frivolous' utilisation of services, and local use of revenue to make improvements in aspects of quality such as drug supplies. While there is as yet little international evidence regarding the effects of user fee systems on financial sustainability, quality and efficiency,[6] potential losses in these areas caused by the removal of user fees in South Africa are also examined.

Maternal health and health care in South Africa

Estimates of maternal mortality in South Africa vary between 156 and 250 deaths per 100,000 births for African women as compared to 3-8 deaths per 100,000 births for white women.[7,8] This signifies a large burden of excess and avoidable mortality within the country. The four main causes of maternal mortality are hypertension, non-pregnancy-related infections (mainly AIDS), obstetric haemorrhage, and early pregnancy losses (mainly septic abortions).[9] There are no national estimates of perinatal mortality, although a few local studies have measured perinatal mortality rates within health services of between 43 and 58 per 1000 live births.[10]

Most pregnant women in South Africa receive some form of antenatal care during pregnancy. White women, however, are far more likely to undertake their first visit early in pregnancy, be seen by a medical practitioner and receive care in the private sector than African women (Table 1).[11] More important, however, is the significant proportion of women who deliver without the assistance of a health professional. In a 1994 household survey, 22 per cent of African women had delivered their last infant at home, a factor which was strongly associated with educational status and geographical location.[11] Fifty-eight per cent and 43 per cent of women who had received no formal education and worked on farms, respectively, delivered their last infant without the support of the health service.

Although a basic infrastructure for maternal care exists in South Africa, there are still many gaps in the quality of care provided. For example, in a national cross-sectional study of 160 clinics in 1997, just over 80 per cent reported providing syphilis testing to pregnant women, but less than 50 per cent of rural clinics had consistently working telephones and only 41 per cent had an ambulance at their doorstep within an hour of an emergency call.[12] Many primary health care services also lack basic supplies and equipment to test urine, measure haemoglobin, or give oxytocics after delivery, all of which are essential for detecting and managing obstetric complications.[7,13]

Table 1: Utilisation of antenatal health services by African and white women[11]*

Indicator	Per cent utilisation for each category: African	White
At least one antenatal visit in last pregnancy	90.2	80.6
Booking visit in first trimester	30.3	88.7
Booking visit in last trimester	11.6	0.8
Use of public sector clinic (nurse-based) for antenatal care	69.3	6.3
Use of private sector (doctor-based) for antenatal care	6.9	77.4

** Data from a national survey of 4000 households of women aged 16-64 years who were asked about their last pregnancy.*

Hostile and judgmental attitudes of front-line providers frequently emerge as a complaint in surveys of community opinion.[7,10,13,14] In in-depth interviews with women attending maternal health services in a peri-urban area of the Western Cape, Jewkes et al[15] uncovered experiences of frankly brutal behaviour towards patients on the part of providers which included 'verbal abuse, beatings, arbitrary acts of unkindness and neglect'.[15] Professional training under a conservative, apartheid regime has socialised many providers into perceiving certain categories of patients (e.g. poor pregnant women, people with STDs) as morally defective,[15,16] and utilisation of services by these patients may even be experienced by providers as a kind of persecution.[16]

In summary, there are vast differentials in maternal health status and in access to and quality of maternal health care within South African society. Access to supervised delivery, safe abortion (despite legalisation in 1996), and emergency referral is still low for many women and together these factors probably account for the bulk of the differentials in maternal mortality within the country. The attitudes of health personnel create additional barriers and increase the marginalisation of certain groups of women, in particular those living in poor rural and peri-urban areas.

Fees collected were remitted to the central level and so facilities had little incentive to enforce payment or refuse care to those who could not pay. This does not necessarily imply that cost of health care was not a barrier in the past. In 1995, Africans in the lowest income quintile made a mean of 1.34 visits to the health service,[19] well below the target of 3-4 visits per annum to primary level services suggested by national and international norms.[14,20] In a 1994 household survey, the cost of health care was the most frequently cited reason for foregoing care among those who had recently experienced an episode of ill health.[11]

The provision of free MCH for pregnant women and children features unambiguously in the earliest policy statements of the African

User fees policies before and after 1994

The health system inherited by the new government in 1994 was characterised by a well-resourced private sector, serving 20-30 per cent of the population, and a fragmented and racially divided public sector for the remaining majority.

Payment for health care in the private sector was mostly (and still is) on a fee-for-service basis, supported by various forms of private health insurance. Prior to 1994, user fees generated the equivalent of 4.5 per cent of public sector recurrent expenditure,[17] collected through a variety of fee structures and recovery systems. In general, however, women receiving maternal care services in the public sector would have paid a relatively low, all-inclusive fee, either as a single, lump sum payment or per day of attendance.[18] In-patient hospital fees tended to vary according to a sliding scale of income, but otherwise operated on the same basis as outpatient fees.

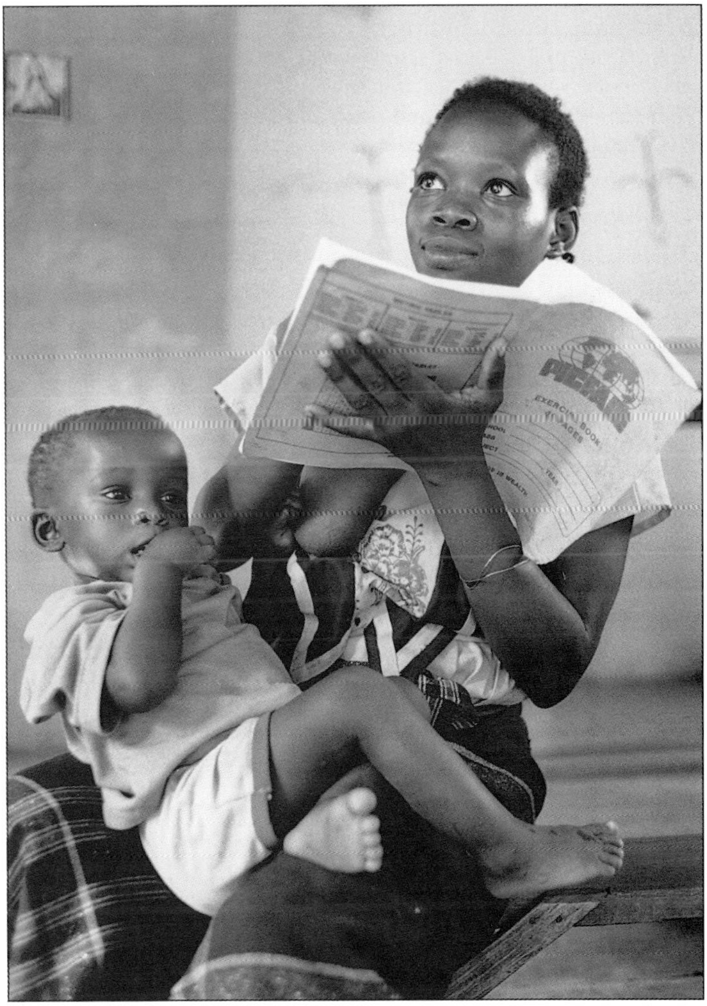

JENNY MATTHEWS

National Congress, prior to its election to the new government in April 1994,[21] and was one of the policies announced by President Mandela in his first State of the Nation speech in May 1994. Included in the free MCH policy were all public services (hospital and primary health care) to pregnant women, from point of confirmation of pregnancy until 42 days after delivery, and children under the age of six years. In April 1996, free care was extended to all public sector PHC services. In parallel to the free care policy, a law was passed in 1996 giving women the right to abortion on request within the first three months of pregnancy.

Removal of user fees is one of several policies supporting the development of accessible, good quality and efficient primary health care. These include the establishment of decentralised district authorities, the building and renovation of clinics, and an essential drugs list. However, the effects of these policies will only be felt in the medium term, and the existing facility and staff infrastructure have thus absorbed the impact of free care.

Impact of free health care on maternal health services

A national evaluation of the free MCH policy was conducted in 1995 by an independent agency.[10] This included assessments of health care utilisation prior to and following free MCH, the financial costs of the policy, and provider and user opinions. Conclusions on the impact of free MCH draw heavily on the findings of this evaluation. An assessment of the medium-term impact of free MCH or of the 1996 policy, which extended free care to all PHC services, has yet to be done. However, some insights are provided in data from two areas in the country: a large network of community health centres in Soweto, Johannesburg, and Hlabisa District in rural KwaZulu-Natal.[22,23]

Utilisation

The national evaluation[10] assessed utilisation of antenatal care in a cross-section of facilities in 13 sites across the country. These sites were purposefully selected to reflect the range of urban, peri-urban and rural settlements, as well

Figure 1: Total antenatal visits before and after free MCH[10]

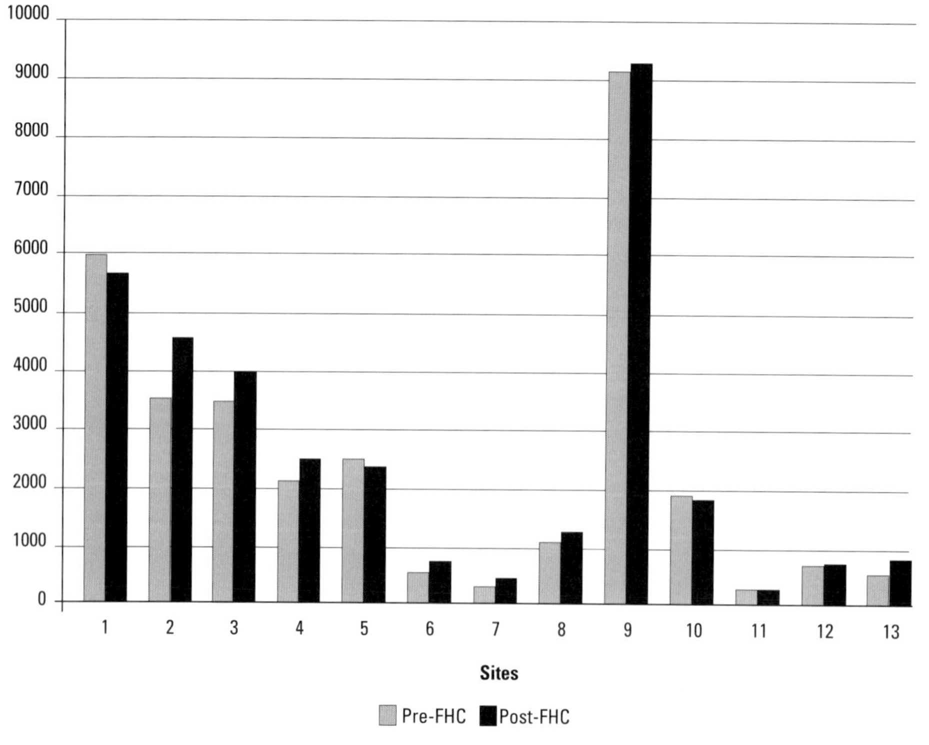

Figure 2: Proportions of deliveries that were 'booked' before and after free MCH in 12 facilities[10]

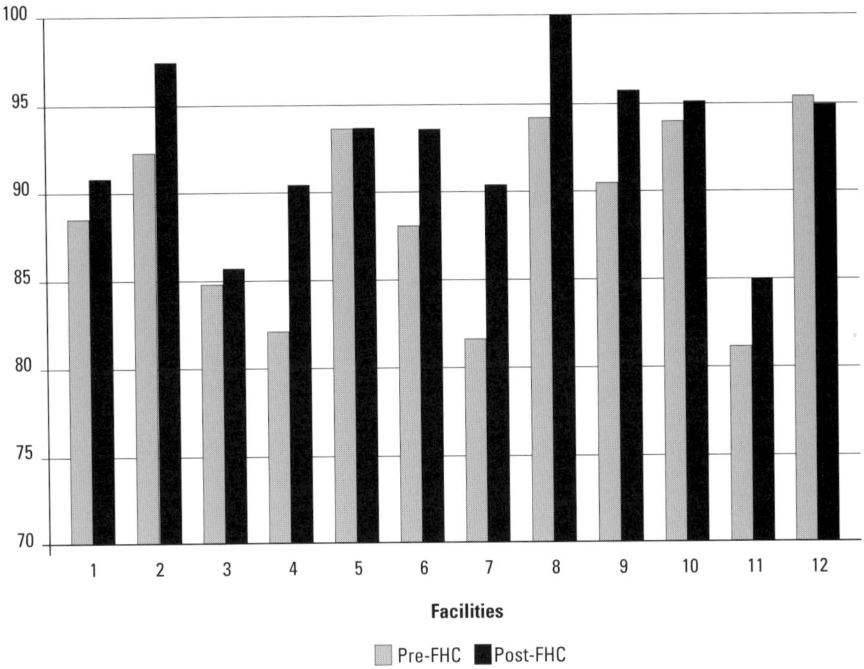

as different levels of care. Total visits over twelve months before (pre-FHC) and after (post-FHC) the introduction of free MCH were compared.

Antenatal attendance increased in 8 of the 13 sites and by a mean across all sites of 14.9 per cent (Figure 1).

Data from birth registers were available in 12 facilities across the sites. In 11 of these 12 facilities, there was an increase in the proportion of deliveries, which were registered as 'booked', i.e. preceded by an antenatal visit (Figure 2). The mean increase in booked deliveries across all 12 facilities was 4.6 per cent. This suggests that women who previously had not accessed antenatal care were now being reached. This is supported by a parallel finding, in the same evaluation, of an increase in the numbers of 'first' visits in antenatal clinics.

The national evaluation has only fragmented information on the numbers of deliveries performed within health facilities. Overall, however, it appears that these did not change. In the rural areas of one province, KwaZulu-Natal, deliveries in the post-FHC period actually declined by 3.9 per cent, and in urban Gauteng, increased marginally by 1.5 per cent.[10]

Have increases in utilisation of antenatal services been sustained? A study of utilisation in a large network of health centres in Soweto, Johannesburg for the 32 months following the onset of free MCH, showed early increases in antenatal attendance followed by a decline to levels lower than pre-FHC (Table 2, Figure 3).[22] This suggests that early gains have not been maintained. However, findings from this relatively privileged urban community cannot be generalised to other parts of the country.

Table 2: Antenatal visits to health centres in metropolitan Gauteng[22]

	Antenatal visits	Per cent change from baseline
Baseline: Nov 1993-May 1994	53,788	–
Nov 1994-May 1995	55,881	+ 3.8 per cent
Nov 1995-May 1996	48,117	–10.5 per cent

Figure 3: Utilisation of antenatal services in the Soweto Community Health Centres, November 1993-January 1997[22]

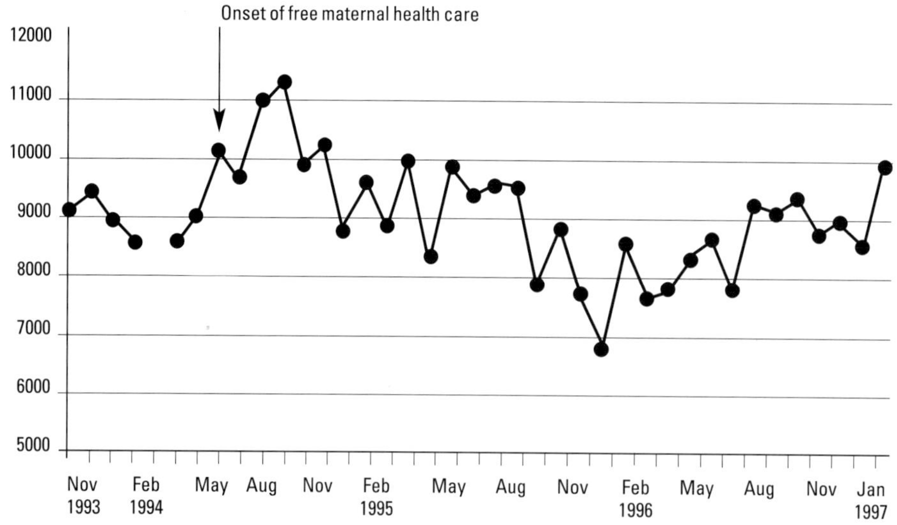

Concern has been raised that incorporating curative services into free care policies (such as for children under six in the 1994 policy and, in particular, following the 1996 free PHC policy) is promoting utilisation that will 'crowd out' preventive services. In the Hlabisa District in the KwaZulu-Natal Province, attendance for curative care at a network of mobile service points between 1994 and 1998 increased by 93 per cent while attendance for antenatal care decreased by 20 per cent.[23] Large increases in utilisation, predominantly for curative services, were also found in the Soweto Community Health Centres following on the announcement of free PHC in 1996. Total attendance was 48.5 per cent higher in the 10 months following the introduction of free PHC, compared to the equivalent 10-month period in the previous year.[22]

One of the more striking aspects of the national evaluation of free MCH[10] was the finding of increased attendance in the paediatric outpatient services of the large, central hospitals. Making both primary *and* hospital care free may have thus stimulated an inefficient use of higher levels of care. One hospital dealt with this by introducing screening procedures and referring patients to primary health care facilities where appropriate.

In summary, the impact of free MCH has been to increase utilisation of existing antenatal services, possibly reaching women who previously would not have attended such services. However, the policy does not appear to have influenced the numbers of deliveries within facilities, and it is unclear to what extent the achievements have been sustained over time.

The greatest impact of free care policies in South Africa appears to have been on the use of curative services. Given the relatively low levels of health service utilisation found in household surveys prior to free care policies, the increases in curative care visits do not necessarily correspond to inappropriate or frivolous use and may reflect a high level of previously unmet need. However, patterns of utilisation in health care services following on free care policies do raise questions about the design of fee systems in ensuring that certain services are protected, in particular, ensuring an appropriate balance between curative and preventive services, and between primary and secondary levels of care.

Financial impact

The financial impact of the free MCH policy was assessed as part of the national evaluation.[10]

Revenue from user fees declined by 27 per cent after free MCH, amounting to 1.5 per cent of the public health care budget. In absolute terms the biggest losses in revenue were in community and regional hospitals. It is possible, however, that these losses were caused by a trend in the reduction of 'private' fee-paying patients in public hospitals, occurring simultaneous to free care policies, rather than to the free care itself. The evaluation estimated that free MCH increased drug costs by 1 per cent of recurrent health sector expenditure. The largest item of expenditure, staff costs, remained constant. The financial costs of free MCH therefore amounted to 2.5 per cent of recurrent public sector expenditure. It is important to note that as revenue is not retained within facilities, these losses were not felt directly at the point of provision.

Relationships between users and providers

In surveys of community opinion, knowledge of and support for free MCH services have been high.[10,11] In certain parts of the country, increased utilisation has been documented in services which historically had always been free,[24] and it appears that the high profile announcements of free care have fostered a general sense of entitlement in relation to public health care services.

However, strong reactions against both the content and the manner of implementation of free care policies have come from front-line providers. The national evaluation[10] and surveys of providers[22,24] have documented the presence of powerful beliefs amongst primary health care workers, namely that:

- free care leads to 'abuse' of services and has removed any constraints to utilisation of services;
- the combination of abortion-on-demand and free care is encouraging women to become pregnant;
- patients attend services to collect free drugs and then resell them to others; and
- foreigners will come to South Africa to use free services.

'Patients in this place are abusing the free health care service...and we don't have control over it. A patient will come on Monday with a headache, on Wednesday with a stomach-ache and on Friday will remember an old sprain he got when he was young and come complaining of knee pain. We have to provide them with a service, we can't chase them...how do we control this?'
(Interview with a professional nurse, Northern Cape, August 1996.)[24]

As part of a broader assessment of the impact of free PHC in Soweto[22] a self-administered questionnaire was distributed to 167 nurses (the main front-line providers in South Africa), to assess their attitudes to and experiences of free PHC. Of the 90 (54 per cent) who responded, only 17 per cent felt that free primary health care should apply to everybody. Pregnant women featured low in the list of groups deserving free care (Table 3).

Nearly three quarters (71 per cent) of respondents first heard about the extension of free PHC in 1996 through the media, 17 per cent were informed by their supervisors and managers and 8 per cent heard about it from colleagues. For one-fifth (21 per cent), their first encounter with the policy occurred at the time of its introduction at their clinic, when increased numbers of patients attended for care.

Both the 1994 and 1996 policies were announced at national level with little prior consultation or preparation of the most decentralised levels of the health system. This has led to the perception that free PHC is being achieved at the expense of service providers (by increasing utilisation), and the policy has therefore had little support from those most directly involved in its implementation. Front-line providers have also developed problematic explanations for the changes occurring around them, which do not necessarily correspond to facts

Table 3: Views of Soweto nurses as to who should benefit from free PHC[22] (n = 90)

Category that should benefit	Percentage of nurses who agreed
Everybody	17
Aged	66
Disabled	53
Children under six years	46
People with chronic diseases	43
Poor and unemployed	37
Pregnant women	11
Nobody	1

of utilisation, and which may reinforce existing prejudices against poor communities, foreigners and pregnant women.

Conclusions

Free care has been one of the most visible policies of the new government in South Africa and is frequently listed amongst its key achievements. It has served as a powerful signal that the state is sensitive to the needs of the poor and disadvantaged, and the policy has had enormous symbolic and political significance. The impact of free care on maternal health and on health care have to be seen within this broader set of objectives.

The available evidence, although incomplete and not fully representative, suggests that gains in maternal health care from removing user fees in South Africa have been relatively modest. They are confined to increases in antenatal attendance, in a context where some degree of utilisation of antenatal care services was already high. Without a concomitant increase in deliveries within health facilities and an improvement in the quality of services, the rise in antenatal visits is unlikely to impact significantly on avoidable maternal and perinatal mortality in the country.

Other measures of equal importance include:

- an expansion in the infrastructure of 24 hour services (to increase access to safe deliveries),
- an increase in the numbers of facilities able and willing to perform abortions,
- improvements in inputs to primary care facilities (drug supplies etc),
- the presence of functioning referral and emergency care networks,
- training in and protocols for obstetric risk management,
- programmes to address the attitudes of providers towards clients, and
- establishing a more women-friendly health care environment.

These measures imply building the capacity of the health care system generally and can therefore only occur over the medium term.

While the policy of free MCH appears to have involved little financial risk on the part of the state, lack of participation by front-line providers in the decision-making process may have reinforced attitudinal barriers to access and utilisation. The experience in South Africa has highlighted the direct and immediate impact of user fee policies on service providers and the need to develop implementation strategies that take this into account. The particular design of user fee policies (preventive vs. curative care, primary vs. secondary level care) has implications for patterns of utilisation, and should also be carefully considered when introducing new policies. Finally, the impact of user fee policies on utilisation needs to be assessed over time, as short-term changes may not be sustained over longer periods of time.

Correspondence

Helen Schneider, Centre for Health Policy, University of Witwatersrand, PO Box 1038, Johannesburg 2000, South Africa. Fax: 27-11-489-9900. E-mail: helens@iafrica.com

References and Notes

1. The per-capita GNP is US$ 3000. World Bank, 1997. *World Development Report 1997*. New York: Oxford University Press.
2. Republic of South Africa, 1997. *Census in Brief: Statistics SA*. Pretoria: Government Printers.
3. May J, 1998. *Poverty and Inequality in South Africa*. Centre for Social and Development Studies, University of Natal.
4. South Africa's population was previously categorised into African, Coloured, Indian and White, and corresponds to a historical gradient of access to wealth and power. In this article, data on 'whites' (14 per cent of the population) are compared with that of 'Africans' (75 per cent of the population) in order to demonstrate the degrees of inequity present in the society. This does not in any way imply endorsement of racist terms or their unsubstantiated use in health research.
5. Reconstruction and Development Programme, 1995. *Key Indicators of Poverty in South Africa*. Pretoria: Reconstruction and Development Programme Office.
6. Gilson L, 1997. Review paper: The lessons of user fee experience in Africa. *Health Policy and Planning*; 12(4):273-85.
7. Fonn S, Xaba M, Tint K et al, 1998. Reproductive health

services in South Africa: from rhetoric to implementation. *Reproductive Health Matters*. 6(11):22-32.
8. Health Systems Trust. *South African Health Review*, 1997. Durban, South Africa: Health Systems Trust/ Henry J Kaiser Family Foundation.
9. Moodley J, Pattinson B, 1998. *First Interim Report on Confidential Enquiries into Maternal Deaths in South Africa*. HST Update, number 38, November 1998.
10. Child Health Unit, University of Cape Town, 1996. *Free Health Care for Pregnant Women and Children Under Six in South Africa*. Durban: Health Systems Trust.
11. Community Agency for Social Enquiry, 1995. *A National Household Survey of Health Inequalities in South Africa*. Washington, California: Henry J. Kaiser Family Foundation.
12. Health System Trust, 1997. Measuring the move towards equity from the site of delivery. In: *South Africa Health Review 1997*. Durban: Health Systems Trust.
13. Fonn S, Xaba M, Tint K et al, 1998. Maternal health services in South Africa. (Special article during the 10th anniversary of the WHO 'Safe Motherhood' initiative). *South African Medical Journal*; 88(6):697-702.
14. Rispel L, Price M, Cabral J, 1996. *Confronting Need and Affordability: Guidelines for Primary Health Care Services in South Africa*. Johannesburg: Centre for Health Policy, University of Witwatersrand.
15. Jewkes R, Mvo Z, 1997. *Study of Health-care Seeking Practices of Pregnant Women in Cape Town. Report Two: Women's Perceptions of Kayelitsha Midwife Obstetric Unit*. Pretoria: CERSA-Women's Health, Medical Research Council.
16. Oskowitz B, Schneider H, Hlatshwayo Z, 1997. *Taking Care of Quality: Perspectives of the Patients and Providers at an STD Clinic*. Technical Report. Johannesburg: Centre for Health Policy, University of Witwatersrand.
17. McIntyre D, Bloom G, Doherty J et al, 1995. *Health Expenditure and Finance in South Africa*. Durban: Health Systems Trust; Washington DC: World Bank.
18. For example, several administrations charged R8,00 (US $1.50) per outpatient visit in 1994, and the poorest patients paid R26 (US$4.40) per admission for inpatient care, with the remainder of the authorities charging rates lower than this. From reference [17].
19. Gilson L, McIntyre D, 1998. Understanding and monitoring health and health care inequity: lessons from South Africa. Case Study for the Global Health Equity Initiative. Johannesburg: Centre for Health Policy. (Unpublished draft)
20. Gish O, 1990. Some links between successful implementation of primary health care interventions and the overall utilisation of health services. *Social Science and Medicine* 30(4):401-05.
21. African National Congress, 1994. *The Reconstruction and Development Programme*. Johannesburg: Umanyano Publications.
22. Schneider H, Kaka Z, Jina S et al, 1997. *A Survey to Assess the Impact of Free Primary Health Care on the Soweto Community Health Centres*. Technical Report. Johannesburg: Centre for Health Policy, University of Witwatersrand.
23. Wilkinson D, Gouws E, Sach M et al, 1998. Does removing user fees encourage attendance for curative services at the expense of preventive services? Paper presented at the 16th Epidemiological Society of Southern Africa Conference, Volkswagen Conference Centre, Midrand, 25-28th October 1998.
24. Schneider H, Magongo B, Cabral J et al, 1998. *Bridging the Quality Gap: Working with Front-line Providers to Improve the Quality of Primary Health in the North-West Province*. Monograph. Johannesburg: Centre for Health Policy, University of Witwatersrand.

A Question of Survival:

I. A Review of Safe Motherhood in Kenya

Wendy J Graham, Susan F Murray

II. Two Years After the Review: Accomplishments, Hurdles and Next Steps

Clare Taylor

Kenya was the birthplace of the Safe Motherhood Initiative and the Call to Action in 1987.[1] It was therefore fitting that Kenya take stock of its own situation ten years on, to identify ways to move forward, given the broader context of current health sector reform and the National Reproductive Health Strategy, which have important implications for the provision of maternity care.[2,3] The emerging picture from multiple data sources reveals a high burden of unsafe motherhood in Kenya, with wide regional differentials. The distribution of causes of direct obstetric deaths is typical, while deaths related to malaria, anaemia, TB and AIDS may be more significant than that reported elsewhere. While 95 per cent of women report at least one antenatal clinic visit, little is known about the quality of this care and its capacity to prevent or treat complications. Conversely, only 45 per cent of women are attended by health professionals at delivery. Life-saving, emergency obstetric procedures are not widely available because human resources are not allocated rationally and the most widely accessible cadre of staff are not trained or permitted to undertake them. Since 1997, comprehensive needs assessment exercises have been carried out in several districts by teams from the Ministry of Health (MOH), non-governmental and donor agencies. A more concentrated, strategic effort is required to prioritise interventions that make a difference, and incrementally and systematically apply them. Many of the obstacles to adequate maternity services are associated with the health system as a whole. In the absence of progress towards health sector reform, support to safe motherhood will be through projects, at least for the time being. In the longer term, government and donors need to be convinced that safe motherhood is a worthwhile investment in Kenya.

I. A Review of Safe Motherhood in Kenya

What is encompassed by the term 'Safe Motherhood' has evolved considerably since 1987. Whilst the focus on maternal mortality has remained, three other outcomes have now been incorporated: maternal morbidity, health of the newborn, and positive health of the mother. As the meaning of safe motherhood broadened, particularly in the early 1990s, so did the range of factors regarded as determinants of poor maternal health, with women's low socio-economic status seen as one of the root causes.

This had three unfortunate effects on the views of policy-makers and planners worldwide:[4] First, safe motherhood was seen as an all-purpose initiative which included any action to improve women's health in the long or short-term. Second, safe motherhood was seen as nothing new, since it included programme activities which had been underway for many years, specifically as Maternal & Child Health/Family Planning (MCH-FP). Third, safe motherhood had goals which were laudable but too vast and daunting to be tackled in resource-constrained settings.

The repercussions of these beliefs – the failure to prioritise maternal health and so commit resources – are now being realised. Almost ten years after the Call to Action, there is still a lack of reliable evidence that maternal mortality or morbidity has declined. However, in this post-Cairo era, the safe motherhood component has returned to its original focus – comprising, primarily, interventions to prevent maternal mortality and life-threatening morbidity. This is the remit adopted in the following review – a remit which is consistent with the Kenyan National Reproductive Health Strategy (NRHS).[3]

The objectives of this review were to:

- describe the levels, trends and differentials in maternal mortality and morbidity in Kenya;
- identify the programme activities in Kenya which have the potential to reduce the burden of unsafe motherhood as well as the barriers to achieving this potential;
- flag the major information gaps on maternal mortality and morbidity in Kenya.

The economic and demographic context

About 17 per cent of Kenya's total land area is suitable for agriculture, which provides the primary livelihood for about 80 per cent of the population.[5] The highest population densities are found in the major urban areas, which contain about 20 per cent of the population.

Since independence in 1963, Kenya's economy has gone through four major phases, with low or negative GDP growth essentially since 1986 – the year when structural adjustment programmes were introduced in various sectors.[5] The economy has been in a particularly difficult phase since the early 1990s, when real GDP continued to fall, inflation rose to unprecedented levels, and there was a decline in real wages and an increase in poverty.[6] Although the indicators for 1994 were suggestive of economic recovery, it was too early to detect any impact on the health and wealth of the general population in 1996-1997. However, the poor overall performance of the economy over many years has clearly affected health status through declining and inadequate expenditure on the health sector as well as increasing poverty, falling living standards, and worsening nutritional status.

Kenya stands out in sub-Saharan Africa with regard to the dramatic decline in the total fertility rate over the past 15 years, from 8.1 in 1975/1977 to 5.4 in 1990/1992[7,8] – with increasing life expectancy, decreasing infant mortality and a slowing down in the rate of population growth (Table 1). These indicators do, however, show marked differences within the country. Although crude death rates have fallen consistently over the last 20 years, uncertainty over the demographic impact of AIDS and over the rate of fertility decline complicates projections for the 21st century.

Table 1: Demographic and economic indicators, Kenya

Population (1995)	27.5 million
Crude birth rate (1995)	42.8/1000
Crude death rate (1995)	11.8/1000
Infant mortality rate (1995)	67/1000
Population growth rate (1995)	3%
Percentage population urban (1994)	16%
Literacy rate (1989)	69%
Real GDP growth (1993)	0.1%
Per capita GOK spending on health (1994)	US$4.50

Data sources on maternal mortality and morbidity in Kenya

The Government of Kenya (GOK) has long-recognised the inadequacy of the routine information system as regards most health outcomes.[2] The completeness of the civil registration system, which involves the official notification of births, deaths and marriages, is largely unknown but suspected to be poor, even in urban areas. Several initiatives have been launched over the years to improve registration, including sentinel surveillance.[9] One recent study of maternal mortality[10] relied upon civil registration data at three district registries, and found that this compared favourably with the completeness of reporting by district hospitals.

As for many other sub-Saharan African countries it is the health services and, in particular, hospitals which have tended to provide most of the information in Kenya on maternal mortality and morbidity until recently. Of the two main approaches used to generate data for the general population, Kenya has experience of both surveys[11] and continuous surveillance,[12] as well as surveys conducted on a local scale, using more intensive methods of data collection.[13]

Levels and trends in maternal mortality

The three main sources used in this review for data on maternal mortality are set out in Table 2. The usefulness of many other studies conducted in Kenya for this overview was limited by the small number of maternal deaths included, though several do provide valuable insights into the factors associated with safe motherhood in Kenya.

At the national level, the official GOK figure for the maternal mortality ratio (MMR) is 365 maternal deaths per 100,000 live births,[3] which was derived from the 1994 national survey[11] for the period 1990-1994. The national average for Kenya obscures the huge differences in levels between provinces and districts. For the three rural districts studied by Makokha et al,[10] the overall MMR was 271, ranging from 219 for Kakamega, 283 for Kirinyaga, to 340 for Kilifi. These figures are not population-based, and will be under-estimates of the level of maternal mortality in the general population. In fact, the figure for Kenya produced by WHO and UNICEF[15] for 1990, using an estimation process, was 670, which is obviously considerably higher.

The UNICEF-funded 1994 national survey[11] was population-based and used the direct and indirect Sisterhood methods[16,17] to give estimates for ten core districts. Wide confidence intervals need to be placed on these estimates owing to the sample sizes. The clear presence of sampling errors is seen in the implausible differences in the MMR – from a high of 2,220 maternal deaths per 100,000 live births for Kwale District to just 19 for Nyeri District; the latter figure based on just one maternal death. By grouping together those districts in the same province, more stable estimates could be produced. Kenya, therefore, still lacks a current and reliable picture of regional differentials in maternal mortality.

Given these difficulties, Kenya has opted to use indicators associated with maternal mortality to gain some idea of regional patterns.[18] Data on two indicators, total fertility rate and trained assistance at delivery are available at the provincial level for 1993 from the Kenya Demographic and Health Survey (KDHS)[7] (*data not shown*). Generally speaking the lower the TFR in a province, the higher the percentage of deliveries with professionally trained attendants. These data give some indication that the level of maternal mortality, as measured by maternal deaths to women aged 15-49 (the maternal mortality rate), can be expected to be highest in Western and Nyanza provinces (high TFR and low professionally-attended deliveries) and lowest in Nairobi and Central provinces (lower TFR and higher professionally-attended deliveries).

This is reasonably consistent with regional patterns of other health and socio-economic indicators seen in the GOK/UNICEF Situation Analysis of 1992.[5] It is, however, important to acknowledge the likelihood of wide differences between districts within each province and the crudeness of this approach, which relies on just two proxy indicators. Thus, the picture which emerges should be regarded as suggestive of regional patterns rather than definitive.

Hospital data can also be used to indicate variations between parts of the country, but their interpretation requires care. In particular, it is often hard to establish whether variation between hospitals in the level of maternal mortality is due to differences in severity of admissions; staff and facilities available to avert death; referral to other hospitals; denominator used (all deliveries or live births only) and reporting procedures. The explanation for any variation is likely to lie in a combination of all these factors.

There have been several studies in Kenya on individual hospitals (*data not shown*). These

Table 2. Selected maternal mortality studies

Locality	Source/Type	Period	Number of events
National[11]	Population-based survey, and hospitals	1990-1994	134 maternal deaths (1990-1994) 292 hospital maternal deaths (1993)
Kakamega, Kirinyaga, and Kilifi districts[10]	District hospitals, and district civil registries	1989-1990	673 maternal deaths
Nairobi[14]	Hospital (Pumwani)	1975-1984	150 maternal deaths

highlight the differences in levels of maternal mortality between district, provincial and national referral hospitals. The 1994 national study[11] also gathered information from 19 district or provincial hospitals, and found 292 deaths for the year 1993. There is a wide range between hospitals both in the numerator (maternal deaths) and in the denominator (live births) for calculating the MMR, and this is reflected in the wide range of estimates – from 1,270 for Kwale District Hospital (based on 10 deaths and 790 live births), and 100 for Pumwani Hospital (based on 18 deaths and 18,040 live births). The low level of maternal mortality at Pumwani will largely reflect the opportunity for referral of serious cases to tertiary hospitals elsewhere in Nairobi.

As regards trends in maternal mortality in Kenya, the availability of a national estimate for the first time in 1994 means that changes over time cannot yet be charted.

Medical causes of maternal mortality

In Kenya most of the data on medical causes of maternal mortality come from hospital studies. Civil registration sources suffer from problems of incompleteness, and population-based surveys which use verbal autopsy techniques have yet to be fully validated.[19] The distribution of medical causes of maternal deaths appears to be reasonably consistent with the findings of hospital-based studies elsewhere in sub-Saharan Africa. There are, however, four points to highlight:

- The pattern of causes reflects both the type of hospital and its location. Thus, for example, eclampsia is a major cause of death even in a provincial level hospital (Pumwani) with easy access to the national referral centre. This hospital is also located in a part of the country where malaria and anaemia are not highly prevalent. The study by Makokha et al[10] was conducted in districts where these indirect causes of maternal mortality are common, and where women travel considerable distances, often arriving in an extremely poor state in the case of haemorrhage.
- Use of the percentage distribution of causes is particularly prone to distortion owing to differential recording between hospitals. The 1994 national study[11] covered 18 hospitals and shows a distribution which is also obscured by the varying representation of different facilities. For example, Coast General in Mombasa contributed almost a fifth of the total maternal deaths, and is located where both malaria and anaemia are prevalent.
- The pattern of causes is broadly consistent with the reported timing of maternal deaths for the two studies where these data are available (*data not shown*), although differential recording of the timing of the category 'abortion' complicates interpretation.
- The data are based on single cause of death reporting. Where both primary and underlying causes are reported, the pattern can look quite different, with indirect causes such as anaemia, hepatitis, tuberculosis, rheumatic heart, malaria and AIDS appearing even more prominently.[20]

There is also a substantial 'unknown' category, which in the case of hospital-based studies usually indicates an omission in reporting rather than a statement that cause was unknown. Both case-reviews using hospital records and interviews with relatives were used together to gain a more complete picture in the study by Makokha et al.[10] Uncertainty over the validity of relatives' reports on medical causes must be borne in mind, however, for all adult deaths and perhaps especially for the sensitive issue of maternal death.[21]

Detailed inspection of hospital notes for 248 maternal deaths revealed a different ranking of diagnoses than that in the hospital admission register and the deaths. Although anaemia emerged as a major diagnosis and cause of death, abortion featured as an important cause of admission but was omitted as a cause in the death register – a fact the authors attribute to the stigma attached to abortion-related mortality:

'During the focus group discussions, it was found that... any woman who was suspected or known to have died from an illegal abortion was not accorded a respectful burial.'[10]

This is a finding consistent with several other studies of induced abortion in Kenya,[22,23] and emphasises the difficulties of obtaining reliable data on what is estimated to be the cause of over a third of all maternal deaths in Kenya and a major cause of maternal morbidity.

Prevalence of maternal morbidity

A crude measure of maternal morbidity is derived by applying the estimated proportions for pregnant women with acute obstetric problems (about 40 per cent) and for life-threatening complications (about 15 per cent). Using the recent figures on the CBR and MMR for Kenya suggests that, every year, over half a million pregnant women suffer acute obstetric morbidity, about 194,000 experience life-threatening conditions and an estimated 4,300 die of maternal causes. These crude approximations do not, however, take chronic or underlying conditions into account.

Data to gauge the prevalence of maternal morbidity in Kenya are limited at both national and sub-national levels, in line with limited experience worldwide of surveys of maternal morbidity.[24-27] Only an incomplete picture for Kenya of selected maternal morbidities can be drawn from a small number of studies of a reasonable size.[23,28-32]

The position of women in Kenya

The discrimination faced by Kenyan women has long been recognised in Kenya. In 1985 the GOK adopted the Forward Looking Strategies for the Advancement of Women, which provided a framework for integrating women into the national development process, but this was never fully implemented. Many of the development projects implemented after the Women's Decade did nothing to improve the lives of Kenyan women and, in some cases, even led to greater marginalisation.[5]

Direct and indirect indicators of discrimination and disadvantage across a woman's lifecycle can be found for Kenya. For example, by the age of 15, 13 per cent of women aged 25-49 were married (compared with 0.6 per cent of men) and by the age of 18, 34 per cent of young women had begun childbearing.[7] Further, the average number of hours spent on domestic work by women over the age of eight was 14.1 hours per day (compared to 1.8 for men),[5] and 27 per cent of women had no formal education (compared to 17 per cent of men).[7]

The socio-economic status of women has a direct impact on safe motherhood through poor health and nutritional status before, during and after pregnancy, limited knowledge and awareness of health, lack of decision-making power and resources for seeking health care, weak negotiating power in terms of sexual and reproductive rights, heavy physical workload regardless of pregnancy status, and exposure to violence.

In the early 1990s, the emphasis given by the GOK, NGOs and UN agencies shifted away from women-in-development programmes and towards a gender-sensitive approach to development, to focus on questions of social justice and power distribution between the sexes, reflected in 1996 in the National Strategy for Reproductive Health Care.[3]

Fertility decline

One of the most significant demographic features of Kenya is the fertility decline over the last 20 years. The explanations for this decline[33] include government policies on education, health, communication, transport and land tenure.[34] Family planning has also clearly played a part.

The GOK's family planning programme is coordinated and implemented by the Division of Primary Health Care/MOH. It was one of the first national initiatives to be launched in sub-Saharan Africa in 1967. Since then there have been several situation analyses of the programme and modifications made to address the weaknesses. According to the 1993 KDHS,[7] almost two-thirds of women interviewed who were modern contraceptive users (representing 20 per cent of all women aged 15-49) had obtained their supplies from government sources. A quarter did so from private medical sources, and the remainder from other sources, such as shops or friends. To maintain current contraceptive prevalence levels in Kenya (around 36 per cent in 1995), will require a 58 per cent increase in contraceptive supplies up to the year 2005.[35]

A huge amount of technical, logistical and financial support has been provided by the donor community to family planning services in Kenya, and supplies are currently highly donor dependent. That this component of reproductive health will continue to dominate resource allocation within the GOK NRHS is clear, and this has implications for the level of resources that will be devoted to reducing maternal mortality and morbidity in the coming years.

Factors related to health care

The provision of care through the formal health sector in Kenya has been the subject of several reviews, with the most recent being completed in 1996 and focusing specifically on health personnel.[6] The GOK Health Policy Framework,[2] launched in December 1994, sets out the agenda for reform over the next 15 years, which aims to build upon the strengths of the current system and address the major weaknesses.

Focusing specifically on maternity care (antenatal, intra-partum and post-partum), there are an estimated 1,900 service delivery points (SDPs) but most of these do not conduct deliveries. Information which would enable classification into Basic Essential Obstetric Care and Comprehensive Essential Obstetric Care facilities is lacking. In terms of personnel, although most hospitals may be adequately staffed as regards the number of doctors, it is unclear how many are trained in obstetrics and gynaecology, and particularly in life-saving skills.

Nurse/midwives are the main providers of antenatal and intra-partum care in the formal health sector, and regulations and standards for nursing practice and education are monitored by the Nursing Council, in collaboration with the Directorate of Nursing in the Ministry of Health. At present, clinical officers do not routinely receive obstetrics as part of their training and they therefore do not play a major role in providing maternity care.

The serious shortage of doctors and clinical officers at health centres is one reason for the public to bypass these facilities, thus creating pressure on hospitals. In terms of intra-partum care, although about two-thirds of health centres have maternity beds and should be able to stabilise serious complications as well as treat minor ones, the lack of appropriately skilled staff forces referral to higher level facilities. The limited capacity for dealing with complications at most health centres encourages some Kenyan women to go straight to hospital and others to remain at home, even in the event of a complication. This situation is further aggravated by outdated guidelines for delivery at health centres, which prevent primiparous women and those of parity three or more, who have no complicating factors, from delivering in these facilities. Many health centres are, therefore, seriously under-utilised in terms of their capacity both to handle normal deliveries and to detect and refer those developing problems.

Although some aspects of utilisation can be assessed from service data, such as distance travelled by users, uptake rates essentially require population-based data which capture both women who do and women who do not use the service. The KDHS[7] is a key resource as regards uptake of antenatal and intra-partum care.

The quality of the service women received, however, cannot be determined from the KDHS, nor can the delays in uptake. There are wide geographical differences in utilisation and the data are confined to surviving women – thus missing those who experienced fatal delays in receiving adequate care. The reasons for delays are numerous, including initial use of home remedies and 'traditional' practitioners, and perceptions of treatment and providers at modern health facilities. Makokha et al,[10] for example, observed from community interviews, a strong fear of caesarean delivery, which was seen as a sign of weakness and a great risk:

'When you sign consent for a caesarean operation, it is synonymous with signing your death certificate.'

There has not in fact been a comprehensive assessment of obstetric services in Kenya, using for example the WHO Safe Motherhood Needs Assessment Guidelines,[36] or the Population Council Situational Analysis Framework.[37] This is surprising, given the extent of assessments of service delivery points for family planning services and, more recently, sexually transmitted infections.

The difference in utilisation rates between antenatal and intrapartum care (Table 3) do, however, give some pointers. In terms of accessibility, there are more service delivery points for antenatal care and thus, in theory, the time and distance involved should be less than for reaching a facility with maternity beds. It is estimated that almost 80 per cent of Kenyans live within a six km walk of a health facility, but walking during pregnancy is a different matter from walking during labour, particularly if a complication has arisen.

The availability of facilities actually providing essential obstetric care in Kenya is unknown, but in urban areas where physical accessibility is less of a constraint, almost a quarter of deliveries still occur away from health facilities. Assuming that hospitals are the only facilities providing essential obstetric care, and in view of the average time between onset and death for selected complications, it is clear that the vast majority of women face a high risk of dying in the event of post-partum haemorrhage.

Cost is known to affect both uptake and delays in seeking care. The GOK introduced cost-sharing in 1989 for specific services, but excluding promotive and preventive services, which includes antenatal care. The Health Policy Framework[2] proposes the extension of user fees, and these are already in operation within private and public maternity facilities in Kenya.

Evidence from other developing countries indicates a direct decline in utilisation of maternity services linked with the introduction of user fees,[38] and this will need to be monitored in Kenya. Fees appear to vary from facility to facility, but generally women are charged in proportion to the service received. A caesarean section for example, is more expensive than a normal delivery. This appears logical in terms of the health service inputs but may also be an important deterrent for poor women seeking care.

Within the international Safe Motherhood Initiative, the skills of the provider are now being placed at the centre of concerns for poor quality care. Puerperal sepsis is a major cause of maternal death in Kenya, and even minor infections can have serious consequences for women with anaemia or those with HIV who are immuno-suppressed. The extent to which some of the complications reported by health services are naturally occurring or due to iatrogenic factors is a subject worthy of urgent attention in Kenya.

The case for discouraging women with normal pregnancies from delivering in overcrowded health facilities with poor infection control, also deserves serious consideration. There are substantial potential benefits from encouraging home

Table 3. Utilisation of maternity services 1993[7]

Variable	**Per cent of births**	
Attendance at antenatal care (at least one visit) by type of provider	**Rural**	**Urban**
Doctor	21.6	29.5
Nurse/midwife	72.9	68.1
Trained TBA	0.4	0
TBA	0.5	0
Other	0.1	0.4
No one/missing	4.4	2.0
First antenatal visit after six months of pregnancy	38.4	
Place of delivery:	**Rural**	**Urban**
Home	59.5	21.2
Government health facility	30.5	58.0
Mission hospital	7.4	12.0
Private hospital/clinic	1.3	7.6
Other	0.8	0.6
Missing	0.6	0.6
Assistance at delivery	**Rural**	**Urban**
Doctor	10.6	23.7
Nurse/midwife	29.7	56.2
Trained TBA	9.4	4.2
TBA	13.8	2.4
Relative	24.6	10.4
Other	0.4	0.2
No one	11.1	2.9
Missing	0.4	0
Median distance (km) to nearest health facility (rural or urban) providing:	**Hosp.**	**H/C**
Antenatal care	17.1	5.0
Delivery care	17.1	7.4
Time (in hours) to reach nearest health facility (rural or urban) providing:	**Hosp.**	**H/C**
Antenatal care		
< 1 hour	42.5	53.3
1-3 hours	24.7	21.6
3+ hours	27.7	10.9
Service not provided	0.8	9.9
Delivery care		
< 1 hour	42.6	34.9
1-3 hours	24.6	16.0
3+ hours	28.0	11.5
Service not provided	0.5	33.8

deliveries in this sense, using birth attendants who are trained on the principle of 'first do no harm' and backed up by a functioning referral system. High quality essential obstetric care will, however, always be needed to manage complications and prevent the majority of maternal deaths in Kenya.

Making motherhood safer

Achieving safer motherhood requires a broad-based approach, and the provision of high quality maternity care must be given priority. Apart from family planning over many years and STIs in the last 5-6 years, however, there is scant evidence of donor support in Kenya for enhancing maternity care on a significant scale. Maternity care comes under the MOH's budget for MCH-FP, but the allocations within this category are hard to disentangle. The amount allocated to family planning, on the other hand, in the 1994/1995 development budget is in excess of Ksh 1 billion;[35] over 80 per cent of which is donor financed.

The Government's recent launch of a National Strategy for Reproductive Health Care is a major step forward in this regard. Developing an implementation plan for these activities will need to take stock of existing initiatives as well as the Health Policy Framework[2] for reform.

Considering the key issue of the provision of high quality obstetric care, what are the significant service-related initiatives underway in the government sector across several provinces? Three should be mentioned in particular:

- extending skills of providers to use manual vacuum aspiration for the management of incomplete abortion;[39]
- re-training and updating the skills of midwives in the use of the partograph;[40]
- training of traditional birth attendants.[41]

Initiatives to upgrade the physical infrastructure of government health facilities in particular neglected areas may also benefit women seeking care during pregnancy and delivery. In addition, there are local-level projects and pilot studies, such as the SIDA-funded safe motherhood demonstration project in Saiya District[42] which aims both to improve the quality of maternal care by early identification of 'risk mothers' and to decrease the number of serious complications during pregnancy, focusing on Ukwala Division.

Several NGOs undertake grassroots activities which are relevant to safe motherhood, such as Maendeleo Ya Wanawake Organisation, which operates in all districts and carries out education on danger signs in pregnancy and labour. Few NGOs, however, provide intra-partum care at more than one site. Population and Health Services, the Kenyan partner of Marie Stopes International, for example, runs one private maternity unit in the low-income area of Eastleigh in Nairobi. The unit has the capacity to function as a Comprehensive Essential Obstetric Care facility (except for blood replacement) and conducted 1,331 deliveries in 1994/1995.[43]

The GOK Health Policy Framework will be encouraging private and NGO providers to play a larger role in the provision of curative care services, and the impact of this on safe motherhood deserves close monitoring. Given appropriate and adequate resource incentives from the GOK, there is no reason to doubt the technical capacity of the private or NGO sector to provide such care on an enlarged scale. However, there are two important concerns: the cost implications for all women and the effectiveness of the referral system. The MOH acknowledges that it may prove hard to maintain efficient linkages between private facilities and those remaining in the public sector – e.g. health centres and dispensaries – and with TBAs supervised by government providers. Given the importance of timely access to emergency care, reassurances are also needed that any shift to private and NGO maternity services will at least improve the current regional inequalities in the geographic distribution of facilities.

There is also a renewed emphasis within the Health Policy Framework on promotional and preventive services, including prevention of unwanted pregnancy; promotion of messages on danger signs in pregnancy and labour; promotion of women's overall health status and well-being; and promotion of clean/safe delivery.

The GOK's proposed decentralisation to district level of the responsibility for the day-to-day running of the health care system is consistent with the major thrust of safe motherhood programming.[44] In contrast, little is known about the impact of opening-up the health insurance market on safe motherhood, though there is evidence, e.g. from Chile,[45] of a dramatic rise in the rate of caesarean delivery after such a reform was implemented.

Recommendations

A realistic and achievable package of recommendations was drawn up, limited to those with clear potential for reducing maternal morbidity in Kenya in the immediate term:

- ***Enhancing national capacity to implement action***

The National Safe Motherhood Task Force should be revitalised and its composition reviewed to ensure adequate representation of government, bi-lateral and multilateral, NGO, private, and parastatal agencies. Terms of reference and conduct of the Task Force should be made explicit, and include: mobilising political commitment; identifying indicators and mechanisms for monitoring reform in maternity services, including the introduction of user fees; liaising with taskforces; and formulating a National Safe Motherhood Programme based on the phased introduction of pilot projects to strengthen maternity services at the district level.

- ***Strengthening maternity services and links with the community***

Commencing in a small number (4-6) of selected pilot districts, projects should be set up to include: a situation analysis of antenatal and obstetric services, following the guidelines developed by WHO[36] or the Population Council,[37] which could build upon the service mapping recently completed in 11 districts for the Ministry of Health, which focused on family planning; provision of essential drugs and equipment; improvements in the clinical and obstetric skills of doctors, clinical officers and nurses/midwives through skills update courses on life-saving skills,[46] improved infection control, interpersonal skills, and supervisory structures; an audit process to review quality of care; TBA training; and strengthening links with the community.

- ***Filling information gaps***

The National Safe Motherhood Task Force will require high quality information not only to plan and monitor the implementation of a rolling programme, but also to fill significant gaps, including minimal reporting systems, initially at facilities in pilot project districts, and enforced notification by District Medical Officers of all maternal and perinatal deaths occurring within health facilities. This reporting system would form the basis of a Kenyan Confidential Enquiry,[47] which would aim to identify avoidable factors.

Opportunities should be sought to gather information on maternal deaths and maternity service utilisation during multi-purpose household surveys, and the Safe Motherhood Task Force should seek to establish a national resource documentation collection on safe motherhood that includes key international reviews and a register of projects completed or in progress. Finally, the facility for supporting small-scale research projects needs to be developed in collaboration with national, research-based groups working in reproductive health.

II. Two Years After the Review

Accomplishments

In 1997, a high profile national launch of the report *A Question of Survival* was attended by key representatives of the Ministry of Health (MOH), donor agencies, parastatal and non-governmental agencies and the private sector. Journalists, female judges and Permanent Secretaries of other government ministries were also invited.

Following the launch, the report was disseminated to provincial and district health managers. As a result there has been increased commitment to and understanding of the far-reaching implications of safe motherhood within the MOH. While safe motherhood is the subject of minimal consideration within the wider political framework, the MOH has succeeded in raising the profile of maternal health issues among its provincial and district managers, and the report has been a vital tool in this endeavour.

A national planning exercise based on the National Reproductive Health Strategy[3] was conducted by all District Health management teams to prioritise and plan for safe motherhood. This exercise was an important achievement for a decentralising and reforming health system and has been incorporated into a National Reproductive Health Implementation Plan.[48] Although these plans prioritise safe motherhood within the reproductive health agenda, they do not prioritise specific safe motherhood interventions; this partly reflects a poor grasp of evidence-based, best practice.

At national level, the MOH, donor agencies and partners have sustained dialogue through the Reproductive Health Advisory Committee which replaced the Safe Motherhood Task Force and meets quarterly. The decision to rename the Safe Motherhood Task Force reflected a re-assessment of its roles and responsibilities in light of the report's recommendations. It was felt that the committee should not hold responsibility for co-ordinating programmes, but rather serve as an advisory committee to the Division of Primary Health Care. The Advisory Committee welcomed new partners, including donor agencies and non-governmental partners. Although the secretariat remains with the MOH Division of Primary Health Care, it is now chaired by the Director of Medical Services, reflecting greater commitment within the MOH. However, its roles and responsibilities remain somewhat ambiguous.

Comprehensive needs assessment exercises have been carried out in several districts by teams of MOH, non-governmental and donor agencies. The needs assessment exercises have been used to develop project documents and, although they have not been published as reports, they have been disseminated to the Reproductive Health Advisory Committee.

Meanwhile the MOH and Reproductive Health Advisory Committee are addressing the wider issues of policy and reform which mitigate against optimal service provision, focusing their immediate attention on policy, standards and guidelines at different levels and among different cadre of staff. A sub-committee of the Reproductive Health Advisory Committee has been reviewing current policy and training against actual needs.

Significant progress has been made to fill the information gaps highlighted in *A Question of Survival*. The 1998 Kenya Demographic and Health Survey[49] included a sibling history from which direct estimates of adult and maternal mortality have been derived using the Sisterhood method. As the number of deaths is relatively small, rates are subject to considerable sampling variation and cannot provide current estimates of regional variations. However, these new data contribute substantially to efforts to measure maternal mortality in Kenya.

For the age group 20-34 years, female adult mortality far exceeds male, and the maternal mortality ratio is 590 deaths per 100,000 live births over the period 1989-1998. This figure is closer to the indirect estimate of 670 proposed by the WHO[15] than to the official figure of 385 (1994).[3,11] The data on reported caesarean section rates confirm that where fertility is high and professionally attended deliveries low, maternal morbidity and mortality can be expected to be highest. The WHO estimates that between 5 and 15 per cent of births will require caesarean section delivery.[50] While the national rate for caesarean section is within the range suggested by the WHO, provincial rates are as low as 1.9 and 3.9 per cent in Nyanza and Western provinces respectively.[49] The inadequate and inappropriate use of the intervention is further suggested by the fact that women with secondary education are three times more likely to deliver by caesarean section than those with no education (11.2 per cent of deliveries compared to 3.6 per cent).[49]

What hurdles remain?

Many of the obstacles to adequate maternity services are associated with the health system as a whole, from policy to personnel. It could be argued that any interventions which are specific to safe motherhood will not be effective, let alone sustained, until the wider issues are addressed, particularly financing and better co-ordination of donor inputs. One of the greatest challenges is to mobilise political commitment to this issue. Progress has been slow, frustrating those within government who are committed to reform, as well as partners outside government.

Largely due to the lack of resources available to maintain basic services and provide adequate remuneration for staff, efficiency remains poor among health managers, planners and service providers. This came to a head in December 1997 when public sector nurses went on strike, paralysing the sector. Management capacity is poor throughout the sector. Medical doctors with administrative and management responsibilities have little, if any, management training. Supervision is virtually non-existent, and staff are rarely held accountable. Confidential enquiry, and other tools for management and accountability, have died out of the public sector. Health sector reform has made some progress in this area, particularly in the area of reproductive health planning, but the benefits have not yet been felt in terms of quality of care.

Life-saving, emergency obstetric procedures are not widely available because human resources are not allocated rationally and the most widely accessible cadre of staff are not trained, or permitted, to undertake them. Kenya has one of the highest doctor-population ratios, yet distribution is highly unbalanced. The current hiring freeze in the public sector exacerbates this problem, while delegation of personnel allocation to provincial level has eased distribution of staff in some regions. Clinical officers are more widely available, but few specialise in obstetrics or anaesthesia. Nurses are the main service providers, but their training and supervision are inadequate, and their roles and responsibilities limit the breadth

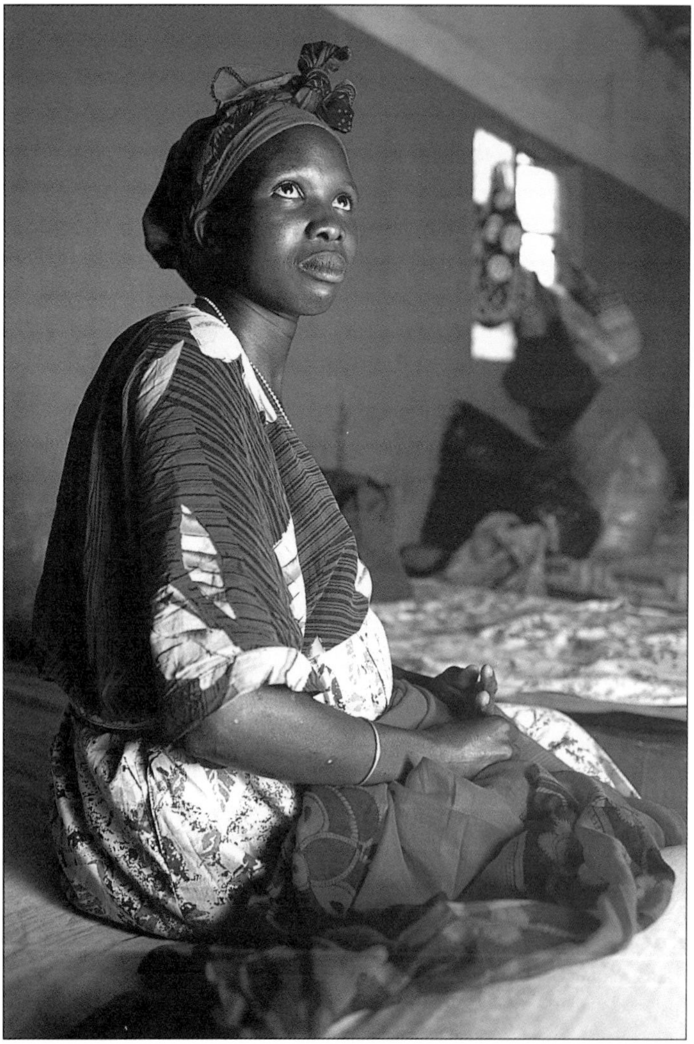

CRISPIN HUGHES / HUTCHISON LIBRARY

and quality of the services they are able to provide. This limits the availability of life-saving procedures such as caesarean section and vacuum extraction.

Within the context of health sector reform, donors are keen to move towards a sector-wide approach to support the government. Before meaningful commitments can be made, the government has faced considerable challenges to lay foundations in terms of policy, accountability and reform. While the policy framework is sound, implementation has not proceeded. The trend of dwindling financial resources from external agencies is likely to continue until progress has been made, even though donors realise that their procedures have contributed to the problematic situation in Kenya, which is reflected in the cumbersome and complicated project portfolio. Donors and government are keen to avoid diverting limited government capacity from the health sector reform agenda to projects that require additional management-intensive support.

Although the non-governmental and private sector cannot replace the public sector provision of services to the poor, they can contribute significant technical expertise as well as services. The building of partnerships between government and non-governmental agencies is a positive response to the current constraints in government-donor partnerships. Linking sectors to their comparative advantage along the lines of health sector reform is critical to the sustainability of any initiative in the current economic environment.

Cross-cutting issues

In a resource-constrained environment, the challenge for policy and programme planners is to maintain a balance of focus, and use every opportunity to integrate services within Primary Health Care. A more concentrated, strategic effort is required to prioritise interventions, such as prevention of severe anaemia, which are going to make a difference, and incrementally and systematically apply them in policy and practice. For example, presumptive treatment of malaria to prevent severe anaemia in pregnancy,[51] a highly cost-effective intervention, is now government policy[52] but is only being implemented in one public sector hospital. Similarly, adequate equipment to perform caesarean section in district hospitals should be prioritised over training of TBAs.

While now an accepted component of reproductive health, safe motherhood is still perceived to be the domain of certain donors (UNICEF, UNFPA, SIDA, WHO, DFID) and has yet to mobilise commitment from most of the bilateral agencies. Few additional donor resources are available to Kenya, where most donors are making no new investments until health sector reform has progressed and good governance has been assured. However, it is likely that new investments in reproductive health will include safe motherhood, according to Division of Primary Health Care priorities.

Lessons learnt have yet to be disseminated and grasped. Opportunities for dissemination and discussion of key evidence, such as that provided by the International Technical Consultation held in Sri Lanka in 1997, have yet to be used to their full advantage. As a consequence, resources are still directed at community level within some projects, without adequate attention paid to essential obstetric care. The importance of evidence-based, best practice such as life-saving skills are under-estimated among service providers and planners alike. This presents a challenge, particularly where medical doctors, who are also managers at district level, need to address their own practices to tackle issues of medical mismanagement.

What next?

In the absence of progress towards health sector reform, support to safe motherhood will be through projects, at least for the time being. Several donors have recently commenced projects in Kenya. UNICEF is implementing an ambitious safe motherhood component as part of its Country Programme, which focuses on the disadvantaged areas of North Eastern Kenya. DFID will support a partnership fund for safe motherhood, including support to a 'demonstration district' and technical and strategic support to partner organisations to encourage the implementation of evidence-based, best practice, without large financial investment elsewhere. UNFPA is supporting a reproductive health project which focuses on safe motherhood best practice in seven districts. It is hoped that these projects, albeit piecemeal, will provide an interim level of support to build capacity and improve service provision at district level. In the longer term, the ambition is for District Health Management teams and their local and national partners to gain increasing autonomy through decentralisation and the reform process, as well as convincing government and other donors that safe motherhood is a worthwhile investment in Kenya.

Acknowledgements

The preparation of this paper was co-ordinated by Katie Chapman, Options Consultancy Services, London, UK. ***Part I*** *is based on the full report,* **A Question of Survival**, *prepared by the authors for Options Consultancy Services on behalf of the Ministry of Health of Kenya and published by the Ministry in 1997. This summary of the report is reprinted here with their kind permission. The original acknowledgements in the full report, slightly shortened here, were as follows: The preparation of this document benefited from wide consultation with individuals and groups in Kenya. The Ministry of Health would like to thank the Division of Primary Health Care, Kenya, who worked extensively with the consultants to ensure the completion of this document. Thanks also to the Kenya Medical Women's Association for their help in distributing the report. In the UK, the report benefited from the assistance of many people, especially Elaine Stirton, Dugald Baird Centre and Sue Bartlett, Options Consultancy Services. Finally, the Ministry of Health would like to thank the Department for International Development UK, without whose support the whole exercise would not have been possible.* ***Part II*** *was written in 1999. The author would like to thank Caroline Sergeant, Department for International Development East Africa, and Caroline Shulman, London School of Hygiene and Tropical Medicine, for their helpful comments on early drafts.*

Correspondence

Katie Chapman, Options Consultancy Services, 129 Whitfield Street, London W1P 5RT, UK. Fax: 44-171-388-1884. E-mail: k.chapman@options.co.uk

References

1 Mahler H (1987): The Safe Motherhood Initiative: A call to action. *Lancet*; 668-670.

2. Ministry of Health (1994): Kenya's Health Policy Framework. Government of Kenya; 1-50.

3. Ministry of Health (1996): National Reproductive Health Strategy 1997-2010. Ministry of Health, Government of Kenya; 3-57.

4. Law M, Maine D, Feuerstein M-T (1991): *Safe Motherhood: Priorities and Next Steps: Forward-Looking Assessment on the Reduction of Maternal Mortality and Morbidity within the Framework of the Safe Motherhood Initiative (SMI).* United Nations Development Programme; 1-40.

5. Government of Kenya/United Nations Children's Fund (1992): *Children and Women in Kenya. A Situation Analysis 1992.* GOK/UNICEF; 1-162.

6. Schwarz RA (1996): *The Health Sector in Kenya. Health Personnel, Facilities, Education and Training.* Development Solutions for Africa; Second edition: 1-19.

7. National Council for Population and Development (NCPD), Central Bureau of Statistics (CBS), Office of the Vice President and Ministry of Planning and National Development [Kenya], and Macro International Inc. (MI) (1994): *Kenya Demographic and Health Survey 1993.* Calverton Maryland: NCPD, CBS, and MI; 1-278.

8. Robinson WC (1992): Kenya enters the fertility transition. *Population Studies*; 46(4):445-457.

9. UNFPA (1992): *Kenya: Programme Review and Strategy Development Report 1991.* UNFPA; 1-75.

10. Makokha AE, Kirumbi LW, Mukolwe JL, Sekadde-Kigondu C (1994): *Causes and Prevention of Maternal Mortality in Kenya.* USAID/FHI; 1-85.

11. Population Studies and Research Institute (1996): *Kenya Maternal Mortality Baseline Survey 1994.* UNICEF; 1: 1-86.

12. Voorhoeve AM, Muller AS, W'Oigo H (1984): The Outcome of Pregnancy. In: *Maternal and Child Health in Rural Kenya.* van Ginneken JK, Muller SA (eds). Croom Helm; 223-240.

13. Boerma JT, Mati JKG (1989): Identifying maternal mortality through networking: results from Coastal Kenya. *Studies in Family Planning*; 20:245-253.

14. Ngoka WM, Bansal YP (1987): Maternal mortality – Pumwani Maternity Hospital – 1975-1984. *East African Medical Journal*; 64 (4): 277-283.

15. World Health Organization (1996): *Revised 1990 Estimates of Maternal Mortality. A New*

Approach by WHO and UNICEF. WHO/FRH/MSM/ 96.11/ UNICEF/PLN/96.1 WHO; 1-16.

16. Graham W, Brass W, Snow RW (1989) Estimating maternal mortality: the Sisterhood method. *Studies in Family Planning*; 20 (3):125-135.
17. Rutenberg N, Sullivan J (1991): Direct and Indirect Estimates of Maternal Mortality from the Sisterhood Method. Paper presented at the Demographic and Health Surveys World Conference, Washington DC; 1-16.
18. Bhat PNM, Navaneetham K, Rajan SI (1995): Maternal mortality in India: estimates from a regression model. *Studies in Family Planning*; 26 (4):203-216.
19. Chandramohan D, Maude GH, Rodrigues LC, Hayes R (1994): Verbal autopsies for adult deaths: issues in their development and validation. *International Journal of Epidemiology*; 23:213-222.
20. Graham WJ (1991): Maternal mortality: levels, trends and data deficiencies. In: *Disease and Mortality in Sub-Saharan Africa*. Feachem RG, Jamison DT (eds). World Bank, Oxford University Press; 6:101-116.
21. Campbell O, Ronsmans C (1995): *Verbal Autopsies for Maternal Deaths*. Maternal Health and Safe Motherhood Programme. Report of a WHO Workshop, London, 10-13 January 1994; WHO/FHE/MSM/95.15. WHO; 1-36.
22. Rogo K (1993): Induced abortion in sub-Sahara Africa, *East African Medical Journal*; 70: 368-395.
23. Lema V, Kamau R, Rogo K (1989): Epidemiology of Abortion in Kenya. Centre for the Study of Adolescence, Nairobi, Kenya.
24. Republic of the Philippines (1994): *National Safe Motherhood Survey 1993*. National Statistics Office, Manila, Philippines/Macro International Inc; 1-172.
25. Graham WJ, Ronsmans CCA, Filippi VGA et al (1995): *Asking Questions about Women's Reproductive Health in Community-Based Surveys: Guidelines on Scope and Content*. MCEU, London School of Hygiene and Tropical Medicine, London, 1995; 6:1-79.
26. League of Arab States (1989): *PAPCHILD: The Arab Maternal and Child Health Survey*. Basic Documentation 2: Model Questionnaires. Tunisia: League of Arab States.
27. Stewart MK, Festin M (1995): Validation study of women's reporting and recall of major obstetric complications treated at the Philippine General Hospital. *International Journal of Gynecology and Obstetrics*; Suppl 48:S53-S66.
28. Aggarwal VP (1980): Obstetric emergency referrals to Kenyatta National Hospital. *East African Medical Journal*; 57(2):144-149.
29. Shulman CE, Graham WJ, Jilo H, et al (1996): Malaria is an important cause of anaemia in primigravidae: evidence from a district hospital in Coastal Kenya. *Transactions of the Royal Society of Tropical Medicine and Hygiene*; 90:535-539.
30. Jenniskens F, Obwaka E (1994): *Syphilis Control in Pregnant Women: Clinic-Based Screening, Treatment and Counselling Services in Nairobi, Kenya*. The MotherCare Project, John Snow Inc/USAID; 7-26.
31. Okeyo TM, Baltazar GM, Stover J, Johnston A (eds) (1996): *AIDS in Kenya: Background, Projections, Impact and Interventions*. National AIDS and STDs Control Programme; Third Edition: 4-49.
32. Mati JKG (1995): Reaching Out with Reproductive Health Care. Experience of the Machakos Project and its Policy and Programme Implications. Institute for Reproductive Health. (Unpublished report)
33. Ndhlovu L, Solo J, Miller R et al (1996): *Kenya: A Situation Analysis Study of the Family Planning Services*. Population Council; 1-50.
34. Brass, W, Jolly CL (eds) (1993): *Population Dynamics of Kenya*, Washington: National Academy Press.
35. Projects and Evaluation Committee (1995): Kenya: Family Health Project (parallel financed with EC). ODA; 95 (17).
36. World Health Organization (1995): *Safe Motherhood Needs Assessment*. Part I: Guidelines. WHO/FHE/MSM/95.1. WHO; 1-133.
37. Sloan NL, Quimby C, Winikoff B, Schwalbe N (1995): *Guidelines and Instruments for a Situation Analysis of Obstetric Services*. Robert H Ebert Program on Critical Issues in Reproductive Health and Population. Population Council; 1-34.
38. Evans I (1995): SAPping maternal health. [Commentary]. *Lancet*; 346:1046.
39. Solo J, Muia E, Rogo K (1995) Testing Alternative Approaches to Providing Integrated Treatment of Abortion Complications and Family Planning in Kenya: Findings from Phase I. Nairobi: Population Council.
40. Division of Nursing, Ministry of Health, World Health Organization (1995) A Report on Needs Assessment on Levels of Knowledge, Attitude and Usage of Partograph in Maternity Units. Nairobi: GOK/WHO: 1-25.
41. MOH (1991) National Curriculum for Traditional Birth Attendants. Nairobi: GOK.
42. SIDA (1995) SIDA-Supported Health Programmes in Kenya. Nairobi: SIDA.
43. Marie Stopes International (1996) A Safe Motherhood Initiative: An Integrated Essential Obstetrics Service Incorporating Maternal, Child Health and Family Planning

Support for Under-Privileged Women in Nairobi, Kenya. Report for the Period November 1994 – October 1995. London: Marie Stopes International.

44. World Health Organization (1994): *Mother-Baby Package: Implementing Safe Motherhood in Countries*. WHO/FHE/MSM/ 94.11. WHO; 1-89.

45. Murray, SF, Pradenas, FS (1997) Health sector reform and the rise of caesarean birth in Chile. *Lancet*, 249:64.

46. American College of Midwives (1991) *Life-Saving Skills Manual for Midwives*. Washington DC: American College of Midwives.

47. HMSO (1994) *Report on Confidential Enquiries into Maternal Deaths in the United Kingdom, 1988-90*. London: HMSO.

48. Ministry of Health (1999) Draft National Reproductive Health Implementation Plan 1999-2003, Ministry of Health, Government of Kenya

49. National Council for Population and Development (NCPD), Central Bureau of Statistics (CBS), Office of the Vice President and Ministry of Planning and National Development [Kenya], and Macro International Inc. (MI) (1999): *Kenya Demographic and Health Survey 1998*. Calverton Maryland: NCPD, CBS, and MI; 1-285.

50. World Health Organisation (1994): Indicators to monitor maternal health goals. WHO Division of Family Health: 20.

51. Shulman CE, Dorman EK, Cutts F, Kawuondo K, Bulmer JN, Peshu N, March K (1999): Intermittent sulphadoxine-pyrimethamine to prevent severe anaemia secondary to malaria in pregnancy: a randomised placebo-controlled trial. *Lancet*; 353 (9153): 632-36.

52. Ministry of Health (1998): National Guidelines for Diagnosis, Treatment and Prevention of Malaria for Health Workers. Ministry of Health, Government of Kenya.

Causes of maternal deaths and morbidity: case studies

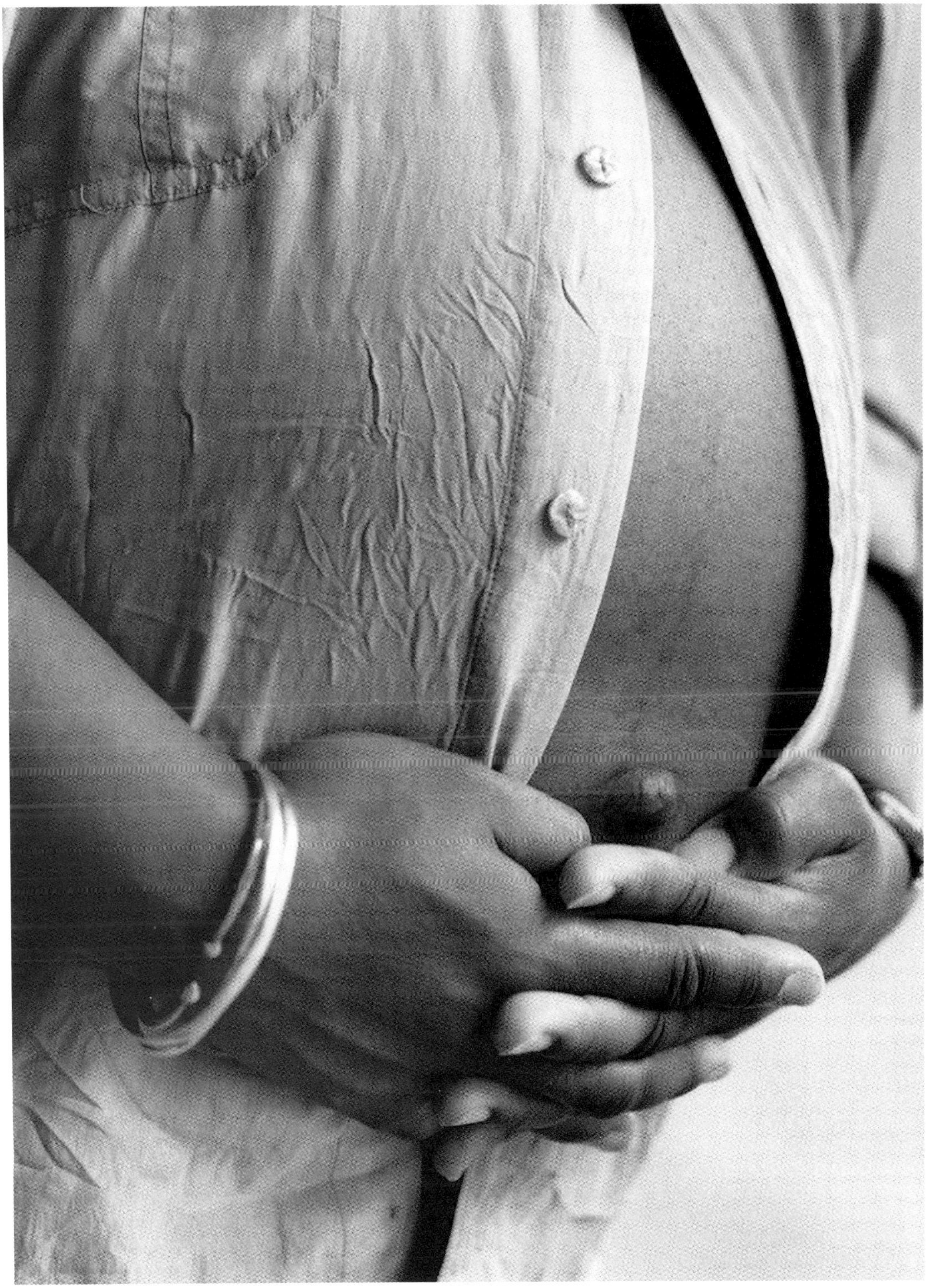

JOANNE O'BRIEN / FORMAT

Maternal Deaths in an Indian Hospital: A Decade of (No) Change?

Vinaya Pendse

This paper examines changes in the profile of women dying in childbirth in Zanana Hospital, a specialist hospital in Udaipur, Rajasthan, India, based on information about 100 consecutive maternal deaths in the hospital during 1983-85 and 1994-96. In the interim, there were significant improvements in the management of obstetric emergencies in the hospital and rapid improvements in Rajasthan's infrastructural facilities. The women who died in childbirth in the hospital in 1994-96 were poorer and in poorer health compared to women who died in childbirth in the hospital during 1983-85, and more of them belonged to socially disadvantaged groups. Almost the same proportion of women in both groups had received inadequate antenatal care. Similarly, the same proportion had been attended by a trained midwife during the initial stages of delivery. Many more had travelled longer distances and spent more money getting to the hospital in 1994-96 than in the previous decade, and more had arrived at the hospital in a moribund condition who could not be saved. Lastly, more of them succumbed to clearly preventable causes of death than in the previous decade – complications resulting from illegal abortions, severe anaemia and malaria. Most of the women who died in hospital in 1994-96 would have died at home in the earlier decade, and their deaths would never have been recorded. To that extent, the changes over the decade may be viewed as positive. However, poverty, gender and social inequalities and lack of access to care and treatment at a point when their lives could have been saved are still bringing as many women to die in our hospital as ten years ago. Until these problems are addressed, women will continue to die needlessly in childbirth, within and outside hospitals.

AFTER more than three decades of work as a specialist in obstetrics and gynaecology in Rajasthan, India, I retired in 1998. During my post-graduate training between 1965 and 1968 and in my early years as a teacher in medical colleges (1969-1980), I witnessed a large number of maternal deaths. The number seemed to be unchanging year after year. I was often gripped by a sense of helplessness.

Rajasthan is one of the poorest states of India, both economically and in terms of health status. The per capita income is much lower than the average for India, and the infant mortality rate is the fourth highest in the country.[1,2] During 1992-93, antenatal coverage in Rajasthan, i.e. at least one contact with a trained nurse-midwife attached to a government primary health centre, was only 23 per cent, the lowest in the country, compared to the national average of 49 per cent.[3] The state also had the lowest proportion of deliveries in a health facility (11.6 per cent) during the same year. More than 40 per cent of births were attended at home by traditional birth attendants (TBAs), and 37 per cent by other untrained persons.[4] The maternal mortality ratio for Rajasthan, estimated to be 938 per 100,000 live births during the period 1982-86, was the second highest in India, almost double the estimated national average of 555 per 100,000 live births.[5]

In 1980, I was appointed as Professor and Head of the Department of Obstetrics and Gynaecology at the RNT Medical College and the Zanana Hospital attached to it, a position I held for the next 17 years. At the time I assumed this position, the emergency maternity care available in the hospital was inadequate. The hospital had been set up in 1959 to accommodate 2,000 deliveries annually. However, the number of deliveries being conducted had crossed 4,000 by

1980, and was continuing to rise rapidly with no concomitant increase in manpower, beds or space. Indeed, the bed capacity was only 150 beds, with 20 beds exclusively earmarked for women having tubal ligation. As a result, there were no beds available for nearly 40 per cent of the women coming in to give birth, who had to lie on mats on the floor. Further, there was no septic ward, and women with sepsis and others were all accommodated in the same ward, with a high risk of cross-infection.

There was also a perpetual shortage of essential drugs and equipment. The labour room had no proper laboratory, store or preparation room attached to it. There was one common operating theatre for obstetric cases, gynaecological cases and sterilisations. The increase in the number of delivery cases, and tremendous increase in the inflow of women with serious obstetric complications from rural areas, contributed to the deterioration of the hospital's obstetric emergency services, resulting in the high rates of maternal mortality observed in the hospital.

It was during 1983-85 that I decided to document the maternal deaths which were happening in the hospital, with a view to drawing public attention to this serious issue. I prepared a report in 1985 on 100 women who had died in Zanana Hospital, which I mailed to government ministers, administrators at the federal and state government levels, the World Health Organization and leaders of local non-governmental organisations. The report did succeed in drawing attention to the problem, and was further helped in 1987 by the launch of the Safe Motherhood Initiative internationally. Eventually, in 1990-91, I received help in the form of government funds to improve the hospital's facilities for dealing with obstetric emergencies. A new operating theatre was constructed, a septic maternity complex was set up and additional staff were employed.

In 1985, I instituted medical audit of all cases of maternal death in the Zanana Hospital, with a view to evaluating care and treatment and bringing about improvements in the hospital's emergency obstetric services. Meetings were held monthly, and all maternal deaths in the previous month were analysed and discussed, and classified as 'avoidable' or 'unavoidable'. The resident post-graduate student who was on duty at the time of any maternal death was responsible for collecting additional details about the woman who died from her relatives, to present at the meeting. Teaching staff as well as non-teaching staff and all post-graduate students would attend the meetings and participate in the discussions.

The analysis and professional interaction in these meetings have led to considerably better management of serious obstetric emergencies and some necessary improvements in services. The setting up of additional facilities has also helped. Even so, several bottlenecks and constraints have remained: power failures, generator failures, ambulance break-downs and strikes in the factory which supplies oxygen are a few examples.

Further, although there have been rapid socio-economic changes in the state of Rajasthan and improvements in the state's infrastructural facilities, these have not been matched by improvements in access to primary health care; in the decade 1985 to 1995, there was only a small increase in the proportion of villages with a health centre – from 14.5 per cent to 20.5 per cent.[6]

In 1994-96, I collected information on a further 100 women who died from maternal causes in Zanana Hospital. I found that despite improvements inside and outside the hospital, the number of maternal deaths seen in the hospital had not declined in the decade 1985 to 1995. At the same time, however, the profile of women who were dying did appear to have changed. The present paper is an attempt to analyse the nature of these changes and the possible underlying factors. It seeks to understand whether or not there has been progress in the prevention of maternal deaths in Rajasthan, or even in the districts served by Zanana Hospital.

The study and its limitations

The first study was based on 100 consecutive cases of maternal deaths at Zanana Hospital, Udaipur, Rajasthan, between 1 January 1983 and 31 July 1985. The follow-up study in the same setting, carried out between 1 March 1994 and 30 June 1996, similarly included 100 maternal deaths.

In both instances, in addition to medical

history, information on each patient's socio-economic status and place of residence, the nature of any care received prior to hospital admission was recorded, the distance covered to reach the hospital, and the nature of and expenditure on getting to the hospital. Cases in which any of these details could not be obtained were excluded from the analysis.

Neither data set has information on the population from which the women who died came. In the absence of this information, it is not possible to make observations regarding changes in the maternal mortality rate or in the relative risk of maternal death based on characteristics of the women. The analysis is only indicative, but it throws up some interesting hypotheses regarding the factors underlying the changes in the profile of maternal deaths in the hospital during the decade concerned.

A context of poverty and gender discrimination

A major factor underlying many avoidable maternal deaths is the combination of gender discrimination and poverty, which begin to have an effect from birth for girls. Higher female infant mortality (92 per 1000) than male (88 per 1000) in Rajasthan (1992), a differential which continues through the adult years, is a clear indicator of this. Rajasathan also has the highest gap within India between female and male mortality rates in the 20-24 age group, with female mortality 1.7 times greater than male mortality.[2] Furthermore, there is also evidence to suggest that gender discrimination, rather than diminishing over time, may in fact be increasing. Thus, the ratio of female to male child mortality rates increased from 1.11 in 1982-84 to 1.16 in 1994.

Education of girls is rare, despite the increase in the number of villages which have a primary school. Rajasthan has the lowest female literacy rate in the country, 21 per cent, while the male literacy rate is 55 per cent.[7] The gender gap in educational status is likely to continue for many more decades, given that the primary school enrolment rate for girls in 1991 was only 50.1 per cent as compared to 106.7 for boys.[8]

Even today, mass child marriage ceremonies arranged by parents, where hundreds of boys and girls wed each other, are very common. The mean age at marriage for women (16.1 yrs) is among the lowest in the country.[1] Once a girl goes to her marital home, it is her duty to beget a child as soon as she can. Her sex life therefore starts immediately or soon after menarche, and in some cases, even earlier.

Forcing early pregnancies and motherhood on teenage girls under the banner of social custom and family is tragic. Not much has changed in Rajasthan in the past decade with respect to frequent childbearing and grand multiparity. Fertility rates remain high, with a total fertility rate in 1991 of 4.7 as compared to 3.9 for the country as a whole. Coming to the hospital in an obstetric emergency will not help prevent the deaths of women who are in a vulnerable state of health to begin with. Maternal mortality is thus, in addition to a health services and poverty issue, also a gender issue.

Yet another factor is the nature of 'development' that has taken place in the state of Rajasthan and the rest of the country over the last decade. Few jobs and income earning avenues appear to be percolating down to the rural areas, but prices of essential commodities and especially food have increased several fold. It would appear that economic inequality has increased, with the lion's share of benefits of technological and economic development cornered by the urban middle and upper classes.

Findings

Demographic characteristics and socio-economic status

There were more maternal deaths (12 per cent) in women aged 18 or less in 1994-96 than in 1983-85 (7 per cent). In both series, nearly one fourth of the deaths were in women over 30 years of age, a trend similar to other Indian states. Twenty-one per cent of deaths in 1983-85 and 24 per cent in 1994-96 occurred in women of gravidity five and above.

A greater proportion of maternal deaths in 1994-96 (68 per cent) occurred in women of the 'very poor' or 'poor' groups, as compared to ten years earlier (55 per cent).[9] Further, a slightly higher proportion of women who died in 1994-96 (88 per cent) were illiterate as compared to those who died a decade earlier (82 per cent), and fewer (4 per cent) had more than five years of schooling than those who died a decade earlier (9 per cent).

There was a statistically significant increase in 1994-96 as compared to 1983-85 in the percentage of those belonging to the 'Scheduled' castes and 'Scheduled' tribes – among the most economically and socially marginalised groups in India (74 per cent vs. 45 per cent). The proportion of maternal deaths among those belonging to higher castes declined to less than half of what it had been in the earlier series.

Interestingly, the decline in the number of maternal deaths was not uniform across the various 'higher' caste groups. The number of maternal deaths among the 'Rajput' caste women remained almost unchanged, from 18 in the 1983-85 study to 14 in the 1994-96 study, while deaths among other 'higher' castes declined from 35 to only 8.

Anaemia

Overall, the haemoglobin levels of women who died in 1994-96 were much worse than those observed in women who died a decade before. Every one of the women (100 per cent) who died from maternal causes in 1994-96 suffered from anaemia (Hb < 10.1 gm %), while the proportion was 83 per cent in the earlier series. In particular, the proportion in the 1994-96 series with very severe anaemia (Hb < 4 gm%) was three times greater, from 11 to 34 per cent.

When the haemoglobin level is less than 4 gm%, the risk of sudden heart failure is very high (up to 40 per cent of all cases).[10] Available blood was preventing some of these deaths in 1983-85. However, administrative and managerial problems related to blood transfusion in acutely anaemic patients have multiplied since 1992, with the advent of newer risks of bloodborne infection – HIV, hepatitis B, syphilis and malarial parasites, and screening for these infections has become mandatory since then. This has frequently resulted in the hospital being unable to provide blood for transfusion because the equipment or supplies to carry out the mandatory tests were not available. Blood donation by relatives continues to be rare. All these factors have contributed to maternal deaths related to anaemia in the 1994-96 series.

Antenatal and delivery care

The proportion of women who had received any primary-level antenatal care had increased statistically significantly during the decade, from 28 per cent to 50 per cent. However, on further exploring the nature of the care received by the two groups of women, we found that the only major change observable was that more women had received tetanus toxoid injections during pregnancy in 1994-96 than in 1983-85 (52 as compared to 32). There was only a very marginal increase (10 per cent vs. 6 per cent) in the proportion who had received adequate antenatal care (comprising four contacts with a health worker, immunisation against tetanus and anaemia prophylaxis). Eighteen per cent had

Table 1. Changes in the profile of women dying in childbirth at the Zanana Hospital, Udaipur, Rajasthan, India, 1983-85 and 1994-96

Characteristics of the women	No. of cases 1983-85 (n=100)	No. of cases 1994-96 (n=100)
Age 18 years and below	7	12
Age 31-40 years	21	22
Gravidity 5 +	21	22
Illiterate	82	88
Belonging to higher castes	53	22 *
Belonging to Scheduled castes/ Scheduled tribes	45	75 *
Poor and very poor	52	68
Moderate to severe anaemia (Hb < 8 gm%)	49	78 *
TBA the main person responsible for antenatal & intra-natal care	68	60
Tetanus toxoid immunisation	32	52
Booked cases	10	5
No primary care	72	50 **
Women from the city	15	7
Women who travelled 100 km to reach hospital	11	20
Transported by jeep	27	62
Transport expenditure Rs. 201- 500	26	38
Transport expenditure Rs. 501 >	3	12
Mortality within 4 hrs of hospital admission	25	34
Eclampsia cause of death	28	13
Haemorrhage cause of death	23	31
Severe anaemia cause of death	4	24
Ruptured uterus cause of death	4	7
Septic induced abortion cause of death	4	15 #

* *p < .01, highly significant*

** *p < .05, significant*

\# *11 cases of sepsis and 4 cases of haemorrhage*

received erratic antenatal care (one or two contacts with a health worker when the latter chooses to make a domiciliary visit) or inadequate antenatal care (falling short of one or more components), while 50 per cent had received no antenatal care at all in the 1994-96 series, as compared to 4 per cent and 72 per cent respectively in the 1983-85 series.

Traditional birth attendants still remained the main people responsible for delivery care for 60 per cent of the women in 1994-96, as compared to 68 per cent in 1983-85.

Distance and mode of transport to the hospital

With the improvement in roads and transport facilities which took place in the years between the two studies, an increased number of women who died in the hospital had travelled from distant places and had arrived at the hospital with the hope of surviving. The proportion of women who had travelled more than 100 km almost doubled, from 11 per cent during 1983-85 to 20 per cent during 1994-96. At the same time, the proportion of maternal deaths from among women from Udaipur city had been halved, from 15 per cent during 1983-85 to 7 per cent in 1994-96.

Because of the hilly terrain and poor (even if improved) roads for the long distances, delays in bringing women to the hospital, leading to deterioration in the woman's condition, were always a strong possibility in the majority of the cases.

As regards means of transport, the most noticeable change was that many more women who died in the 1994-96 group (62 per cent) had travelled in by jeep as compared to those in the past (37 per cent). This vehicle, suitable for rough and bumpy roads, has gained popularity as a mode of private transport because it is far less expensive than a private taxi, and faster than other traditional modes of transport available at the village level. There was not much change in the other modes of transport used, which included buses, trucks and the age old bullock-cart. Three-wheeler taxis (auto-rickshaws) were available for transport in Udaipur city.

Eight women in the 1994-96 group were carried manually on a cot or on someone's back. More than one third of the women had used more than one mode of transport to reach the hospital. Often, a woman would be carried on a cot or on someone's back from her village to the nearest motorable road. From there a passing private bus, minibus or truck would be flagged down and asked to transport her to some part of Udaipur city, and then a three-wheeler would be hired to reach the hospital. Distance and lack of transport together may have contributed to far more maternal deaths in the community than among women who reached the hospital.

Only 8 percent of the women in the 1994-96 study and 6 per cent in the 1983-85 study were transported by hospital ambulance. Despite the passage of ten years and repeated requests and reminders from us at Zanana Hospital, there has as yet been no policy directive from the Health Department regarding the transport of emergency maternity cases from rural areas to hospital. Transport is not provided by the government, even for serious cases referred from primary health centres in the district.

Expenditure on transport

All but those who used hospital ambulances had to hire private transport and pay for it. The exorbitant amounts they had to pay are of great concern, given that the majority of them were extremely poor.

The average expenditure on transporting the dying woman in each case had doubled in the period between the two studies, from Rs. 150 to Rs. 300. This may partly be due to the increased cost of fuel and the longer distances travelled. However, more families in 1994-96 had ventured to come to the hospital from longer distances, in the hope of saving the woman's life. We gathered that many of the families had to borrow from a local moneylender or pawn some of their belongings before undertaking the journey. The whole experience left them poorer both materially and emotionally, especially when, despite their desperate efforts, the woman's life could not be saved.

Interval between hospital admission and death

Twenty-one per cent of the women in 1994-96, as compared to 13 per cent in 1983-85, died within two hours of admission, which indicates that their condition was so bad that nothing could be done for them in the way of hospital emergency care. While this was also true in the past, the number of women arriving in a moribund condition was much higher in the 1994-96 series.

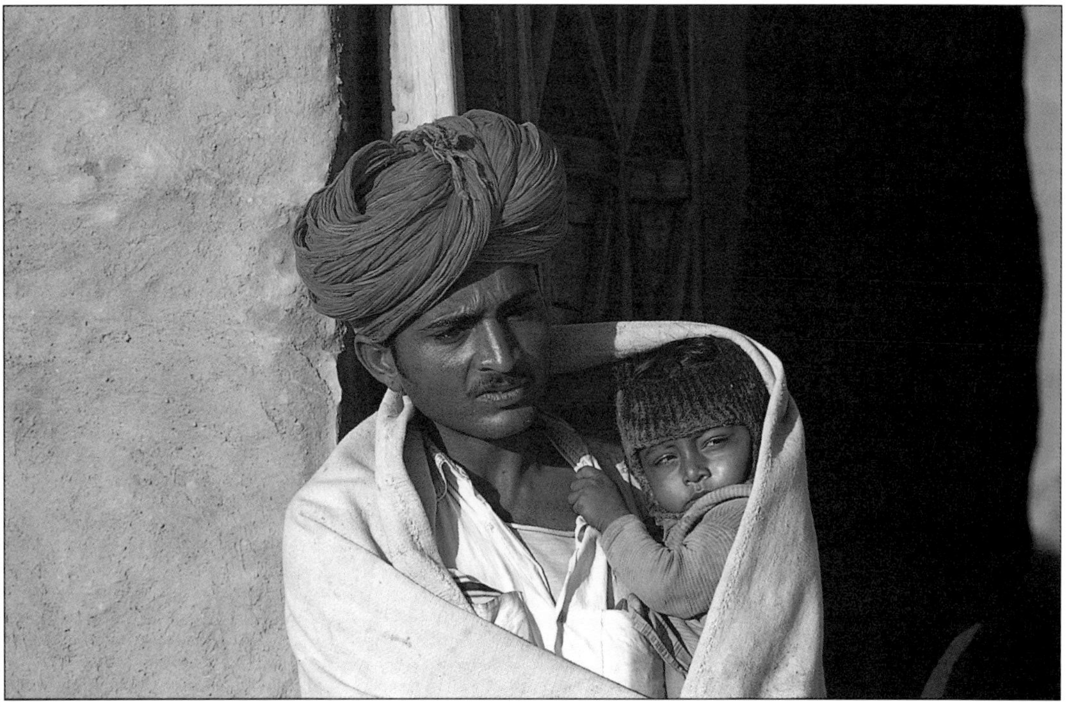

HUTCHSON LIBRARY

Causes of death

Some changes in the pattern of direct causes of death over the period from 1983 to 1996 can be observed. Some of these are positive. For example, although the number of women admitted with pregnancy-induced hypertension remained more or less the same, the proportion of deaths due to eclampsia dropped from 28 per cent in 1983-85 to 13 per cent in 1994-96. This is directly due to hospital policy since 1990 of timely administration of magnesium sulphate to all women with suspected cases of eclampsia except those who had received other drugs prior to admission.

On the other hand, it was disturbing to find that malaria was probably responsible for the deaths of 17 women in the 1994-96 series, of whom 9 women had a confirmed diagnosis of malaria. In contrast, there were no deaths related to malaria in the 1983-85 series. Further, there was a six-fold increase in the number of deaths due to severe anaemia (Hb < 6 gm%), probably all related to malaria. Deaths due to ruptured uterus were also slightly higher (7 per cent as compared to 4 per cent), but this was not statistically significant.

An equally disturbing finding was a significant increase in the proportion of deaths from complications of induced abortion. There were 15 maternal deaths related to induced abortion during 1994-96, as compared to only 4 during 1983-85. Of these, cases of septic abortion were three times higher in 1994-96 than in 1983-85 (11 vs. 4), and four women died from haemorrhage following induced abortion in 1994-96 as compared to none in 1983-85. All the abortion deaths in both series resulted from abortions carried out by unregistered and unskilled practitioners, sought because of the absence of proper abortion services, even at district referral hospitals.

A decade of (no) progress?

Since it opened in 1959, Zanana Hospital in Udaipur has remained the only tertiary care hospital in southern Rajasthan to render proper, specialist emergency obstetric services to the women not only of Udaipur city, but also Udaipur district, adjacent districts and the adjoining state of Madhya Pradesh. Although there are two other government health centres in the city, these only provide outpatient services and have not been upgraded to offer emergency obstetric care.

What have we at the Zanana Hospital learned from this comparison of the profile of women dying from complications of pregnancy, birth and induced abortion during the mid-1990s with those who died in the mid-1980s? A larger proportion suffered from infections and were severely anaemic than their counterparts in the mid-1980s. Nearly half of them did not receive any antenatal care, and the care received by most of the rest was erratic and inadequate. Many more had travelled longer distances and their families had spent more money getting them to the hospital. Many more arrived in a condition where nothing could be done to save them. Finally, more of them lost their lives from clearly preventable causes than the women who died in the decade before them, i.e. complications resulting from illegal abortions, and severe anaemia and malaria.

As regards socio-economic status, the women who died in 1994-96 were less educated and poorer, and more of them belonged to socially disadvantaged groups compared to those who had died in 1983-85, with one exception. There was a continuing high representation of Rajput women among maternal deaths both during 1983-85 (18 per cent) and 1994-96 (14 per cent), while that among other caste groups declined dramatically (from 35 per cent to 8 per cent).[11] Rajputs are a comparatively affluent and politically powerful caste group, but the women are subject to more restrictions than in other higher caste groups. This includes norms of *purdah*, segregation of women at social gatherings, *sati* (self-immolation at the death of the husband), female infanticide and non-acceptance of widows remarrying, which are still very commonly practised among them. The relationship between these manifestations of a high level of gender discrimination and the continuing high proportion of maternal deaths among Rajput women, warrants further scrutiny.

As regards causes of death, the increase in anaemia is directly related to an increase in the frequency of malaria caused by *Plasmodium falciparum*, which is more often fatal than other kinds of malaria, and is becoming increasingly resistant to chloroquine.[12]

It is not possible to determine from the data whether more women were having induced abortions than in the past, or whether more women who developed complications were able to reach the hospital or were being brought in for treatment in 1994-96 than in the past. Although there is little hard data, access to induced abortions from trained providers is mainly available only in large public and private hospitals in India, which means that poor, rural women have little or no easy access and continue to rely on unskilled providers and dangerous methods.[13] In any case, the proportion of deaths due to illegal abortions in recent years is unacceptable in a country where abortion has been legal since 1972.

These problems must be added to the fact that the health services at primary and referral level have not been improved sufficiently to safeguard women's lives until they can reach our hospital in cases of emergencies. Hence, although our efforts within the hospital to improve emergency obstetric care have made a difference in terms of saving some women's lives, we are able to succeed only up to a point.

These observations, based on experience, are mostly corroborated by data available for the state of Rajasthan, and suggest the following. The health status of the population has not improved in crucial aspects, including maternal mortality. The resurgence of malaria has taken a heavy toll of lives during the present decade and is especially dangerous in pregnancy. Further, since 1993-94, the state has also witnessed a resurgence of viral hepatitis which has also been associated with maternal deaths in recent years, although precise figures for these are not available.

Health service infrastructure has improved only marginally. Access to antenatal care has improved mainly with respect to immunisation against tetanus. The overall quality of antenatal care remains poor or is inaccessible. Worse still, abortion services as well as emergency obstetric services remain almost unavailable to the vast majority of rural women. Women who want to space pregnancies do so at great risk to their lives. This also points to the failure of the family planning programme to meet women's need for birth spacing methods.

The only positive change brought about by 'development' has been improvements in the network of roads and access to public transport.

In addition, there has been a general improvement in the level of awareness of the people, probably because of seasonal migration to urban areas in search of work, as more of them seem to know about the emergency obstetric services available at our hospital.

The consequence is what is reported here: many of the women who would have died at home in the past, and whose deaths would never have been counted, are now arriving at our hospital. However, because the problems of transport, money and distance remain so large for them, we are unable to prevent their deaths. Hence, the number of maternal deaths taking place in the hospital remains unabated after a decade.

To the extent that more women are now coming to the hospital from farther away and from poorer and lower caste groups, the changes in the profile of women dying over the past decade may be viewed as positive. However, unless and until all the factors contributing to the continuing high numbers of maternal deaths are put right, starting from the social and economic inequalities which place women at a disadvantage even before they become pregnant, women will continue to die needlessly in childbirth, both within and outside hospitals.

Correspondence

Dr Vinaya Pendse, 10/11 Banera House, Fatehpura, Udaipur 313004, Rajasthan, India.

References and Notes

1. The per capita income for Rajasthan was Rs. 3983 in 1990-91 (current prices), as compared to Rs. 4325 for India as a whole. Department of Family Welfare, 1992. *Family Welfare Programme in India – Year Book 1991-92.* New Delhi, , Ministry of Health and Family Welfare, Government of India.
2. The infant mortality rate for the state was 90 per 1000 live births in 1992, the fourth highest in the country. Office of the Registrar General, Vital Statistics Division, (various years). *Sample Registration System: Fertility and Mortality Indicators.* New Delhi, Ministry of Home Affairs, Government of India.
3. International Institute for Population Sciences, 1995. *National Family Health Survey: India, 1992-93, Introductory Report.* Bombay.
4. International Institute for Population Sciences, 1994. *National Family Health Survey: India, 1992-93.* Bombay.
5. Mari Bhat PN, K Navaneetham, S Irudaya Rajan, 1992. *Maternal Mortality in India: Estimates from an Econometric Model.* Dharwad, Population Research Centre, Working Paper 24 (January).
6. During 1981-1991, there were several major improvements in the state's infrastructure and in that of Udaipur district. The proportion of villages in the district connected by public transport increased from 21 per cent to 37 per cent. Villages with a primary school increased from 46 per cent of all villages to 73 per cent. Office of the Registrar General, India, 1993. *Census of India, 1991.* District Census Abstract, Udaipur district. New Delhi, Ministry of Home Affairs, Government of India.
7. Office of the Registrar General, India, 1991. Provisional Population Totals, *Census of India, 1991.* Paper 1 of 1991, Series 1. New Delhi, Ministry of Home Affairs, Government of India.
8. Department of Education, 1993. Selected Educational Statistics: 1990-91. New Delhi, Ministry of Human Resources Development, Government of India.
9. The definitions of 'poor' and 'very poor' are as follows: Those who are very poor are those with no regular employment or source of income and no assets. The 'poor' are defined as those whose household income is less than Rs. 1600/- per month (US$ 40) in 1994-96, which is below the 'poverty line' income specified by the Planning Commission of India as Rs. 2600/- per capita per month (US $65). For 1983-85, the poor were defined as those with a household income of less than Rs. 500 per month at current prices.
10. World Health Organization, 1992. *The Prevalence of Nutritional Anaemia in Women: A Tabulation of Available Information.* Geneva. WHO/MCH/MSM/92.3.
11. Rajputs are a warrior caste who rank immediately below the Brahmins in the caste hierarchy and form the top rung of the economic and political hierarchy.
12. World Health Organization-South East Asia Regional Office, 1999. *Health situation in the South East Asia Region 1994-1997.*
13. See for example Gupte M, Bandewar S, Pisal H, 1997. Abortion needs of women in India: a case study of rural Maharashtra. *Reproductive Health Matters.* No. 9(May):77-86.

Identifying Interventions to Prevent Maternal Mortality in Mexico: A Verbal Autopsy Study

Ana Langer, Bernardo Hernández, Cecilia García-Barrios, Gloria Luz Saldaña-Uranga and the National Safe Motherhood Committee of Mexico

In order to identify factors associated with maternal mortality that could be modified through concrete interventions, the National Safe Motherhood Committee in Mexico carried out a verbal autopsy study of all maternal deaths in 1995 in the states of Guerrero, Querétaro and San Luis Potosí. These deaths occurred mainly among poor, uneducated women. A physician provided care during delivery to only half the women who died; 44 per cent died in the community and 71 per cent during delivery and the puerperium. Causes of death identified through verbal autopsy were mostly consistent with those on death certificates, except as regards induced abortion. Health-seeking behaviour was analysed using the 'three delays' conceptual model. Lack of timely recognition of the severity of the condition, tolerance of a high threshold of pain, the belief that some complications are natural, cost, and perception of the quality of services as poor deterred women from seeking help. A comparison group consisted of women with similar complications to the women who died and were attended at the same hospitals, but who survived. The women who survived were five times more likely to be referred for and get the help they needed than those who died; they also had more years of schooling. The relationship between these warrants further study. Delays interacted with the nature and severity of complications and occurred at all levels. It might be valuable to develop standards and recommendations for avoiding and reducing delays at both household and primary and secondary care levels, within acceptable time limits for each of the major medical complications. These results were presented to local and national stakeholders who developed an extensive agenda for addressing maternal mortality at the state level.

MEXICO has one of the highest levels of maternal mortality in Latin America. According to official records, the maternal mortality ratio (MMR) decreased from 95 per 100,000 live births in 1980 to 53 per 100,000 in 1995,[1] the year when our study was conducted. In the 1990s, however, there was stagnation in the rate of improvement during the first years of the decade followed by an increasing ratio of deaths in 1994-95. This increase could reflect improvements in the identification of maternal deaths, but it could also be a consequence of the economic crisis and structural adjustment occurring in the country since the 1980s, which has had a particularly negative impact on the poorest sectors.

According to the World Health Organization (WHO), maternal mortality is on average 15 times higher in developing countries than in developed nations.[2] Far from disappearing, this gap may be increasing. In 1970-75, maternal deaths in middle-fertility countries in the Latin American region, Mexico included, were 8.65 times more likely to occur than in Canada (with the lowest MMR in the continent) but they were 15 times more likely to occur in 1985-89.[3] As with infant mortality, maternal mortality is an extremely sensitive indicator of the socio-economic conditions of the population, and probably the most revealing of social inequality in relation to the risk of death.

To analyse the factors leading to maternal

mortality in Mexico, the National Safe Motherhood Committee developed a verbal autopsy study of all maternal deaths in 1995 in three states with differing socio-economic characteristics – Guerrero, Querétaro and San Luis Potosí.[4] Later, the women who had died were compared with women with similar complications who were attended at the same medical centres, but who survived.

District and tertiary level health care facilities in these three states are concentrated in their capital cities, and are not easily accessible from the poorest areas. Criteria used to select the study sites included high maternal morbidity and mortality, professionals able to carry out the research, and willingness on the part of research groups, health institutions and non-governmental organisations to translate the knowledge generated into concrete activities directed towards a reduction in maternal deaths.

The objectives of the study were:

- to determine the actual maternal mortality ratio after adjusting for under-recording of maternal deaths in the three states;
- to characterise maternal deaths according to medical causes;
- to identify the personal, family and community factors that influenced health care seeking patterns and provision in the event of complications during pregnancy, labour and puerperium.

Conceptual framework

One useful classification of the factors contributing to a maternal death is as 'distant' or 'intermediate' determinants (following a model used for analysing child survival), according to the way they affect the process that potentially leads to death.[5] In this framework, 'distant' determinants (socio-economic conditions and cultural factors) have varying degrees of influence on 'intermediate' determinants (the woman's health, reproductive history, access to and use of health services and self-care). The intermediate determinants have a direct effect on the obstetric complications (i.e. haemorrhage, infection, unsafe abortion, toxaemia and so on) which are the eventual cause(s) of death.

The factors associated with maternal mortality may also be classified according to their origin as biomedical – health problems associated with the death, which are usually stated on death certificates or in hospital records - and non-biomedical – women's life conditions (largely affected by socio-economic and gender issues), the circumstances under which the maternal death happened and the accessibility and quality of health care. In many cases, there are no specific sources of information on the non-biomedical factors.

A third conceptual model is that of the three delays: delay in the decision to seek care, which includes delay in recognising an obstetric complication; delay in reaching the medical facility; and delay in obtaining the care needed to manage the problem.[6] This model is particularly useful for analysing the information obtained through the verbal autopsy technique. Biomedical and health-related factors identified in this study were classified according to the first two models, while social factors were ordered according to the three-delay model.

Study population and methodology

In order to define the study population, we prepared a list of all maternal deaths for each state, by selecting those death certificates coded as maternal deaths according to the WHO 9th International Classification of Diseases.[7] Because of the limitations of official statistics, an effort was also made to identify any maternal deaths that were not coded as such and add them to the list. For this purpose, we reviewed all death certificates for women aged 12 to 49 who had died due to complications likely to be related to reproduction, such as embolism, infection with no further specification, complications of anaesthesia, etc. Relatives of these women were visited, and the women's deaths were classified as maternal if their relatives confirmed that they had been pregnant in the year prior to their deaths.

For women who had died in a hospital, a comparison group was included with the aim of identifying factors that affected the risk of dying from maternal causes. This group was made up of women who had experienced obstetric complications similar to those faced by the women who had died and who had received care in the same hospital and season of the year, but who had survived.

The verbal autopsy technique

The verbal autopsy technique uses a structured and open-ended questionnaire with a close relative or friend of the deceased person, and asks them about the biomedical and social circumstances which led to the person's death, with special emphasis on the medical causes of death.[4] This technique has been used successfully in studies of both maternal and infant mortality.

In this study, the instrument included three close-ended sections in which the following groups of variables were recorded:

- women's socio-economic conditions, which included age, education, occupation and household characteristics, and reproductive history, such as number of pregnancies, miscarriages, deliveries, caesarean sections, stillbirths and live births;
- factors that allowed a medical diagnosis to be reached;
- non-clinical factors that contributed to the death (i.e. factors associated with the search for care and access to services).

The instrument also included an in-depth interview with the relative, during which they were asked to reconstruct in their own words the entire process from the beginning of the pregnancy until the woman's death. A detailed description of the qualitative component of this study will be published elsewhere.[8]

We preferred to administer the questionnaires to a woman relative who was also willing to be interviewed in depth and who had been in contact with the deceased woman during the process that led to her death. We interviewed the relatives of the women in the comparison group, too, rather than the women themselves, in order to avoid bias and increase comparability between the two groups.

All interviews were conducted in the homes of the informants by a trained interviewer. The study objectives and procedures were explained and consent was obtained by signature on a letter. For non-literate interviewees, a fingerprint was sufficient. When interviewing someone whose mother tongue was other than Spanish, a translator known in the community was invited to help the interviewer.

Maternal mortality ratios and underestimation

Our inspection of death certificates and community searches allowed us to identify 164 maternal deaths during 1995 in the participating states. This included 37 deaths in addition to the 127 reported in the vital statistics. Table 1 shows the number of recorded maternal deaths and the corresponding maternal mortality ratio (MMR), as well as the additional deaths we found in each state and the corresponding MMR. The under-recording of deaths in the official MMRs was obtained by comparing our figures with the vital statistics.[1]

The additional maternal deaths significantly increased the maternal mortality ratio from 49 per 100,000 births (vital statistics) to 64 per 100,000 (study data estimate) (p=.03). The extent of under-reporting – 23 per cent in the three states (27 per cent in Guerrero) – was less than that found some years ago in other sites in Mexico, which could be a result of improvements in the recording of vital statistics.[9-11]

Socio-demographic and reproductive characteristics of the women

Information about 145 maternal deaths was collected from interviews, with some differences

Table 1. Maternal mortality by state, Mexico, 1995

State	Recorded maternal deaths	MMR *	Maternal deaths found	MMR*	Under-recording (%)
Guerrero	64	44	88	60	27
Querétaro	24	58	26	63	8
San Luis Potosí	39	57	50	73	22
TOTAL	127	49	164	64	23

** Maternal Mortality Ratio = number of maternal deaths per 100,000 recorded live births*

in the response rate to certain questions. These differences did not vary by state. The socio-demographic characteristics of the women who died are presented in Table 2. On average, the women were 28.6 years old and 93 per cent had a steady partner. They had a low level of formal education: 20 per cent had never gone to school and 39 per cent had not finished primary school. A large majority (88 per cent) did not have a paid job and were not entitled to social security (84 per cent); these proportions are far below the national and state averages for adult women for years of education, employment and entitlement to social security.

Almost half the women (42 per cent) had been living in extremely poor conditions and crowded households (an average of 3.7 persons per room). As in most studies on maternal mortality in developing countries, the group with the highest concentration of maternal deaths were poor, uneducated women with limited financial independence.

As many as 24 per cent of the women who died were primiparae, 34 per cent had had one to three pregnancies, and 42 per cent four pregnancies or more. The average parity of 3.6 in this sample is high given that the total fertility rate in Mexico in 1995 was 2.6.[12] In 51 per cent of cases, the period of time between the pregnancy that led to the woman's death and the previous pregnancy was shorter than two years. A quarter of the sample had had a miscarriage or an induced abortion in previous pregnancies. These women's deaths left an average of 3.2 children motherless at home.

Table 3 presents selected variables related to maternal health care prior to the women's deaths. Seventy-one per cent of the women received antenatal care in the pregnancy that ended in their deaths; that included 2.5 antenatal visits on average, 2.1 with a doctor and 0.4 with a

Table 2. Socio-demographic characteristics of women who died due to maternal causes*

Variables	Guerrero		Querétaro		San Luis Potosí		Total	
	%	(no.)	%	(no.)	%	(no.)	%	(no.)
Age (years)	27.5		28.9		30.4		28.6	
Average (S.D.)	(8.4)		(8.5)		(7.8)		(8.4)	
Schooling								
None	20.0	(14)	25.0	(6)	16.0	(7)	20.0	(27)
Incomplete primary school	40.0	(28)	25.0	(6)	27.0	(20)	39.0	(54)
Complete primary school	20.0	(14)	21.0	(5)	23.0	(10)	21.0	(29)
Secondary school or higher	20.0	(14)	29.0	(7)	14.0	(6)	20.0	(27)
Occupation								
Housewife	88.0	(66)	88.0	(21)	89.0	(40)	88.0	(127)
Worker	11.0	(8)	12.0	(3)	9.0	(4)	11.0	(15)
Student	1.0	(1)	0.0	(0)	2.0	(1)	1.0	(2)
Entitled to social security services	15.0	(11)	16.0	(4)	18.0	(8)	16.0	(16)
Marital status								
Living with a partner	29.0	(22)	15.0	(4)	23.0	(10)	25.0	(36)
Married	62.0	(46)	81.0	(21)	73.0	(32)	68.0	(99)
Dwelling condition index								
Very low	22.0	(16)	8.0	(2)	14.0	(6)	17.0	(24)
Low	26.0	(19)	23.0	(6)	25.0	(11)	25.0	(36)
Medium	52.0	(37)	69.0	(18)	61.0	(27)	58.0	(82)

** Numbers in parentheses indicate the number of women in each category*

midwife. It is not possible to say whether the antenatal care was of poor or good quality, as a formal assessment has never been carried out in these settings. A physician provided care during delivery for only 51 per cent of the cases, while for 26 per cent traditional birth attendants (TBAs) were in charge and for 23 per cent the women was attended by 'others' during birth.

Place of death was a hospital for 36 per cent of the women in the sample, while the rest died in their own or a TBA's house, in the road or the street while trying to get help, or while being transported to hospital.

Most of the women died around the time of delivery. Nine per cent died in the first half of pregnancy, 20 per cent in the second half, 25 per cent during delivery, 25 per cent on the day after giving birth and 21 per cent between day two and day 42 of the post-natal period. The low proportion who received medical attention while giving birth, the high proportion who died in the community, and the fact that 71 per cent died as a consequence of a delivery-related complication or in the six weeks thereafter, reflects a lack of access to, inadequate utilisation of and poor quality of delivery and emergency obstetric services in these communities.

The verbal autopsy instrument included a section on medical complications. This information was analysed by two experts who established the cause(s) of death. In the 99 cases where there was information from both the death certificate and the verbal autopsy, there was an 80 per cent concurrence on the cause of death between the two sources. Since death certificates are usually a reliable source of information in Mexico, this level of concurrence supports the validity of verbal autopsy for establishing biomedical causes of death when analysed by experts.

It is noteworthy that induced abortion was the cause of death responsible for making the discrepancy between the two sources as high as it was, since fewer deaths were classified as abortion-related on the death certificates. Legal restrictions on induced abortion in Mexico, and the implications of recording an abortion-related death for the woman's family and the health care provider, can explain this discrepancy.

Delay in the decision to seek care

Key factors which contribute to a delay in seeking care are the ability of the woman and/or her family to recognise that her symptoms are serious enough to justify medical care, concerns about the quality and cost of health services, and the distance they would have to travel to obtain care.[6] In this study, the severity of the woman's condition was recognised in only 56 per cent of the cases during the first 24 hours after problems arose; between the second and seventh day in 17 per cent of cases, and only after a week or more in 11 per cent of cases. In 16 per cent of the cases, the presence of complications was not recognised at all (Table 4).

Table 3. Reproductive health care of women who died of maternal causes (selected variables)*

Variables	Guerrero		Querétaro		San Luis Potosí		Total	
	%	(no.)	%	(no.)	%	(no.)	%	(no.)
No antenatal care for this pregnancy	22.0	(16)	38.0	(10)	33.0	(14)	29.0	(40)
Personnel at delivery								
Midwife	39.0	(15)	4.0	(1)	27.0	(9)	26.0	(25)
Doctor	42.0	(16)	58.0	(14)	56.0	(19)	51.0	(49)
Other	19.0	(7)	38.0	(9)	13.0	(6)	23.0	(22)
Place of death								
Community	56.8	(42)	69.2	(18)	73.3	(33)	64.1	(93)
Hospital	43.2	(32)	30.8	(8)	26.7	(12)	35.9	(52)

** Numbers in parentheses indicate the number of cases in each category*

The in-depth interviews provide some insight into why in a considerable proportion of cases the severity of symptoms was recognised only very late or not at all. Firstly, women in poor settings tolerate a high threshold of pain and other health problems. Secondly, people believe that complications during pregnancy and delivery are normal or natural events.

'In the fourth month she started to have severe headaches. We did not visit the doctor because we thought it was normal. She had also had these headaches in previous pregnancies.' (Husband)

In 90 per cent of cases where the severity of symptoms was understood to be serious, a decision to seek help was made: 70 per cent sought help immediately or in less than four hours, 10 per cent took a day and the remaining 20 per cent took longer (Table 4). Again, the perception of services as being of poor quality, and concerns about the cost, were shown to be deterrents to seeking help more quickly.

'She never visited a doctor because she thought that hospitals killed people.' (Mother)

'She got heavier and heavier, and she had great pain in her left arm. But they did not seek any help because doctors charge too much and they had no money.' (Mother-in-law)

Women's lack of autonomy in decision-making was also identified as an obstacle to seeking timely care: one woman had never had a check-up during her pregnancies because her husband did not allow it.

There is no recognised rule by which to establish whether help was sought early enough. Obviously, the time that elapses before a woman seeks help has different implications according to the type and severity of the complication.

'They sought help only when she got very sick. The doctor said it was too late, that she had died because she had lost so much blood.'

Delay in arriving at a health facility

The time it took for the women to get to the first health facility was under an hour in 56 per cent of cases, between one and four hours in 33 per cent, and longer than four hours in 11 per cent of cases (Table 4). In the qualitative interviews, relatives identified the lack of adequate means of transport as the main barrier. Because obstetric emergencies usually require immediate treatment, the time it took half of the women to get to the health facility may have been an important contributory factor in their deaths. Distance and other geographic barriers are even worse in other regions of Mexico than those found in the three states where this study took place.

To reduce delays, health providers could use the opportunity offered by antenatal care to teach women to recognise complications that require care. Innovative means of transport could be discussed and information could be provided about the appropriate institution to attend. Sensitising women and their families during antenatal visits to seek delivery care early in labour, and emergency care when they or others first suspect there may be a problem, may be one of the most important roles antenatal care could play in reducing maternal mortality.

Delay in the provision of adequate care

Arrival at a health facility does not ensure that a woman will receive the treatment necessary to save her life. Half the women in this sample (51 per cent) went to a facility where the required care was not available. They then decided to go or were referred to another facility, with substantial delay resulting. For 37 per cent of the women, the time that elapsed between the first and the last facility they attended was longer than 12 hours (Table 4). The availability and quality of care are clearly lacking; although health facilities may be within a reachable distance, they may not be able to offer adequate care.

'Her husband walked for 15 minutes to find a car. He picked up his wife and took her to the health centre, which was closed at the time. From there, they went to a larger town, Amealco, where providers told them they would transfer the woman to San Juan del Río, because they were short of equipment and drugs. There, she got intravenous fluids but nothing else. A police car finally transported her to the general hospital in Querétaro, but by then she was dead.' (Neighbour)

Table 4. Delays in the search for, access to and provision of adequate care

Variables	Guerrero		Querétaro		San Luis Potosí		Total	
	%	(no. of women)	%	(no. of women)	%	(no. of women)	%	(no. of women)
Time required to recognise complication								
1 day	53.0	(25)	72.0	(18)	49.0	(21)	56.0	(64)
2 - 7 days	13.0	(6)	8.0	(2)	26.0	(11)	17.0	(19)
8 days or more	17.0	(8)	12.0	(3)	7.0	(3)	11.0	(14)
Never detected	17.0	(8)	8.0	(2)	18.0	(8)	16.0	(18)
Decision to seek help[a]	92.0	(36)	87.0	(20)	89.0	(31)	90.0	(87)
Time elapsed between realising there is a complication and asking for help								
Immediately	50.0	(17)	38.0	(9)	40.0	(14)	43.0	(40)
$<$4 hours	24.0	(8)	21.0	(5)	34.0	(12)	27.0	(25)
$\leq$1 day	14.0	(5)	8.0	(2)	6.0	(2)	10.0	(9)
$>$1 day	12.0	(4)	33.0	(8)	20.0	(7)	20.0	(19)
Time to arrive at first health care facility								
$<$1 hour	63.0	(22)	56.0	(13)	49.0	(13)	56.0	(48)
1 - 4 hours	31.0	(11)	18.0	(4)	48.0	(13)	33.0	(28)
5 hours or more	6.0	(2)	26.0	(6)	3.0	(1)	11.0	(9)
Sought help in another place[b]	46.0	(16)	30.0	(6)	72.0	(21)	51.0	(43)
Time elapsed between first and last care provision[c]								
$<$1 hour	24.0	(6)	37.0	(9)	11.0	(3)	23.0	(18)
1 - 4 hours	28.0	(7)	25.0	(6)	0.0	(0)	17.0	(13)
5 - 12 hours	12.0	(3)	8.0	(2)	46.0	(13)	23.0	(18)
$>$12 hours	36.0	(9)	30.0	(7)	43.0	(12)	37.0	(28)
Waiting time for care provision[c]								
Immediately	40.0	(9)	67.0	(12)	68.0	(13)	58.0	(34)
$<$1 hour	14.0	(3)	6.0	(1)	16.0	(3)	12.0	(7)
1 - 4 hours	32.0	(7)	16.0	(3)	11.0	(2)	20.0	(12)
$>$4 hours	14.0	(3)	11.0	(2)	5.0	(1)	10.0	(6)
Number of facilities visited[c]								
1	46.0	(13)	67.0	(12)	34.0	(10)	47.0	(35)
2	43.0	(12)	33.0	(6)	52.0	(15)	44.0	(33)
3 or more	11.0	(3)	0.0	(0)	14.0	(4)	9.0	(7)

(a) Among those who detected the complication;
(b) Among those who arrived at the first care facility;
(c) Among those who sought care.

The more time women had to spend going from one health facility to another, the greater the risk of death; in this study, more than 50 per cent of the women had to go to two or more health facilities. However, it is also the case that referral to a second health facility, although time-consuming, may also be life-saving in a critical way, if the referral centre is able to provide the treatment that the woman needs.

In hospitals, too, there were problems of quality of care even though, theoretically, well-trained staff and essential equipment and drugs are available.

'They only visited her the morning after the baby was born. They got scared when they realised that her face and nails were blue, very dark. The resident left the room saying nothing. I looked for the doctor. He and a nurse transferred my daughter to another section of the hospital, and they did not let us in. After an hour they came out to tell us that my daughter had died of a haemorrhage.' (Mother)

Waiting time at the health facility was another important component of this delay: 28 per cent of the women in our sample had to wait to be seen for an hour or more, which may well be too long in an emergency, especially given other delays.

Type of delay in relation to cause of death

Our data highlight the various complexities involved in seeking care, but separating the data by type of delay may over-simplify the reality from women's point of view. Usually, a chain of delays takes place that interacts with the nature and severity of obstetric complications. For example, the women who died from sepsis were the ones who recognised they had a complication at a later stage, who spent more time making up their minds to look for help, and who were among those who had to wait longer to be treated. On the other hand, women who died due to haemorrhage were those who tended to need more time to reach a health care facility, and who more often did not receive care in the first facility they attended. Finally, women who died as a consequence of complications of induced abortion were the ones who more often spent more than four hours getting from the first to the last health care facility.

Comparison between women who died and women who survived

By comparing the women who died in a hospital with those who survived similar obstetric problems, we hoped to identify specific circumstances or behaviours which increased the chances of survival, and which might help us to identify interventions based on these findings, to help to extend awareness of protective behaviours in the community.

The desire to be pregnant, the utilisation of antenatal care, the length of pregnancy at the first antenatal appointment and the type of provider were not significantly different between the two groups, even after adjustment for age and parity.

The only socio-economic variable that was statistically significant in the comparison between the two groups was the number of years of schooling of the woman and her partner. Among the deceased women, 16 per cent had never gone to school and 37 per cent had not finished primary school, as compared to 8 per cent and 18 per cent among those who survived, respectively ($p<0.05$). Similarly, 21 per cent of the deceased women's partners had never gone to school and 45 per cent had not finished primary school, as compared to 9 per cent and 19 per cent in the partners of survivors, respectively ($p<0.05$).

There was only one statistically significant difference in the variables used to describe the 'three delays' - the lack of referral to another health care facility when referral was called for. The women who died were five times more at risk of not being referred than those who survived (OR 5.27, CI 1.06-26.16). There might have been an association between schooling and referral. Indeed, based on our results we can formulate the hypothesis that a higher level of schooling helped women to take the decision to go on to another health centre, or encouraged a different attitude amongst health providers, who more often referred women with more education on to facilities where they received the care they needed.

Discussion and conclusions

On the one hand, this study confirms the findings of similar studies: first, maternal deaths occur mostly among poor, uneducated women with limited decision-making power and autonomy;

and second, that maternal deaths are the consequence of a long and complex chain of delays, and only in a few cases can a death be attributed to one specific event. Furthermore, it confirmed that maternal mortality ratios are under-estimated, though in this case, under-recording was lower than in previous studies conducted in other regions of Mexico.[10,11] This might be due to measures that the government has established in recent years, such as the inclusion of a question about pregnancy status on the death certificates of women of reproductive age.

On the other hand, the study has produced some new findings. First, we were able to demonstrate that in settings where death certificates are reliable as sources of information, such as Mexico, verbal autopsies do not add much to the classification of biomedical causes of maternal deaths. However, both sources of causes of deaths have important limitations: death certificates only record primary causes of death and therefore do not indicate other important and related medical complications, while the validity and reliability of the information obtained through verbal autopsies varies according to the quality of the information each interviewee provides. Based on these findings, we would not recommend verbal autopsies as a way of exploring biomedical causes of maternal death in countries where vital statistics are of an acceptable quality.

We found the three-delays framework extremely useful as a conceptual basis for data collection and analysis. However, it was difficult to draw conclusions and specific recommendations based on this approach. The development of standards, based on the type and urgency of the medical complications, would be an important contribution towards understanding the role of the different factors that lead to maternal deaths, and would provide grounds for specific recommendations for women and their families, as well as for health care providers at primary and secondary level, e.g. the amount of time within which help should be accessed for specific complications.

In this study, we included a comparison group, expecting this to provide useful information, especially regarding protective behaviours, which could then be translated into specific recommendations. Unfortunately, this previously untested approach produced very few clues. Although from a conceptual point of view we chose the best possible controls, the information found in the medical records was very poor. As a consequence, a group that in theory would have been well suited for comparison, in practice may have been very different from the women who died in terms of medical diagnosis and severity of complications. In spite of these limitations, we were able to confirm the crucial role played by years of schooling (both the woman's and her partner's) as a protective factor. Although the study design does not allow us to draw definitive conclusions, we hypothesise that more schooling positively influenced maternal outcomes; those with more schooling were much more likely to be referred for help to a facility that was equipped to provide them with the care they needed.

Probing the type of delay in relation to cause of death provided some interesting leads. In-depth analysis of this interaction would give important clues as to what complications women and their families recognised as severe and worth treating, and what problems received priority attention from health care providers, which are grounded in socio-cultural and medical factors.

As regards interventions to reduce maternal deaths, two specific recommendations arose from this study. First, further research is called for on our hypothesis that level of schooling affected women's ability to seek and be referred for care. If this proves true, then empowerment of women and their families to feel entitled to access care, and sensitisation of health care workers regarding potential biases in their treatment of the poorest women, are both important. Second, we suggested it might be valuable to develop standards and recommendations for avoiding and reducing delays at both household, primary and secondary care levels, within acceptable time limits for each of the major medical complications.

Finally, one of our main objectives with this study was to raise awareness among national and state-level key players about maternal health as a priority public health problem, and to suggest relevant and feasible interventions to decrease maternal deaths. To this end, we presented the findings of the study in conferences in all three states where the research was conducted and in a national workshop. Participants in these included policy-makers responsible for matters related to women's health (health services, education, transport and communications, among others), as well as local non-governmental organisations and researchers.

As a result of these sessions, a long list of relevant interventions were identified by the research teams and local collaborators, some more feasible than others, but all of them recognised internationally as important. These included epidemiological surveillance and medical audit of maternal deaths; better roads and transport systems; education at community level on danger signs that mean care is needed; promotion of health-seeking behaviour; ensuring that all women have access to free obstetric and emergency obstetric services; upgrading health facilities and linking them through an efficient referral system; training health care providers; and elaborating institutional norms and guidelines. These recommendations have since been adopted as an agenda at the state level, an acknowledgement by local stakeholders that maternal mortality is a pressing problem that cannot be ignored.

Acknowledgements

Members of the state Safe Motherhood Committee who participated in this study include: Asencio Villegas and Hugo Alarcón (Guerrero); Enrique Hidalgo and Ramón Macillas (Querétaro); and Maribel Martínez and Andrea Saldaña (San Luis Potosí). We thank María del Carmen Elu, co-ordinator of the National Safe Motherhood Committee, for continuous help and support; Sofía Reynoso for training of interviewers; Minerva Romero for help in the collection of death certificates, and personnel from the Directorate of Evaluation and Statistics of the Ministry of Health for the coding of death certificates. We also appreciated the collaboration of the Ministry of Health and the Instituto Nacional de Estadística, Geografía e Informática (INEGI) for access to mortality statistics. We are grateful to the World Bank (and especially Anne Tinker) for their financial support for this project and their commitment to the cause of safe motherhood in developing countries.

Correspondence

Dr Ana Langer, Population Council, Escondida 110, Coyoacán, Mexico DF 04000, México. Fax: 52-5-554-1226. E-mail: alanger@mpsnet.com.mx

References

1. Dirección General de Estadística e Informática Estadísticas Vitales. Mexico: Secretaría de Salud, corresponding years.
2. World Health Organization, 1990. Focus: maternal mortality. A silent tragedy. *International Journal of Gynecology and Obstetrics*. 31:295.
3. Rajs D, 1996. Maternal mortality. *Adult Mortality in Latin America*. Timaeus I, Chackiel J, Ruzicka L (eds). Clarendon Press, Oxford, 276-94.
4. Ronsmans C, Campbell O, 1994. *Verbal Autopsies for Maternal Deaths. Report of a Workshop*. London School of Hygiene and Tropical Medicine, London.
5. Mosley WH, Chen L, 1984. An analytic framework for the study of child survival in developing countries. *Population and Development Review*. 10(Suppl):191-214.
6. Thaddeus S, Maine D, 1990. Too Far to Walk. Maternal Mortality in Context (Findings from a Multidisciplinary Review).
7. World Health Organization, 1978. *International Classification of Diseases*. 9th edition. Washington DC.
8. Castro R, Campero L, Hernández B, Langer A. "She started with intense headaches, but we thought it was normal": A study of maternal mortality in Mexico through verbal autopsies. (Submitted for publication).
9. Langer A, Hernández B, Lozano R, 1994. La morbi-mortalidad en México: niveles y causas. In: *Maternidad Sin Riesgos en México*. Langer A, Elu MC (eds). Comité Promotor por una Maternidad sin Riesgos, Mexico City, 23-29.
10. Langer A, Elu MC (eds), 1994. *Maternidad Sin Riesgos en México*. Comité Promotor por una Maternidad sin Riesgos, Mexico City.
11. Reyes S, 1994. *Mortalidad Materna en México*. Mexican Institute of Social Security, Mexico City.
12. Consejo Nacional de Población, 1997. *La Situación Demográfica en México*. Mexico City.

Nutrition in Pregnancy in Rural Vietnam: Poverty, Self-Sacrifice and Fear of Obstructed Labour

Do Thi Ngoc Nga and Martha Morrow

Maternal and infant mortality and morbidity continue to be of concern in Vietnam, where nutritional surveys have found low weight gain in pregnancy to be widespread. Fear of obstructed labour as one explanation of voluntary food restriction ('eating down') remains untested. Qualitative methods were used in this preliminary study in rural Vietnam to investigate influences on women's intake of food in pregnancy. Results show that 'eating down' was a contributory factor in low intake of nutritious food in pregnancy, but is best understood in the context of social, cultural, economic and environmental circumstances. Against a backdrop of poverty, other major influences were normative role expectations of self-sacrifice by women, ignorance about the physiological demands of pregnancy and lack of appropriate reproductive health services and education for women and their families on the part of health workers. Long-term, multisectoral approaches are needed, including discussion of normative and gender-based role expectations; education for women, their families, health workers and the community on women's nutritional and other health needs in pregnancy and how these also benefit infants; improvements in health facilities and services for women; addressing poverty as it affects pregnant women in relation to access to food and heavy workloads; and programme planning based on research results that takes a broader view of maternal and infant health, particularly as Vietnam undergoes rapid social change and development.

NUTRITIONAL status is a crucial component of reproductive health. Previous surveys in Vietnam have found that chronic energy deficiency (body mass index below 18.7) affects 40-50 per cent of reproductive-age women, with the highest rates in rural areas, where 80 per cent of the population resides. Up to 79 per cent of pregnant women are deficient in iron.[1] Vegetables and rice comprise the bulk of intake among rural women, who consume only one-third of their calcium and iron requirements.[2] Even in an area receiving World Food Programme supplements, only 37 per cent of women gained eight kilos or more during pregnancy.[3] Nationwide estimates in 1990 put the rate of low birth weight (under 2500 grams) in Vietnam at 17 per cent.[4] In the words of a recent UNICEF working paper:

The birth weight of a newborn child is a sensitive indicator of both the child and the mother. For the child, it is also an indicator of future health status throughout childhood and even into adolescence and adulthood.[5]

There has been debate about the impact of pregnancy food supplementation on birth weight.[5,6] While some argue that pre-pregnancy anthropometric measurements are better predictors of preterm delivery[7] and birth weight,[8,9] a recent 5-year randomised, controlled trial in the Gambia recorded increases in maternal and fetal weight when chronically malnourished women ate a high-energy biscuit daily.[10]

Maternal health status is closely linked to dietary intake during pregnancy; anaemia may shift a woman's balance towards death during delivery.[5] Inadequate nutrition is related directly or indirectly to most maternal deaths; along with anaemia, stunted growth leads to obstructed labour and vulnerability to infection.[5] The detached intellectual debate about women's ability to survive pregnancy on very low intake by nutrient 'efficiency' has little relevance to the reality of poor outcomes and loss where serious undernutrition is the norm.[11]

Low pregnancy weight gain in some societies has been attributed to 'eating down', ie. deliberately restricting consumption for fear that a larger baby will cause obstructed labour.[12,13] Nutritionists have posited that this takes place in Vietnam, where anxiety about parturition is natural given high rates of maternal mortality (estimates of 107-576 per 100 000 live births).[1,2,14]

Obstructed labour is dangerous and is directly implicated in about 11 per cent of maternal deaths worldwide,[5] though its exact role in Vietnam is unknown. Some commentators argue that efforts to increase fetal birth weight may be irresponsible if safe, effective surgical delivery options are unavailable.[15] However, the Gambia study concluded that increases in fetal head circumference in the group receiving supplements were not large enough to influence complication rates.[10] Low birth weight, on the other hand, unquestionably endangers offspring, who may face poor health along with impaired pelvic development, setting up a cycle of risk for the next generation of mothers[5] and is probably implicated in widespread malnutrition and stunting among Vietnamese children under the age of five (up to 49 per cent in 1990).[1] There is an unassailable moral imperative to address the health needs of infants, girls and women, and to avoid setting up a competitive value scale between these population groups.

Since Vietnam moved to a modified market economy in 1986, many have benefited from rapid economic growth. However, the transition from collectivised farming to household-based production has put pressure on rural families, who now need cash to purchase previously subsidised public services.[1] Poor rural women are least likely to have the training and capital to take advantage of the new system.[16,17]

Approximately 86 per cent of women are employed, mainly in physically arduous occupations, particularly agriculture,[18] where they form the majority of unskilled labour.[19] Total fertility rates were about 3.1 in 1993 (higher in rural areas),[18,20] reflecting lack of adherence to the official two-child policy. About half of rural women had had no antenatal care in the five years preceding a recent national survey.[18] Within this context, poor maternal nutrition is of concern. The Seventh Congress of the Communist Party of Vietnam (1991) set targets for reducing the rates of maternal mortality and morbidity and infant mortality by half, by the year 2000. Food and micronutrient supplementation, health education and the home garden movement are widely promoted within reproductive health interventions.

While Vietnamese surveys give ample proof of nutritional inadequacies in pregnancy, the suggestion that women practice 'eating down' has not been investigated. This preliminary study aimed to contribute to reproductive health interventions in Vietnam by exploring constraints on food consumption in pregnancy. Health interventions often fail because of over-reliance on the conventional wisdom or simple statistical associations in determining causality.[21] Women's health behaviours are grounded in specific socio-economic and cultural complexities; qualitative or combined research methods can facilitate investigation of attitudes and practices from the perspective of those being studied, particularly in the context of rapid development.[22-24] These methods have been used successfully to explore fertility decisions in Vietnam.[25] Results from this type of study can be used to inform larger-scale surveys to determine population prevalences of particular findings.

The study

The study, undertaken during 1996, aimed primarily to explore social, cultural, economic and environmental influences on the food intake of pregnant rural women. The study site was a typical farming commune, located about 50 km from Hanoi, which had not yet benefited from a nutrition education programme. Most women in the commune were working in agriculture, some as daily labourers, and many had extra jobs (vending, basket making and brick making). In 1995 the population included 917 women with at least two children. About 500-600 men had migrated to the cities for work. Prior to meeting the respondents, the principal researcher visited commune health workers to obtain information about the site, including patterns of maternal health care.

Selection of participants was based on health centre records, which indicated that there were about 70 pregnant women in the second or third trimester of pregnancy. Those in the second trimester (54) were selected for the study on the grounds that this period of pregnancy is usually characterised by relatively good appetite and less fatigue compared with the first and third trimesters. Ethical clearance for the study was given by the Institute of Sociology, National Center for Social Sciences and Humanities of Vietnam in Hanoi. Potential respondents were assured of their right not to participate and the confidentiality of their responses. Ten were invited to join a focus group discussion (FGD), of whom nine accepted. It later emerged that one participant was found to be in her third trimester. The remaining 45 women were invited for in-depth interviews and all agreed to participate. Thus, all but one of the 54 women actually in their second trimester of pregnancy either participated in the FGD or an individual interview.

The women in the focus group discussion were asked to identify publicly-expressed norms and attitudes, clarify terminology and modify a list of possible influences on women's dietary intake during pregnancy, which was to be used for individual interviews. The modified 'theme list' included: income, food availability, distance from home to market, time for shopping and cooking, personal food preferences, forms of food avoidance, knowledge about dietary and rest requirements in pregnancy, family food distribution, 'eating down', living in an extended family, migration of husbands, views of health care, doing extra jobs and pressure to bear sons.

Individual in-depth interviews, held in women's homes in May-June, included basic demographic questions (age, occupation, parity) and open-ended questions drawn from the theme list to stimulate discussion. Standard qualitative methods of thematic analysis were used. Discussion over several days between the authors led to a shared interpretation of patterns.

All the respondents worked primarily in agriculture, with secondary jobs in vending or handicrafts. Their ages ranged from 19 to 40, and all but 15 were multiparous. Half had husbands working in Hanoi. The names used in this paper are not their real names.

Socio-cultural influences on food consumption

Analysis of FGD and interview data revealed that eating habits in pregnancy were best understood to result from the interaction of sociocultural influences aggravated by poverty, ignorance about pregnancy needs and inadequate health services. 'Eating down' could not fully account for nutritional practices.

While Vietnamese woman are equal to men in law, in practice their position is often distinctly lower in terms of education, wages and customary practices.[26,27] Traditional norms dictate that a married woman should produce children (including at least one son), endure hardship without complaint, be frugal and industrious, and acquiesce to the wishes of husbands and parents-in-law, with priority accorded to the young and old.[28]

Questions about diet in pregnancy evoked smiles and the response, 'We eat as usual in pregnancy', which means rice, vegetable and pickles, rarely accompanied by (more costly) meat or tofu. Meals were taken together, and special items such as meat were offered to young children, the elderly and less commonly to husbands. As part of the woman's body, the growing fetus is accorded no special treatment. Women ignored their own needs while undertaking the bulk of household work and caring for the young, the old and the sick. This suggests that traditional gender roles remain normative, even during pregnancy.

'Sometimes I want to eat this or eat that but I am afraid my in-laws would think I just want to satisfy my mouth.' (Kim)

Occasionally women were urged to eat if they showed an aversion to food during pregnancy, but only to maintain their energy and their ability to work. Otherwise, even though they were pregnant, they still got the least good food.

'My child is nearly two and always sick, so if we have any tasty (ie. high-calorie) foods we give them to her. If there's anything left over, my old, weak father-in-law and my disabled sister-in-law get some. My mother-in-law and I are the main labour force in the family but we hardly ever get anything tasty to eat.' (Lan)

Daily patterns were virtually unchanged in pregnancy. Farming has periods of intensity and crucial seasonal demands. The typically heavy, lengthy labouring day continued unabated during pregnancy for most of the women, and working hard remained the principal descriptive feature of their lives. Questions about taking rest provoked much laughter in the focus group discussion, and responses such as this were typical:

'We live in the countryside, so we usually work until the day we deliver. And some women deliver in the field or in the road!' (Huong)

Some women even argued that regular work until delivery would facilitate childbirth.

'It is said that if pregnant women continue to work until delivery it will be easy in delivery.' (Anh)

Multiparas had worked until delivery in the past and that had not changed. Linh, in her ninth month of pregnancy said, when encountered on her way to the fields:

'How can I rest when other family members are working, even my old father-in-law? I knew you were coming to see me today but… everyone else in the family went to the field. I didn't want them to think I was lazy.'

'My husband told me if I felt tired I should rest, but being a daughter-in-law I feel ashamed if I do.' (Chi)

'I'm always the first to get up. I make the fire, boil water and cook breakfast. When the others get up breakfast is ready.' (Loan)

Most women worked 16-18 hours per day, as elsewhere in Vietnam,[1] depending on the season. Socially constructed definitions of the good wife, mother and daughter-in-law were reflected in a sense of shame about letting up, even in pregnancy, unless someone like a new sister-in-law could be enlisted to take up the workload, which happened in one case until the sister-in-law too became pregnant.

After breakfast, most women went to the fields, which might involve a long commute on foot or bicycle. The poorest hired out their labour for 5 000 – 10 000 dong (about USD 0.50-1.00) per half-day. Field work usually resumed after lunch. Kept busy with housework, childcare, cooking or extra jobs like embroidery, few took the customary noontime nap. Some worked part time in brick-making or as market vendors. These results are consistent with the Viet Nam Living Standards Survey, which found rural women worked an average of 1.4 jobs.[29] Respondents apparently accepted exhaustion as normal.

'My father-in-law and my husband can have a short sleep at noon but my mother-in-law and I have much that remains to be done. How can we rest?' (Du)

'Sometimes I want to stay at home to rest but thinking of the rice being ripe I force myself to go to the field.' (Phuong)

A long working day leaves little time for cooking, which may indirectly influence food consumption. Relentless work and insufficient rest also predisposed the women not to eat very much, further compromising nutrient intake. Many felt inclined to eat only light, watery meals:

'I know crab is good for pregnant women but it takes time to prepare so I don't eat it'. (Phuong)

'Sometimes I feel too exhausted to have food. I only want something to drink and I always feel sleepy.' (Huong)

The influence of poverty

The women's low status is reflected in their lack of control over household expenditure, including on food. Spending was ordained by mothers-in-law and/or husbands, a custom that was not openly questioned by respondents, as with other issues related to role and status.

'Sometimes I want to buy some more food for meals but I feel embarrassed to ask my husband for money.' (Anh)

The role of gender differences, while important, however, should not be seen in isolation but against a backdrop of financial insecurity, a reality of rural life for many. The women are the first to work hard and the last to be self-indulgent with food or rest in the context of the wider stresses of poverty, including the demands of the market economy – and it is this that makes pregnancy more perilous.

Vietnam is one of the world's poorest countries, and still suffers from the legacy of years of war and the destruction of its infrastructure and environment. Following the 'liberalisation' of the economy and reductions in public services, schooling became more costly. There is evidence of declining enrollments, especially for girls, at primary and upper secondary level.[30] Paltry wages for unskilled work and rural unemployment are driving many men (and some women) to seek work in the cities.[31]

Rural women are less likely than men to receive agricultural training or credit that would allow them to invest in improved crop yields or small-scale enterprises,[27,31] and new needs for cash are forcing women to work extra jobs during the time they might have been able to rest, with negative health consequences. Further, women's labouring wages are lower than men's.[27] Poor rural women are doubly squeezed; they must work harder, on the one hand, and reduce expenditure on the other. Struggling to repay debts at usurious interest rates is also an issue raised by several respondents, as elsewhere.[1] The consequences for purchasing ability, including for food, are negative.

'I can earn 4,000 dong (about US$0.40) per day taking bricks from the kiln...I know it's not much but I need the money to buy rice.' (Mai)

'My husband and brother-in-law can earn 500,000 to 600,000 dong (about US$50) per month, but it all goes on making payments on our debt, so I have had to look for an extra job.' (Lan)

Half the sample had husbands working in the cities, which appeared to have a largely negative impact on their ability to purchase food. Inheriting their husbands' tasks and faced with increased dependency on in-laws, they found their autonomy over food purchasing further eroded.

'Before going to the city my husband told me not to work so hard. But no matter how exhausted I am, my circumstances don't allow me to rest.' (Mai)

'Sometimes I want to buy some fruit, but I have no money.' (Phuong)

'If I would like to have some fruits my mother buys them for me, because she knows I don't have money.' (Xuan)

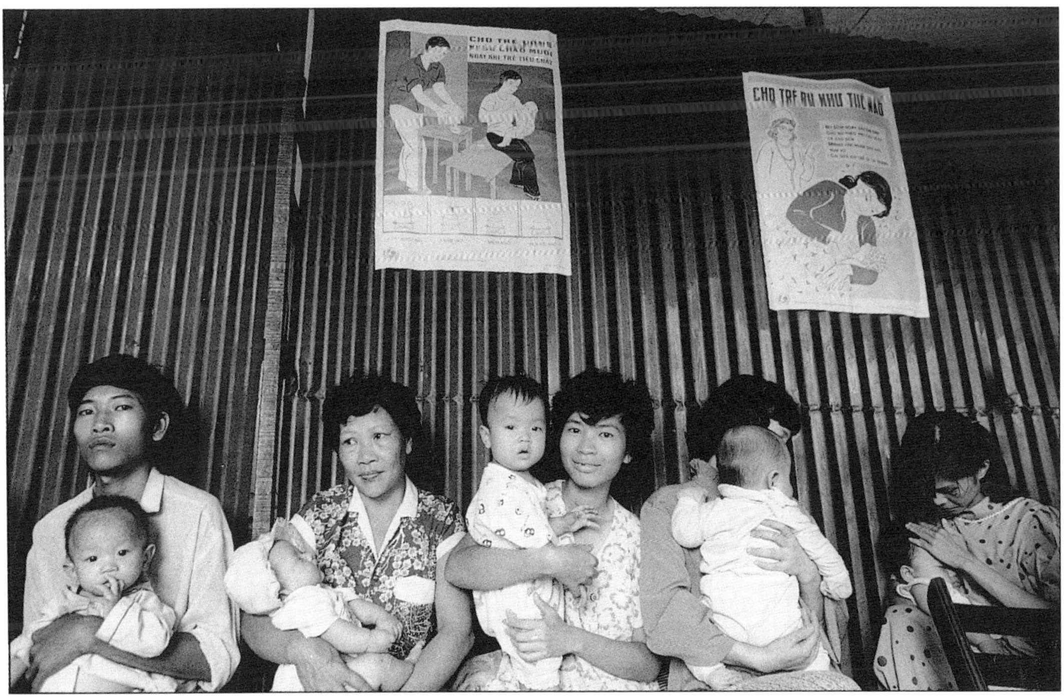

JENNY MATTHEWS

Male migration has positive effects on income and therefore diet, however, if extra earnings allow families to repay loans or purchase rice when prices are lower, or if the husband buys special foods for the family. However, earning ability is not consistent, rural life is precarious, and an unexpected crisis can mean disaster.

'Sometimes he brings some hundred thousand dong, but often he only gets enough for his two meals a day.' (Huong)

'Every week I go to the market twice... Usually I buy vegetables, small fish, soup, fat and fish-sauce. But if somebody in the family gets sick, we have to sell our rice stocks, and then buy rice later on.' (Minh)

While Vietnam officially has a two-child policy, women in this commune, as elsewhere, were found to exceed the sanctioned number if they had only living daughters.[32,33] Poverty may largely explain this practice: first, male wages are higher, and second, sons traditionally support their parents in old age, while daughters move to join their husbands' families. The substantial potential benefits of male offspring clearly outweighed, for many poor women, the risk of having another mouth to feed (even possibly a girl), as well as other potential risks related to maternal health and official opprobrium.

'Before going to the city my husband told me to try to give birth to a son but he didn't tell me anything about eating. As he knows, I always give food to my children first.' (Mai)

'I know to have one more child is very hard for us, but we want to have at least one son. Three daughters are still three daughters.' (Uyen)

Nutritional needs in pregnancy: knowledge and practice

It has been suggested that pregnant women practice 'eating down' during pregnancy.[2,14] Some of the women, especially primiparas, said they did so, but generally only in the third trimester of pregnancy, when their abdomens were perceptibly larger. 'Eating down' occurred even among relatively affluent women with some knowledge of nutritional needs. Restrictions varied, with a few avoiding food in general, and others avoiding only high-calorie or *bo* (nourishing) foods.

'I know when I'm pregnant I should eat bo *foods ...But everybody tells me that the first child is always difficult in delivery, so I dare not have too much good food.'* (Phuong)

'I find my belly is getting big, so I dare not eat so much bo *food as before.'* (Uyen)

'My mother-in-law told me: "...after delivery you are free to eat what you like".' (Loan)

Respondents were mostly unaware of the need to eat adequately and to refrain from physiological strain. Few knew anything about optimum weight gain, claiming that no one had advised them of this.

'For each meal if I can have two or three bowls of rice I feel very happy... I don't think I need to have more high calorie or nourishing foods.' (Ha)

'I have no feeling about eating for the child in my belly, but I know one thing: I have to try to eat to be able to work.' (Tuyet)

Some of the women felt they should eat certain *bo* foods, such as stewed chicken, eggs and *la ngai* (a leafy vegetable), which are expensive, but only when they felt 'uncomfortable'.

'Some days ago, I carried fertiliser to a distant field. It was heavy and the field was far away, so I felt uncomfortable inside afterwards. I ate two eggs in order to make my baby all right.' (Lan)

The impact of inadequate health services on nutrition

Health service delivery in Vietnam is moving towards 'user fees'. Local communities now fund many services; this exacerbates regional disparities. Low wages in the public health sector have further eroded standards.[34] Recent commentaries cite acute difficulties for rural women in accessing good quality health care, as this would force them into debt to cover any major medical expenses.[16,17]

There were several ways in which reproductive health services were inadequate. There is limited contraceptive choice and this probably accounts for some unwanted pregnancies.[33] The local commune health centre does no pregnancy testing, abortions or sterilisations. Women said they could ill-afford to lose work time and travel costs to procure these at district level.

'We have one boy and one girl – that's enough. But this time I wasn't using any family planning method. By the time I managed to get to the district hospital, I was very big.' (Huong)

Low rates of antenatal screening are the norm outside most urban centres,[1] which means that advice about health and nutrition during pregnancy is often not being obtained. It appeared that non-attendance by the respondents at the local clinic was due primarily to limited awareness of the value of antenatal visits. Most women only attended if they had an acute problem, such as bleeding. Those who did attend did not always receive appropriate care, however. For example, health workers themselves said women need gain only 6-7 kg in pregnancy, well below the 10-12 kg amount recommended internationally. Women were rarely weighed or monitored, and the quality of advice varied considerably.

'I don't know how much I weighed before I got pregnant and I don't know how much I weigh now.' (Mai)

'Last week I went to the health centre because I had a bad backache. They gave me some medicine to take. I don't know what kind of medicine it was, but I took it. They didn't advise me at all about eating or working.' (Linh)

'Once I went to the health centre because I felt uncomfortable in my stomach. The health worker said my belly was too small and advised me to take more nourishing food.' (Ha)

In one instance, the health worker had less influence than the woman's mother-in-law:

'I went to the health centre because I was bleeding and the head of the health centre advised me to stop pulling water from the well. But I'm afraid of my mother-in-law, so I haven't stopped.' (Oanh)

The World Food Programme (WFP), which used to operate in this area, had come to the end of its cycle and was terminated. Health workers thought that some women no longer attended for antenatal care because of community beliefs that attendance had only been a WFP bureaucratic requirement. If this is true, it illustrates the need for all relevant groups to understand the rationale for such interventions.

Finally, the poor quality of local equipment and the presence of only one trained midwife meant that cases of pregnancy and delivery complications were being referred to the district hospital. The women were not only aware of local service delivery problems; they also voiced anxiety about what would happen if they were referred for care at district level, where they were afraid of the costs involved as well as of death or disability from surgical interventions. Thus, 'eating down' was a way of avoiding not only obstructed labour but the medical consequences.

'I've heard that the first delivery is…even more difficult if the baby is big. For this reason I don't dare eat much nourishing food, because I'm afraid of being operated on at the district hospital.' (Loan)

Discussion

This study reveals that food consumption in pregnancy in the rural north of Vietnam cannot be attributed to a single cause. Adherence to normative expectations of women's subordination (unmodified in pregnancy) put poor rural women and infants at risk. While children are deemed most deserving of nutritious food, it is not understood that the need for nutritious food in pregnancy satisfies more than the expectant mother's taste buds.

Exacerbating the effects of these norms are harsh economic realities, particularly as a market system replaces the planned socialist economy. With the household now the basic unit of production, poor women bear the brunt of marshalling family capacity to purchase goods and services. At the same time as they work extra jobs instead of resting, they also cut food consumption to reduce expenditure. When men migrate for jobs, women replace them in the fields and continue to carry their own workload as well. Pregnancy is seen as no excuse for altering daily patterns of work, rest or eating. Loss of appetite often accompanies exhaustion, further jeopardising food intake at a time of extra nutritional demand. Poverty is the context in which role expectations are transmuted into distinct health risks for women and their offspring.

In addition, 'eating down' is practiced by some women who fear both the risks of obstructed labour and the surgical interventions intended to overcome it, and who wrongly attribute obstetric complications to increased maternal food intake. Yet 'eating down' endangers not only pregnant women but also the next generation of mothers, whose low birth weights predispose them to inadequate pelvic development.

These reproductive health issues must be viewed against the background of rapid social and economic transformation in Vietnam. The poor are least able to avail themselves of market opportunities or to purchase formerly subsidised services, and women are especially vulnerable because their reproductive and productive roles are essential for family financial security. This preliminary study suggests that inadequate maternal intake emerges from the nexus between traditional norms and contemporary life circumstances.

Implications for programme and policy development

Although the generalisability of this study's findings, as with much qualitative research, are limited (eg. by a small sample size), the issues that emerged have been identified in other recent social health investigations as well.[16,17,27] Hence, the results are worthy of consideration in formulating reproductive health policies and interventions in Vietnam.

The complex aetiology of nutritional behaviour in pregnancy calls for long-term, multi-sectoral approaches, which include the following:

- ***Normative and gender-based role expectations***

Normative role expectations do not disappear quickly even in the presence of rapid social change. Greater awareness of the health consequences of traditional female role expectations could facilitate the development of protective strategies. The media, the Vietnam Women's Union and academic centres could further expand their activities[35] to encourage discussion of gender issues. At present in Vietnam, if not in most societies, women are unlikely to accept food supplements if these are not also available to other family members. This often-overlooked constraint may explain why there has been a limited or even non-existent impact of such programmes on weight gain in pregnancy among women elsewhere.[6]

- ***Educational programmes***

Ignorance about women's nutritional and health needs in pregnancy can undermine interventions. Health workers must understand essential obstetric care and be able to communicate that knowledge locally. Small incentives to encourage antenatal attendance might be cost-effective. Loudspeakers, radio, or home visits could be utilised for health promotion. Norms of self-sacrifice, meanwhile, could be turned to advantage in reproductive health programmes. For example, messages for women could be presented in terms of the imperative to begin nurturing their children before they are born by eating well and resting. Given women's lack of autonomy, such messages should also be targeted at husbands and parents-in-law. Everyone in the community should be informed that proper nutrition will not cause obstetric complications and that 'eating down' is dangerous. Because pre-pregnancy weight is linked to healthy childbearing, nutrition education for girl children should be for the entire community.

- ***Improving health facilities and services for women***

A better resourced health service and better quality of reproductive health care would, over time, help to improve outcomes and counteract the kinds of fears that contribute to 'eating down'.

- ***Addressing poverty: income generation and food production***

The ability to afford abundant, nutritious food and to reduce heavy workloads during pregnancy would mitigate some of the adverse effects revealed in this investigation. Poverty is not easily eliminated, particularly during economic restructuring, but the health consequences should be publicly acknowledged so that even limited changes can be made. The complex and mutually reinforcing interaction of gender and poverty led Walker[36] to conclude that 'interventions to improve the nutrition of women are unlikely to be successful unless these underlying and basic conditions are also addressed'; this study supports this observation. Skills training and credit programmes for women would assist in breaking the cycle of poverty. Training in the home-based garden system pioneered by the National Institute of Nutrition could enhance family nutrition while generating cash income.

- ***Future research and dissemination of findings***

An accurate understanding of nutritional patterns and influences requires both bio-medical and qualitative research. Both methods are also needed to formulate effective interventions to address maternal and infant health in a rapidly changing environment. Researchers should disseminate their findings widely to stimulate debate about the impact of economic and social policies on rural women and infants, who are among Vietnam's most vulnerable groups. In the case of this study, following the compilation of findings, the researchers returned to the study site to give some nutrition education sessions. In conjunction with the Institute of Sociology, a public seminar is planned to report the study findings to researchers, health officials and members of community groups in Hanoi.

Acknowledgments

This project was developed in a workshop supported by the Australian Agency for International Development (AusAID) and the UN Population Fund (UNFPA-Hanoi). UNFPA-Hanoi also provided funding for the study. The authors are grateful to these agencies and to Dr Phan Thu Ha for assistance in study design; Dr Dao Minh An (research assistant); Dr Wendy Holmes and UNFPA for useful comments on this paper; Pr Tuong Lai and Dr Pham Bich San, Institute of Sociology, Hanoi, for facilitating the project; and the People's Committee, commune health workers and pregnant women who so generously shared their views.

Correspondence

Dr Pascale Allotey, Key Centre for Women's Health, University of Melbourne, 720 Swanston Street, Carlton, Vic 3053, Australia. Fax: 61-3-9347-9825. E-mail: p.allotey@kcwh.unimelb.edu.au

References and Notes

1. *Women's Health Profile: Viet Nam*. World Health Organization Regional Office for the Western Pacific, Manila, 1995. (Principal contributors: Morrow M, Nguyen Thi Thom and Rayner-Smith J)
2. Pham Thuy Hoa, Cao Thi Hau, Le Thi Hop et al, 1994. Daily food intake of pregnant and lactating women in some northern rural communes and Hanoi city. *Y Hoc Viet Nam*. 182(7):42-45.
3. *Analysis: a number of PHC indicators through reports of 16 provinces and cities*. PAM Project. Health Statistics and Information Centre, Ministry of Health, Hanoi, 1993.
4. *Human Development Report 1995*. United Nations Development Programme, New York, 1995.
5. Gillespie S, 1997. *Improving Adolescent and Maternal Nutrition: An Overview of Benefits and Options*. UNICEF Working Paper, Nutrition Series 97-002, New York.
6. Kramer MS, 1997. Balanced protein/energy supplementation in pregnancy. In Nielson JP, Crowther CA, Hodnett ED et al (eds). *Pregnancy and Childbirth Module of the Cochrane Database of Systematic Reviews* (updated 4 March 1997). Cochrane Collaboration; Issue 2. Cochrane Library, Oxford.
7. Siega-Riz AM, Adair LS, Hobel CJ, 1996. Maternal underweight status and inadequate rate of weight gain during the third trimester of pregnancy increases the risk of preterm delivery. *Journal of Nutrition*. 126:146-153.
8. Johnson AA, Knight EM, Edwards CH et al, 1994. Dietary intakes, anthropometric measurements and pregnancy outcomes. *Journal of Nutrition*. 124 (6 Suppl):936S-942S.
9. Achadi EL, Hansell MJ, Sloan NL et al, 1995. Women's nutritional status, iron consumption and weight gain during pregnancy in relation to neonatal weight and length in West Java, Indonesia. *International Journal of Gynaecology and Obstetrics*. 48(Suppl):S103-19.
10. Ceesay SM, Prentice AM, Cole TJ et al, 1997. Effects on birth weight and perinatal mortality of maternal dietary supplements in rural Gambia: 5 year randomised controlled trial. *BMJ*. 315:786-90.
11. Winkvist A, Jalil F, Habicht JP et al, 1994. Maternal energy depletion is buffered among malnourished women in Punjab,

Pakistan. *Journal of Nutrition.* 124:2376-85.
12. Nichter M, Nichter M, 1983. The ethnophysiology and folk dietetics of pregnancy: a case study from South India. *Human Organization.* 42(3):235-6.
13. Brems S, Berg A, 1989. 'Eating down' during pregnancy: nutrition, obstetric and cultural considerations in the Third World. Population and Human Resources Department, World Bank, New York.
14. Tu Giay, Ha Huy Khoi, Chu Quoc Lap, 1991. Food intake and nutrition status of the Vietnamese. In UNICEF, Proceedings from International Symposium on Nutrition in Primary Health Care in Developing Countries, November 14-20, 1991. Hanoi.
15. Garner P, Kramer M, Chalmers I, 1992.Might efforts to increase birthweight in undernourished women do more harm than good? *Lancet.* 340:1021-22.
16. Le Thi Vinh Thi, 1997. Social policy towards rural women. *Vietnam Social Sciences.* 2(58):33-48.
17. Do Thi Binh, 1997. Some problems concerning social policies towards rural women in the period of economic restructuring. *Vietnam Social Sciences.* 2(58):3-13.
18. Viet Nam Inter-censal Demographic Survey, 1994. Major Findings. Statistical Publishing House, Hanoi.
19. Ungar E, 1994. Gender, land and household in Vietnam. *Asian Studies Review.* 17(3):61-72.
20. *Contraceptive Requirements and Logistics Management Needs in Viet Nam.* Technical Report No. 16. United Nations Population Fund, Hanoi 1994.
21. Yach D, 1992. The use and value of qualitative methods in health research in developing countries. *Social Science and Medicine.* 35(4):603-12.
22. Grybosky K, Gross R, Schultink W et al, 1995. The importance of qualitative methods for field-based nutritional research. [Letter]. *American Journal of Clinical Nutrition.* 62(July):153-55.
23. Leslie J, 1992. Women's lives and women's health: using social science research to promote better health for women. (Part of 'Family structure, female headship and maintenance of families and poverty'.) International Center for Research on Women. Population Council, New York.
24. Van Landingham M., Knodel J, Saengtienchai C et al, 1994. Aren't sexual issues supposed to be sensitive? *Health Transition Review.* 4(1):85-90.
25. Johansson A., HT Hoa, LT Nham Tuyet, et al, 1996. Family planning in Vietnam – women's experience and dilemma: a community study from the Red River Delta. *Journal of Psychosomatic Obstetrics and Gynecology.*17:59-67.
26. Le Thi, 1994. Family and its educational role. *Viet Nam Social Sciences.* 4:81-87.
27. Thai Thi Ngoc Du, Nguyen Thi Oanh, Truong Thi Kim Chuyen et al, 1994. *The Role of Women in Agricultural Production in the Mekong Delta.* Women Studies Department, Open University of Ho Chi Minh City, Ho Chi Minh City.
28. Jamieson N, 1993. *Understanding Vietnam.* University of California, Berkeley.
29. State Planning Committee, 1994. *Viet Nam Living Standards Survey 1992-1993.* General Statistical Office, Hanoi.
30. Truong Thanh-Dam, 1997. Uncertain horizon: the women's question in Vietnam revisited. In Beckman B, Hansson E and Roman L (eds.) *Vietnam: Reform and Transformation.* Conference proceedings, Center for Pacific Asia Studies, University of Stockholm, Stockholm.
31. Le Ngoc Van, 1997. Labour change in rural families: new roles of males and females. *Vietnam Social Sciences.* 2(58):21-34.
32. Goodkind D, 1995. Vietnam's one-or-two-child policy in action. *Population and Development Review.* 21(1):85-111.
33. Johansson A, Nguyen The Lap, Hoang Thi Hoa et al, 1998. Population plicy, son preference and the use of IUDs in Vietnam. *Reproductive Health Matters.* 6(11/May):66-76.
34. Chalker J, 1995. Viet Nam: profit and loss in health care. *World Health Forum.* 16(2):194-95.
35. Center for Women Studies, 1994. A participatory approach to gender responsiveness policy research. Strengthening the role of Vietnamese rural women in development. *Results of the Project VIE/90/WO1.* UNIFEM and Center for Women Studies, Hanoi.
36. Walker SP, 1997. Nutritional issues for women in developing countries. *Proceedings of the Nutrition Society.* 56:345-56.

Where There's No Tradition of Traditional Birth Attendants: Kassena Nankana District, Northern Ghana

Pascale Allotey

The philosophy underlying the Safe Motherhood policy of training traditional birth attendants (TBAs) assumes the existence of TBAs who are recognised and accepted by their communities and accessible to women in those communities. This paper describes a TBA training programme implemented in remote, highly dispersed communities in the Kassena Nankana District in northern Ghana, where there were previously no TBAs and where most births were not attended or were attended only by kinswomen. Thirty women who were not previously TBAs were chosen by community elders to be trained by midwives as birth attendants. A study among 245 pregnant women, the trained attendants and other traditional and modern health care providers in the district showed that few women were willing or able to make use of the trained attendants. This programme introduced a new service provider into the community whose role was not clearly defined or incorporated into the existing modern or traditional maternal health services. Only when the specific needs of the Kassena Nankana District are addressed can a workable solution be developed that has some chance of reducing maternal deaths and morbidity there.

IN most rural societies women giving birth are assisted by other women, often their kinswomen, outside of modern health services.[1] These women, known as traditional birth attendants (TBAs), are responsible for assisting approximately 60 to 80 per cent of births in developing countries. As members of the local community, their role is an integral part of the culture in their societies.[2-5] The recognition of the potential for TBAs to improve the coverage of assisted births and to contribute to the improvement of maternal health care led to an international initiative begun in the early 1980s to train TBAs and upgrade their skills.[2,6] However the adoption of such a policy with little consideration for the diversity of local birthing practices can result in a waste of resources and a failure to recognise and take advantage of local knowledge and solutions.

This paper describes a TBA training programme in a remote and highly dispersed rural community in Northern Ghana with endemic malaria, lymphatic filariasis and schistosomiasis.The findings were part of a larger anthropological and epidemiological study on maternal and morbidity, and traditional and modern interventions in the district, which was conducted from June 1993 to March 1994. The main aim of the study was to investigate the 'burden of illness' in pregnancy, defined to include the relationship between disease and illness, marginalisation, ethnicity, gender and culture and how these mediate the experience of pregnancy and affect access to various systems of health care. [7]

The study

The study followed a sample of 245 pregnant women from 28 weeks of pregnancy to six weeks post-partum. The women were recruited from the population of pregnant women in villages within the catchment area of modern maternal health services (that is, within a radius of seven km of the district hospital). All the women living in this area, identified through a pre-existing demographic surveillance system, who were 28 weeks' pregnant during the sampling period and who agreed to participate, were included in the study. Seventeen women were excluded; ten were going to leave the area before the end of the follow-up period and seven were not allowed to participate by their husbands. Data were also obtained from trained birth attendants and traditional healers and soothsayers living in the study area who were accessible to the women, and from Ministry of Health staff, using a combination of focus group discussions, in-depth interviews, observation and participant observation. Four focus groups were conducted with 30 trained birth attendants,[8] in groups of 6 to 11 participants. Two focus groups were held with Ministry of Health staff, one with 8 public health nurse/midwives on the District Health Management Team (DHMT), and the other with 5 midwives on the maternity ward. Two traditional healers and two soothsayers were interviewed, as were five key informants from the Ministry of Health. Participant observation data were collected at the antenatal clinics and consultations with the soothsayers and traditional healers were also observed.

Each woman in the sample was visited at least once every four weeks by the researcher (myself) or by one of two research assistants. They were interviewed about any illnesses they had experienced, healers they had consulted, treatment measures they had taken, reasons for their choice of healers and treatment, and their perceptions of the quality and efficacy of the intervention. Data were supplemented with physical examinations, laboratory investigations and network analysis data from carers and other family members.

The community

The Kassena Nankana District is a remote rural district in Northern Ghana covering an area of 1675 square kms. The climate is tropical monsoon with a wet season characterised by erratic and torrential rainfall, and a dry season influenced by the Saharan northeast trade winds, creating heat that scorches most of the vegetation and causes recurrent bush fires. For most of the 160,000 people in the rural parts of the district, roads are opportunistically created by the tracks of vehicles that have previously cut their way through the vegetation. These routes become impassable with flooding in the rainy season.

Settlements are highly dispersed with extended family groups living in compounds one to five kms apart. A typical compound consists of several one-room, flat-roofed adobe huts enclosed by a low mud wall. As a general rule, each adult male member of a family has a hut and may build another for each wife he acquires. However, it is also common for several women to share a hut with other women and their children. Most compounds house three generations of an extended family, with the oldest man acting as head of the compound. A village in this area consists of a number of dispersed compounds of related families, with village boundaries discernible mainly by the people who live within it.

Pregnancy and childbirth – the traditional perspective

The most recent community-based survey in the district[9] estimated a maternal mortality rate of 813 per 100,000 live births, one of the highest in the country.[10] The main causes of maternal deaths were post-partum haemorrhage, infections, obstructed labour and severe anaemia, all preventable with good management.

The remoteness of most of the communities in this region has ensured that adherence to traditional practices and cultural belief systems, particularly those associated with pregnancy and childbirth, has remained strong. Traditionally, a woman was not recognised by her family as being pregnant until the pregnancy was officially announced by *lingeru*, a complex and colourful ritual performed by the mother-in-law. This would usually occur after abdominal distension was evident (generally about 20 weeks into the pregnancy). The head of the compound was then informed and he would consult a *vuru* (soothsayer)[11] who, with the aid of ancestors and other spirits, would foretell the development and outcome of the pregnancy. During pregnancy and childbirth the *vuru* would offer advice about treatment of illness and utilisation of various health services, although he was not directly responsible for the intervention. It was not uncommon for women to cite edicts from the *vuru* as their reason for not attending antenatal clinics.

Should a woman become ill during pregnancy, there were a range of *tindana* (traditional healers) to consult, each with a specific area of specialisation, depending on the perceived cause of the illness. The *vuru* would often provide advice on which particular *tindana* should be consulted.

Labour was recognised by the waters breaking and the appearance of the presenting part of the infant in the vagina. Contractions alone were not considered a definitive sign of imminent birth because they mimicked a number of other culturally-defined conditions.[7] This has implications for the time required to call for assistance. Birth was considered the exclusive domain of women, who usually gave birth on their own or assisted by one of the older women in the compound. Births usually took place in the area of the compound where the livestock were tended overnight – over a bed of evenly spread, dried cow dung which was soft enough to be comfortable but ensured that the placenta and other products of conception would remain in the part of the compound that was considered unclean.

Two types of *tindana*, both of them men, would be called in to manage difficult births. One specialised in the removal of retained placentae and the second in the management of obstructed labour. The principal role of the latter *tindana* was to perform ritual genital excisions (removal of the prepuce, clitoris and labia minora) at puberty. During prolonged second stage births, however, he would also perform incisions to widen the vaginal opening.

In general, the status and popularity of *tindana* would be determined by the conditions they treated and the people who consulted them. Because of the low status of women, *tindana* who specialised in conditions related to childbearing, though important, were not perceived as particularly powerful in the community. The *vuru* on the other hand, were very powerful members of the community because of their involvement in almost every aspect of people's lives.

Role of the District Health Management Team

Maternal health services, provided mainly at the District Hospital, consisted of an antenatal clinic twice a week and a 21-bed maternity unit. These services were considered inaccessible by many women because of hospital charges, the cost of drugs and transport where available. These were prohibitive in a community that essentially operated a non-cash economy. In addition, because of the lack of transportation, women who did use the antenatal clinic had to walk the whole distance and were therefore more likely to attend only on days when there were other activities in the vicinity, such as the food markets which were held every three days. A little over half of pregnant women would attend the clinic at least once during a pregnancy but only one quarter of the births in the district took place in the hospital.[10]

The Kassena Nankana District TBA training programme

In response to the international Safe Motherhood Initiative, TBA training was adopted as part of the maternal health policy in Ghana in the 1980s.[5,12,13] There had been several trials of the 'TBA model' with some success in regions in southern Ghana, where traditional birth attendants existed within the community.[12] These TBAs had skills which they had learnt through apprenticeships with older, experienced women in their communities. It was therefore a relatively simple task for staff of the Ministry of Health to identify them and train them to assess gestational age, recognise the potential for infection and cross-infection, recognise complications, refer women to health centres, practise good hygiene and advise mothers on breastfeeding, family planning and the care of their infants. The training sessions were conducted mainly in classrooms and in the community in order to make the TBAs feel comfortable.[13,14]

The implementation of a similar programme in Northern Ghana was delayed largely due to the political neglect of the northern regions.[15,16] However, in response to persistent reports of high maternal morbidity and mortality in the northern regions and the difficulties Ministry of Health staff reportedly had in gaining access to remote communities, government training of TBAs in the District was started in the northern regions in the late 1980s.[17]

For the introduction of the programme to the villages in the study area, the elders were approached by the DHMT and asked to nominate 30 traditional birth attendants to be trained by the Ministry of Health.[7] The advantages of trained birth attendants to the community were explained to the elders. The elders were also told that the community would have to negotiate remuneration with the women once they were trained.

The requests presented a problem for the elders for two main reasons. First, they were not sure whom to nominate for training. There was no tradition of one experienced woman serving a whole village or collection of compounds as a 'birth attendant'. The *tindana* who managed complicated births were men and were not considered by the elders to be appropriate candidates for what was being proposed, which was essentially a woman's responsibility. Second, the criteria for the selecting the women applied to at least one woman in every compound in an area that had in excess of 1,000 compounds.

The elders were therefore faced with the task of selecting a limited number of women who would not only be respected by the people living in compounds other than their own, but who would also be prepared to travel vast distances between compounds on a regular basis. The elders [18] (all of whom were men) resolved the problem by selecting women according to the status of their compound head in the community. Those women who were related to a chief, *vuru* or *tindana* were the ones most likely to be selected.

The 30 women who were chosen underwent two weeks of training, which was provided by midwives from the DHMT. The training programme was similar to the ones used previously for training TBAs in southern Ghana. The practical sessions involved the examination of pregnant women attending the antenatal clinics and the observation of births on the district hospital maternity ward. The trainees graduated as Ministry of Health trained and registered TBAs. They were expected to conduct normal births in the community, refer to the hospital antenatal clinic any pregnant women who were grand multiparas or primiparas, those who appeared to have non-cephalic presentations, multiple births or an unusual obstetric history, and to give advice on good diet and personal hygiene. They were also given a notebook in which to keep a record of their work. Since most of the women being trained were illiterate, it was incumbent upon each of them to find someone in the community to update their records for them.

The performance of the trained attendants was monitored through supervisory visits from the staff of the Maternal and Child Health Unit.[17] They were each given kits with a supply of cotton wool, soap, gentian violet, a new razor blade and some ligatures. They were advised by the midwives who trained them that these items were to be replaced by each pregnant woman they assisted. At the community level, it was decided by the elders that any other payment that they received for attending a birth was to be negotiated with the head of the compound where the birth took place.

On completion of the course, the trained attendants had a meeting with women in the community. Their training and the services they could provide were detailed and it was agreed that when a woman became pregnant, an attendant would be informed at the same time as the traditional announcement of the pregnancy. The pregnant woman was expected to consult the trained attendant for a review during pregnancy and advice about whether it was safe to give birth at home. The trained attendant would also be sent for when the woman was in labour.

Perceptions of the attendants following their training

Most of the trained attendants had found the training very difficult but reported that they had been too embarrassed during the sessions to ask questions. They found that the midwives assumed that they would 'know a lot of things even though they had never been to school'. The attendants reported that they had enjoyed the practical sessions that taught them about the assessment of gestational age and determination of the lie of the foetus, and general examination to determine if the woman had anaemia. Although they had observed births on the maternity ward, they stated that it was not possible for them to assist in the way the midwives did because women gave birth in different positions in the compound. However, in their practice, they were more confident about assisting in births, recognising when to assist in third stage, diagnosing excessive blood loss, and recognising when to refer real or potential complications to the hospital. These were the services that they offered to women in their community.

Overall, they felt their opportunities to practise since training were limited. They complained about poor community support and a lack of appreciation of their skills. They explained that they were seldom informed when a woman became pregnant, and they only found out a woman was pregnant if they happened to run into her in the food market. They also reported that, although their selection for the training was based on recognition of their importance in the community, they were not always treated with the respect they believed they deserved. Some said they had been met with hostility in some of the compounds they visited and others said that on occasions, 'they were not even offered *flour water*' (a drink given to welcome visitors to a compound). Some of them wanted the government to give them more power to 'control' pregnant women and to force them to do what they were told.

They also complained about the financial burden of their work. They expected some form of remuneration from the families of the women they assisted, or at least the replenishment of their birthing kits. They reported that remuneration, when given at all, was always given with a great deal of reluctance, and they invariably had to replenish their kits themselves.

Both the *vuru* and *tindana* interviewed reported that although they participated in community consultations with the district health staff, they had not been invited by the community or the district health staff to play a role in the TBA programme, as they had expected. Although they did not want to do the work of a trained attendant in normal births, they felt they should have been included in the training programme to learn how to improve their skills and provide added assistance to the women they did attend.

Utilisation of the trained attendants

From one rainy season to the next (one year), the trained attendants had hoped to attend an average of 30 women each; however, they did not have their own catchment areas because of the way they had been selected and there was a considerable overlap in their potential clients. In fact, only 16 per cent of women in the present study were attended by a trained attendant. The proportion was even less in a study of the whole district, where only three per cent of women interviewed were attended by trained attendants.[10]

Of the 30 trained attendants, the two identified by the pregnant women as being the most popular assisted a maximum of four births each over the one-year period. Nine attendants only assisted women in their own compounds, whom they would have assisted with or without training.

Of the 245 women in the study, only eight women had reported to a trained attendant outside their own compounds during their pregnancies, of whom five were subsequently referred to the antenatal clinic because it was their first pregnancy or because they had had more than five previous births. A total of 164 of the 245 women attended the antenatal clinic at least once during their pregnancies.

Approximately 44 percent of the 245 women gave birth in the hospital, which is a substantially higher proportion than the 25 percent reported in the study mentioned above of the whole district.[10] However, the sample for the current study was selected from among women who lived relatively close to the district hospital, unlike the study of the whole district.

Of the 137 women who gave birth at home, only 22 were assisted by one of the trained attendants, of whom one was subsequently referred to the hospital in the post-partum period for a vulval haematoma.

Women's perceptions of the trained attendants

The pregnant women in the study generally thought that it was a good idea to train local women to assist in pregnancy and birth, because they were closer to their own homes and could provide a service that was cheaper than the services provided in the hospital. The women who did use the trained attendants reported that they would otherwise have given birth on their own because there was no one in their immediate compounds whom they thought could assist them. In addition they tended to be women who had some access to household finances through trading, albeit infrequently, in the local market, and could therefore afford to pay for the services provided. The trained attendants also tended to live relatively close to their compounds or to have family ties with their compound heads.

Both women who had and had not used a trained attendant reported that it was not always easy to locate a trained attendant when one was needed, because the trained attendants had their own domestic responsibilities; when a woman was sure she was in labour it was often too late to get help from someone who lived outside the compound. The women were also reluctant to call trained attendants out during the night, because most of the attendants were older women and they considered it disrespectful to disturb their night's sleep. They also noted that, given the distances between compounds, the trained attendants often lived too far away. As one woman observed:

'If I send for a trained attendant when I go into labour, the baby will be born and weaned by the time she arrives to assist in the birth!'

Most of the women agreed that an important skill of the trained attendants was their ability to recognise complications that required outside help more quickly than untrained women in their compounds. However, they also said that because the trained attendants could not deal with the complications themselves, a woman would have to go to hospital or call in one of the *tindana* anyway. Consequently, the women felt that although important, the services provided by the trained attendants were almost as limited as the assistance they got from women in their own compounds who had had no training, and who did not require any payment. In addition, the decision whether or not to use a trained attendant was not solely that of the pregnant women. It also depended on the availability of funds and the moods of their husbands or compound heads. If a husband or any of his family members were not pleased with the pregnant woman or if the newborn baby was a girl, the trained attendant might not be paid and this would have been a source of embarrassment for the women. Most of the pregnant women, therefore, felt that they could not always justify calling in, let alone paying, a trained attendant.

A further reason given for not using the trained attendants was that the trained attendants expected the women to purchase razors, soap and cotton wool in readiness for the birth, in spite of the general knowledge that there was a taboo against it. The proverb *'Ba ba mon sore lom ye ba po bu'* ('It is testing the gods to buy herbs for the ritual bath before you have given birth') was cited. A few women also claimed they did not use trained attendants because they did not know who the trained attendants were.

Discussion

One of the major aims of the Safe Motherhood Initiative has been to increase the number of births attended by skilled attendants,[19] including TBAs. Obstetric coverage by TBAs in other parts of Ghana was reported in 1993 to be approximately 29 percent and increasing steadily.[13,20] However, unlike other Ghanaian tribes, the people in the Kassena Nankana District did not have a tradition of women servicing entire villages or areas. Therefore the title of traditional birth attendant was a misnomer in their case.

This meant, in effect, that a new service provider was being introduced to the community; one who required remuneration, even if the amount was token. In addition the trained attendants' roles were not clearly defined within the local traditional medical system nor indeed in relation to the existing modern health services. This raises the question of the adequacy and effectiveness of the TBA programme for the Kassena Nankana District.

With the TBA training programme, the government of Ghana has promoted a basic non-technical approach to maternal health care at the grassroots level which incorporates TBAs. This was originally intended as a stop-gap measure until there were more skilled personnel to provide quality care in the rural areas. If the health services are committed to the longer-term use of TBAs in the maternal health programme for the district, a number of steps need to be taken.

The health authorities need to negotiate the inclusion of women and other traditional healers – as well as the elders – in the planning and implementation process, in spite of the poor status of women in the social structure of the community. Not only would this improve the knowledge of the community about the skills the trained attendants have to offer, but also, with greater input the choice of trainees would be more appropriate and acceptable to a wider section of the community. Furthermore, the involvement of the community would improve their general knowledge of maternal health issues and involve the men in efforts to improve maternal health.

On a broader policy level, the role of trained birth attendants within the Primary Health Care programme needs to be revisited. In Ghana, as elsewhere, skilled health personnel prefer to remain in urban areas,[21,22] a phenomenon that has been described as the 'inverse care law'. Even in highly industrialised countries, such as Australia, which report an overall excess of trained medical staff, providing enough skilled medical staff in remote rural areas remains a problem. If TBAs are to be made a permanent fixture in the northern regions of Ghana, their role in the modern health system and their training need to be formalised and incorporated with a clear commitment to ensuring quality services for women in rural areas.

Evaluations of TBA programmes in other West African countries suggest that people would prefer TBAs to have more skills, particularly in the identification and management of problems specific to the post-partum period.[23,24] Data from India suggest that in order to improve the outcome of home deliveries, particularly of the third stage of labour, which has the highest potential for fatalities, it is necessary to equip TBAs to provide first aid and other curative skills.[25] There is ample evidence to suggest that procedural skills can be taught to health workers at the basic level of primary health care, irrespective of their level of education.[26-29] Although the trained attendants in the present study reported some difficulties of understanding during their training, it is possible to design skill-based training targeted at people with little or no formal education.

There clearly is an urgent need for improved access to quality maternal health services in the Kassena Nankana District. The training of birth attendants may have seemed an appropriate intervention because it appeared to be effective in other regions of Ghana. However, due to culture, geography and the social organisation of communities in the North, their needs for trained birth attendants and the type of training required are clearly different. Only when the specific needs of the Kassena Nankana District are addressed can a workable solution be developed that has some chance of reducing maternal deaths and morbidity there.

Acknowledgements

Funding for this project was provided by the Community Health Research and Training Unit of the University of Western Australia, Clinipath Laboratories and The St John of God Health System. I am grateful for the support of Anne Read, Peter Underwood, Scott Bamber, Lenore Manderson, the staff of the Ministry of Health in Bolgatanga and Navrongo and the Navrongo Health Research Unit and last but not least, the women of the Kassena Nankana District.

Correspondence

Pascale Allotey, International Programs, Key Centre for Women's Health in Society, Faculty of Medicine, Dentistry and Health Sciences, University of Melbourne, 720 Swanston St, Carlton 3053, Australia. Fax: 61-3-9347-9824. E-mail. p.allotey@kcwh.unimelb.edu.au

References and Notes

1. Alto W, Albu R, Irabo G, 1991. An alternative to unattended delivery – a training programme for village midwives in Papua New Guinea. *Social Science and Medicine*. 32(5):613-18.
2. Stephens C, 1992. Training urban traditional birth attendants: balancing international policy and local reality. *Social Science and Medicine*. 35(6):811-17.
3. Camay X, Barrios C, Guerrero X et al, 1996. Traditional birth attendants in Mexico – advantages and inadequacies of care for normal deliveries. *Social Science and Medicine*. 43(2):199-207.
4. *Traditional Birth Attendants: A Joint WHO, UNFPA and UNICEF Statement*. World Health Organization, United Nations Fund for Population Activities, United Nations Children's Fund. Geneva, 1992.
5. Eades C, Brace C, Osei L et al, 1993. Traditional birth attendants and maternal mortality in Ghana. *Social Science and Medicine*. 36(11):1503-07.
6. Pigg S, 1995. Acronyms and effacement: traditional medical practitioners (TMP) in international health development. *Social Science and Medicine*. 41(1):47-68.
7. Allotey P, 1995. The burden of

illness in pregnancy in rural Ghana: a study of maternal morbidity and interventions in Northern Ghana. PhD Thesis, University of Western Australia. Perth.

8. Women who underwent the Ministry of Health TBA training programme in the Kassena Nankana District are referred to in the paper as trained birth attendants for clarity of terminology. However they are referred to by the Ministry of Health as traditional birth attendants and were trained with the protocol of the national TBA training programme.
9. The Sisterhood method was used in the assessment of maternal mortality.
10. Dollimore N, Odoi-Agyarko H, Owusu-Adyei O, 1993. *A community based study of risk factors in maternal mortality in the Kassena-Nankana District of Northern Ghana*. Safe Motherhood Initiative of WHO, Accra.
11. The traditional medical system consists of the *vuru* (soothsayers) who are the guardians of the spiritual well-being of the people of the Kassena Nankana district and the *tindana* (traditional healers) who provide physical healing. Soothsayers are believed to have the ability to communicate with ancestors and an individual's personal gods and to give advice based on the communication to ensure well-being, provided the advice is taken. The soothsayer is usually able to provide a 'preliminary diagnosis' of an ailment and recommend the type of traditional healer that should be consulted. The traditional healers usually specialise in particular areas of healing, so that one would see one healer for ailments caused by offending a spirit and another for ailments associated with a 'bad' pregnancy. The choice of healer did not necessarily depend on symptoms and was often dictated by soothsayers.

12. Ampofo D, Nicholas D, Amonoo-Acquah M et al, 1977. The training of traditional birth attendants in Ghana: experience of the Danfa rural health project. *Tropical and Geographical Medicine*. 29:197-203.
13. *National Consultative Seminar on the Safe Motherhood Initiative*. Ministry of Health, Ghana. Accra, 1993.
14. Cabral M, Kamal I, Kumar V et al, 1992. *Training of Traditional Birth Attendants (TBAs): A Guide for Master Trainers*. Program of Maternal and Child Health and Family Planning, Division of Family Health, World Health Organisation. Geneva.
15. Nugent P, 1993. *The Flight Lieutenant and the Professor: The Road to Ghana's 4th Republic*. Occasional Paper No. 43. Centre for African Studies, Edinburgh University. Edinburgh.
16. Ardayfio-Schandorf E, 1982. *Rural Development Strategies in Northern Ghana: Problems and Prospects for Reaching the Small Farmer*. Vol 18. Geo Books, Swansea.
17. *Ministry of Health. War Memorial Hospital Navrongo. Annual Report 1992*. District Health Management Team Navrongo, Ministry of Health, Ghana. Accra,1992.

18. All major decisions were taken by the elders in the community and although this was a women's health issue, it was considered a sufficiently important departure from custom to warrant a decision by the elders.

19. *Maternal Health and Safe Motherhood Programme. Progress Report 1991-1992*. Division of Family Health, World Health Organization. Geneva, 1993:
20. Neumann A, Nicholas D, Ammonoo-Acquah et al, 1986. Evaluation d'un programme de formation des accoucheuses traditionelles au Ghana. *WHO Offset Publication*. 95:56-67.
21. Hart J, 1971. The inverse care law. *Lancet*.1:405-12.
22. Gilson L, 1995. Management and health care reform in Sub-Saharan Africa. *Social Science and Medicine*. 40(5):695-710.
23. Akpala C, 1994. An evaluation of the knowledge and practices of trained traditional birth attendants in Bodinga, Sokoto State, Nigeria. *Journal of Tropical Medicine and Hygiene*. 97:46-50.
24. Wollast E, Renard F, Vandenbussche P et al, 1993. Detecting maternal morbidity and mortality by traditional birth attendants in Burkina Faso. *Health Policy and Planning*.8(2):161-68.
25. Sawhney H, Gopalan S, 1994. Home deliveries and third stage complications. *Australia and New Zealand Journal of Obstetrics and Gynaecology*. 34(5):531-34.
26. Godwin P, 1983. Training health workers: what needs to be taught and who should teach it? *Social Science and Medicine*. 17(22):1819-25.
27. Chowdhury S, Chowdhury Z, 1975. Tubectomy by para professional surgeons in rural Bangladesh. *Lancet*. 2:567-69.
28. Sutter E, 1983. Training of eye care workers and their integration in Gazankulu's comprehensive health services. *Social Science and Medicine*. 17(22):1809-12.
29. Sheffield V, 1983. Training for primary and preventive eye care. *Social Science and Medicine*. 17(22):1797-1808.

Lakshmiben: A Case Study of a 'Near Miss' Obstetric Event, Gujarat, India

Emily Fatula

This is a case study of the childbirth experience of Lakshmiben, a woman from a village in Gujarat, Western India. The village is served by the Deepak Medical Foundation, founded in the early 1980s to provide medical assistance and health care services to 20 villages in the Nandesari area of Gujarat. The Deepak Medical Foundation runs a clinic staffed by a gynaecologist and has facilities for conducting normal deliveries. It also provides an ambulance service to the community, and training for traditional birth attendants and community health workers. The case study described in this paper was documented through direct observation, as part of a larger study carried out in 1996 to explore childbirth practices in the area and Deepak's role in improving these practices.[1] It illustrates the obstacles to obtaining appropriate medical care for a woman developing complications during delivery. The problem is less one of lack of awareness or unwillingness to seek medical help on the part of the woman or her family, and more the consequence of a non-functioning health care system.

I had gone with my research assistant to interview Induba, one of the *dais* (traditional birth attendants). She was not at home because she had gone to attend to Lakshmiben, a woman in labour. We arrived at Lakshmiben's parents' house with a Deepak field supervisor in the Deepak clinic ambulance about 11:10 a.m. The mud and cow dung house was on one side of a small courtyard; it was one room deep and about three or four rooms wide. Running the width of the house was a covered, semi-enclosed veranda-like area with a mud floor. Induba was sitting there with Lakshmiben.

Lakshmiben, a young woman probably in her early 20s, was in the customary position for a woman in labour, lying on her back on a blanket on the floor. She was in the front area of the house, behind an overturned cot, which served as a screen, surrounded by about six neighbourhood women. This was her first delivery and she had come to her mother's house in her seventh month of pregnancy. It is common practice in this part of India for women to return to their natal homes for the first, and sometimes subsequent, pregnancies. While at her husband's house, she had had one tetanus toxoid shot, and she had been given iron tablets but had not taken them.

Induba had been called when the pains began at 7:00 am. Dr. Shah (a local homeopathic practitioner) had been called when the birth was deemed to be 'delayed', but no one remembered exactly when he arrived. He had given Lakshmiben two injections soon after he arrived; it was not clear what these injections were or why they were given.

By the time we arrived, Lakshmiben was agitated, which the women said was due to the presence of a 'spirit', so they said a special prayer and waved a handful of wheat flour over her head. At this point, they also moved her inside because they felt the exposed area was not appropriate for giving birth.

The neighbourhood women also were advising that Lakshmiben be taken to the Deepak clinic but the mother, father and Lakshmiben were resistant. The father was worried that if Lakshmiben were to go to the Deepak clinic, she might be referred to another more expensive hospital. He said that he could not afford to pay the costs charged by the Deepak clinic or any other hospital. Lakshmiben's mother also was worried about the expense. Lakshmiben herself was resistant to outside intervention. It was difficult to figure out who was going to decide where Lakshmiben would deliver.

After some time, the Deepak field supervisor was able to convince the father that Lakshmiben should be taken to the Deepak clinic. By then, it was 2:15 pm. Lakshmiben was taken to the Deepak clinic in the ambulance which had brought us to the village. She was accompanied by Induba, the health worker and her infant, six village women and a small girl, and three others, as well as myself.

At the Deepak clinic, Lakshmiben was examined by the gynaecologist and taken into the labour room. She could not deliver the baby. By 3:45 pm, it was clear she needed to be referred to another hospital because she had obstructed labour and needed a caesarean section. The Deepak clinic staff had done what they could in a timely manner, but they were just not equipped to handle the operation and had no choice but to refer her. The Deepak gynaecologist called ahead to the large government hospital in Baroda and everyone got into the ambulance to go with Lakshmiben to Baroda.

We arrived at Baroda at about 4:30 pm. Fifteen minutes after we arrived, the lights went off due to a power cut. Lakshmiben was taken into an examining room and at 5:00 pm we were told that Lakshmiben needed blood. There was blood available in the hospital, but the hospital did not permit patients to have blood until a donor was found to replace what would be used. My research assistant and I went to arrange for a donor. When we arrived back to tell the doctors that a donor would appear the next day, we were sent to the blood bank to get blood. The blood, however, was unavailable due to the power cut.

We then had to go to the drugstore, which was located on the hospital grounds, to buy needles, syringes and solution for the IV. None of these were provided by the hospital. Next we had to go to the admissions office to get Lakshmiben's admission papers. Only after completion of all these formalities would the doctors attend to Lakshmiben.

When we arrived back at 6:30 pm, Lakshmiben was in a critical condition. We were told that there was no chance that the supply of electricity would resume soon. Her father was given two choices: either agree that the doctors perform the caesarean section in the dark with flashlights, with no blood and no electrical equipment, or take Lakshmiben to yet another hospital half an hour away by a three-wheeler taxi.

The father opted to have the operation performed at this hospital in the dark. The operation began and my research assistant and I went to collect blood from a children's hospital across town. When we got back with the blood, the operation was already over. Lakshmiben and the baby girl had survived even without the blood.

This case illustrates the numerous structural and institutional barriers to safe childbirth for many women in developing countries. Lakshmiben's family recognised the need for medical help and their delay in seeking help was due to a fear of the medical expense. However, once the decision was made to seek treatment, there was a lack of basic infrastructural and treatment facilities at hospital referral level and a series of bureaucratic hurdles that got in the way of timely treatment. The hospital's rules and regulations required those who had brought a patient to the hospital to run around collecting blood, drugs and necessary medical equipment before she could be operated on, even though she was in a potentially life-threatening condition. Lakshmiben survived the ordeal. Hundreds of thousands like her are not as lucky.

Acknowledgements

Thanks to Aruna Lakhani and Sunanda Ganju (Deepak Medical Foundation, Deepak Charitable Trust); the Mehta family (Deepak Nitrate Limited); Deepak health and administrative staff at the Nandesari office; Lajwanti Mirani (translator); Dr Bert Pelto; and the dais, health care providers, and women of the Nandesari villages.

Correspondence

Emily Fatula, 1835-C Corcoran Street NW, Washington DC 20009, USA. Tel: 1-202-265-4350. E-Mail: efatula@erols.com

References

1. Fatula E. Changing Patterns of Childbirth Practices. Working Paper: Deepak Medical Foundation/Deepak Charitable Trust. January 1997. (Unpublished report)

A Comprehensive Approach to Vesico-Vaginal Fistula: A Project in Mwanza, Tanzania

Maggie Bangser, Balthazar Gumodoka, Zachary Berege

This article discusses vesico-vaginal fistula (VVF), a form of maternal morbidity arising from obstructed labour, which typically affects girls and women who are poor, young and have limited access to obstetric care in emergency situations. VVF leaves girls and women leaking urine, and sometimes faeces, uncontrollably through the vagina. The severe social stigma associated with VVF often makes it difficult, or impossible, for girls and women with the condition to live a normal life in their families and communities. This paper describes the problem of VVF, an innovative VVF project at the Bugando Medical Centre in Mwanza, Tanzania, findings of an exploratory study among 50 women patients who came to the Centre for VVF repair, and makes recommendations on prevention and treatment for VVF on the part of health systems.

VESICO-vaginal fistula (VVF) is a serious form of maternal morbidity and often leaves those who experience it – some as young as 12 years old – to live a life of isolation and shame. VVF is a hole that develops between the vagina and the bladder of a pregnant woman during prolonged and obstructed labour. This hole typically results from necrosis of the vaginal tissue caused by constant pressure from the head of the baby pushing through the birth canal, often due to cephalo-pelvic disproportion. In some cases, the fistula develops between the rectum and the vagina, causing recto-vaginal fistula, or RVF. These holes, or fistulae, leave girls and women leaking urine, faeces or both uncontrollably through the vagina. VVF also causes ulceration of the genital area from the constant leaking. 'Foot drop', or neurological damage to the lower limbs, sustained during childbirth from the same causes, can make it difficult or impossible for some patients to walk.

Current data on the incidence of VVF are practically non-existent, although the problem has been reported throughout Africa and the Indian sub-continent. Research and the observations of health professionals in Africa and Asia indicate that girls and women with VVF tend to have malnutrition and chronic anaemia, often come from extremely poor families, and encounter weak health and transport systems during an obstetric emergency[1-11] Health providers in Tanzania and Ethiopia report that the lack of financial resources stops women from seeking care for VVF[5,7,8,12] and is also likely to play a role in women's inability to access health services during childbirth.

Over 90 per cent of all VVF in Africa is caused by obstructed labour.[10,13,14] In Tanzania, where the maternal mortality ratio is estimated at 529 per 100,000 live births,[15] obstructed labour is a leading cause of maternal mortality and morbidity. Rough estimates in Nigeria suggest that the prevalence of VVF may be 50-80 per 100,000 live births.[2]

High levels of malnutrition in girl children may have serious consequences for future pregnancies; in 1994, one-third to three-quarters of children in various districts of Tanzania were under-nourished or malnourished.[16] Malnutrition can lead to increased risk of obstruction due to stunting which affects both height and the size of the pelvis, and can cause cephalo-pelvic disproportion.[2,17,18] Among VVF patients at Dodoma Regional Hospital in Tanzania, 72 per cent were 150 cm or below in height;[10] similarly, in a Nigeria study over half were below 150 cm.[19]

Data from Ethiopia also suggest that VVF patients are small.[17]

The social consequences of VVF include divorce by husbands and ostracism by others due to the smell and the stigma of leaking.[9,17,19,20] In nearly every case of obstetric fistula, the baby will have died undelivered,[17,21] leaving many women to face the social stigma of childlessness as well, with consequences for remaining in their familes and communities and maintaining their marriages. In northern Nigeria, as the condition persists, women are significantly less likely to be living with their husbands and more likely to return to living with their parents. The social isolation compounds the woman's own belief that she is a disgrace and has brought shame on her family. Women with VVF often work alone, eat alone, use their own plates and utensils to eat and are not allowed to cook for anyone else.[9] In some cases they must live on the streets and beg.[8]

The Bugando Medical Centre Project on VVF

In March, 1997 a group of health and human rights professionals in Mwanza, Tanzania began a project to address VVF. The Project was created to provide treatment to girls and women with VVF, raise awareness of this neglected issue of reproductive health and rights, promote prevention, and advocate for increased resources and attention to the problem. The Project was based at Bugando Medical Centre (BMC), the second largest referral hospital in Tanzania, which serves a catchment area of eight million people. The Project was designed to address VVF in the context of girls' and women's right to health, emphasising both the social and medical dimensions of the problem.

The first phase of the Project operated for 18 months. A key activity sought to strengthen the skills of BMC doctors and nurses and to establish a VVF clinic. During 1997 and 1998, approximately 150 girls and women with VVF were treated at the hospital. Training focused on sending one doctor and two nurses to the Addis Ababa Fistula Hospital (AAFH) in Ethiopia for intensive, hands-on experience with VVF repair and care. In addition, the Project was able to bring a team of three specialists from AAFH to BMC to do training and help to set up the clinic.

When VVF services were available, women overcame immense obstacles to seek care. Despite the high cost of transport and the devastation of roads and railway lines from the rain during El Niño, a significant number of women arrived. Radio, rather than written announcements, was the most effective and efficient way to reach women, particularly those living in remote areas and those with low literacy. When the first announcements were made in August 1997, over 50 women came to the hospital immediately.

The Project conducted an exploratory study on the impact of VVF on girls' and women's lives, reported below. Educational outreach activities included a workshop on VVF and women's right to health for approximately 70 doctors, nurses, midwives and community health workers from the districts in Mwanza region. The Tanzania Midwives Association, which collaborates closely with the Project, designed and directed this outreach effort. In addition to taking information back to their districts, workshop participants mobilised women, men and young people in their communities to develop picture images on the health and rights of girls and women. These images, re-produced by the VVF Project in a 1999 calendar, formed part of the Project's public education materials.

Workshop participants also developed simple workplans for addressing women's health at the district level. Unfortunately, the Project was not in a position to ensure the implementation of the workplans, which, if this could have been started immediately, would have reinforced local health initiatives and reduced the frustration of health workers at the delays.

The Project also sought to break the silence surrounding VVF by stimulating open discussion among health workers and the public on girls' and women's right to health. In addition to the calendar, the Project collaborated with the kuleana centre for children's rights to produce 50,000 copies of a popular, pocket-sized booklet narrating the story of a young girl with VVF. Patients and staff at BMC were actively involved in developing the booklet. In addition, simple information sheets in Swahili on VVF and urinary stress incontinence were developed for all VVF patients at BMC and shared with other health facilities. All the Project's public education materials were distributed throughout the country in partnership with the Tanzania Ministry of Health.

Provocative wall murals, based on the picture images developed for the 1999 poster, were painted in six districts of Mwanza region. The murals were a popular and effective mechanism for increasing awareness about the determinants of VVF, including early marriage, and the responsibility of families and communities to assist women during pregnancy.

Other advocacy efforts sought to include VVF on the health agenda in Tanzania, Africa and internationally, including participation of the Project Team in medical and professional meetings, and collaboration with the media. In addition, as a result of regional collaboration, colleagues in other East African countries are interested in adapting the Project's public education materials.

Project staff placed a priority on establishing an efficient and streamlined project management system, with weekly meetings. Overall management of the Project was time intensive and often demanding for BMC staff, who had multiple commitments within and outside the hospital. Given the extensive demands on staff in many health settings, a project like this one may well require a person whose time is dedicated solely to its management.

A continuing challenge was to ensure that no girl or woman with VVF was turned away because she could not pay. Although some colleagues were concerned about providing free services, the Project was successful in raising money for the exclusive purpose of direct patient care. Institutions with religious affiliation and selected individuals committed to women's health have been particularly supportive in this regard. But unless and until there is a secure funding base for VVF repair in Africa, treatment may be sporadic and limited.

The study

The Bugando Medical Centre VVF Project conducted an exploratory study to document the impact of VVF on the lives of girls and women, and to use the findings for service delivery and advocacy. The first 50 patients who arrived at BMC for care at a VVF clinic between August and October 1997 were invited to participate. All 50 women agreed to take part. It is not known how representative the findings of the study are for women overall in Tanzania, given the relatively small size of the study population, the short study period and the limited catchment area. Nonetheless, discussions with VVF care providers in Tanzania point to similarities among women across the country.

All the participants in the study were Tanzanian, and the interviews were conducted in Swahili or the patients' first language. The primary interviewer was a Tanzanian woman who was experienced in conducting interviews for research and was aware of VVF through her own family and acquaintances. The interviews were conducted while the women waited for VVF repair and in the post-operative period. Follow-up interviews were not possible as patients returned to their homes.

Given the highly sensitive nature of VVF, confidentiality was assured and every attempt was made to interview patients in privacy. A semi-structured questionnaire comprising 61 questions was administered in one sitting; each interview took about 60-75 minutes. Questions covered the patient's socio-demographic background, marriage and children, her life before and after having VVF, the labour and delivery that resulted in VVF, previous attempts to get treatment, and experience at BMC. Computer analysis of the data was done by staff at the National Institute of Medical Research in Mwanza.

Who are the girls and women with VVF?

Research has shown a relationship between early marriage/childbearing and the risk of obstetric complications, including VVF. In Africa and South Asia many VVF patients are in their teen years and primiparae.[17,22-24] Sixty-four per cent of new VVF patients in a Nigeria study gave birth to their first child by the age of 17 and 33 per cent by the age of 16.[9] Nearly 20 per cent of VVF patients in Pakistan were between the ages of 15 and 19 and most were primiparae.[25]

Early marriage and childbearing were a common factor in this study; 25 per cent of the girls were married by the age of 16. Over three-quarters of study participants were aged 20 or less when they first became pregnant (Table 1) and 38 per cent were primiparae. Despite some encouraging signs that women are now marrying later in Tanzania, national data still show that

Table 1. Age at first pregnancy (n=49)

Age	Number	Per cent
< 15	1	2
15-20	37	74
21-25	9	18
26-30	1	2
N/A	1	2

in 1996, over a quarter of all teenagers had already begun childbearing[15] and there is evidence in some parts of Tanzania of a dramatic decrease in age at marriage due to parents' fears that girls may become pregnant outside of marriage.[19]

Approximately two-thirds of the patients and nearly three-quarters of their husbands in the BMC study had completed some or all of primary school. Slightly over half of the participants reported having currently living children before developing fistula, which is higher than in a Nigeria study, where approximately one third of patients had living children before developing fistula. The latter study found that having living children might have contributed to the stability of patients' marriages,[9] and this may have been the case in Tanzania as well.

Although questions on socio-economic status were not asked, the women reported a low level of income after acquiring VVF, and their anxiety regarding the costs of treatment and transport suggested that most came from backgrounds marked by poverty. Of the 80 per cent who responded as to their current earnings since having VVF, nearly half were unable to estimate any cash income; about a quarter had 'been unable to work for a long time' and 10 per cent reported that their income was 'too little in relation to their needs'.

About three-quarters of the women paid as much as US $9 for transport to the hospital for treatment, which represents about five per cent of the official annual per capita gross national product (GNP) in Tanzania. The appearance of patients upon arrival further confirmed their poor economic status – most brought only one *khanga* (cloth covering) and a bowl for food, but few had cash, soap, toothpaste or body cream to last during their hospital stay.

Experience and attendance in labour and seeking assistance

Nearly every patient in the BMC study began her labour at home, compared to about 50 per cent of women delivering at home in the general population.[15] Nearly all the patients (92 per cent) were eventually referred to a health facility, almost half of them to a site up to one hour away, and approximately one fifth to sites five to eight hours away.

Fewer than 12 per cent of the women were assisted by a trained health worker during childbirth and six per cent by a traditional birth attendant (TBA). Six per cent of the study participants laboured alone, and others were assisted primarily by a family member or other person (Table 2).

Poverty is likely to affect the ability to reach a health facility during the obstructed labour that can eventually lead to VVF. Often living in rural areas far from health care,[9,17] pregnant women with complications must travel long distances for obstetric care and, if they get VVF, for eventual treatment. In Tanzania, some people must walk up to 45 kilometers to reach a health facility.[16]

Studies from other countries indicate that some women with fistula experienced prolonged and obstructed labour for up to four days.[17,25,26] Almost two-thirds of the girls and women in this study were in labour for two or three days and eight per cent reported that labour continued for over three days. None of the study participants reported that the people around them understood the problem of obstructed labour or how it related to the age of the mother, reinforcing the need for basic education on these issues.

At the health facilities to which the study participants were transferred, 42 per cent had a caesarean section and another 42 per cent had an assisted

Table 2. Assistance during childbirth (n=47)

Assistant	Number	Per cent
Mother	15	30
Mother-in-law	7	14
Trained health worker	6	12
Husband	5	10
Alone	3	6
Traditional birth attendant	3	6
Friend	1	2
Other	7	14

vaginal delivery. Over three-quarters reported that the baby was dead at delivery, exacerbating an already traumatic situation. In some studies of VVF, the rates of fetal death are much higher.[17] Once women in the study began leaking urine, only two were given catheters to manage the VVF, highlighting the absence of adequate services and information at the peripheral level.

After being treated at BMC, approximately 80 per cent of the 50 women were cured of their fistulae. Patients who were not cured were given follow-up appointments and counselling. Information sheets on VVF printed in Swahili were given to all patients and a specific sheet explaining pelvic floor exercises was given to patients experiencing stress incontinence after repair.

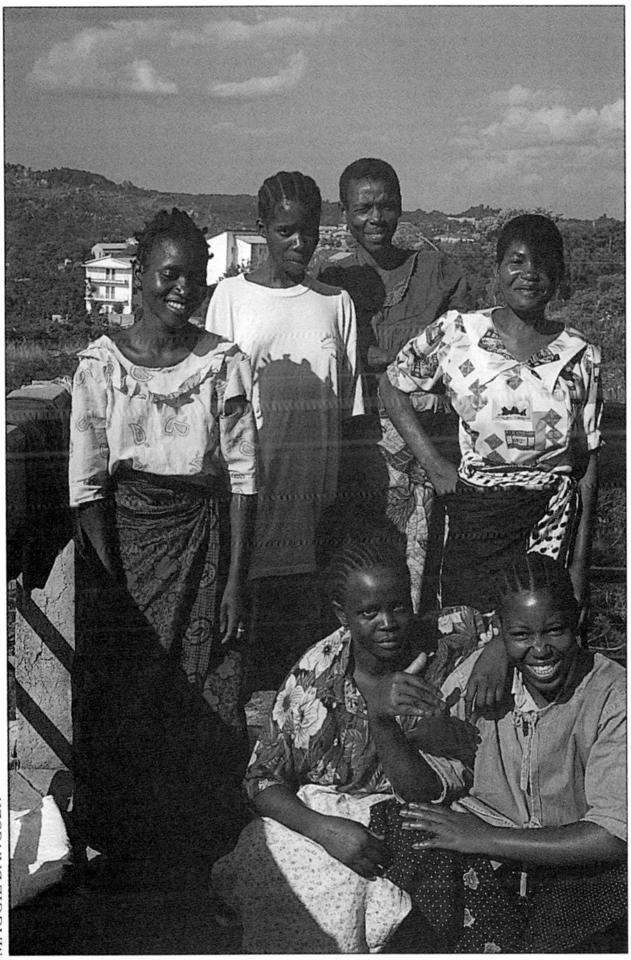

MAGGIE BANGSER

VVF patients, Bugando Medical Centre

Effect on inter-personal relationships

Leaking urine may significantly affect the inter-personal relationships between women with fistula and their husbands. Nearly all of the women in the study were, or had been, married. Approximately half of them were still living with their husbands when they came to the hospital for treatment. However, among those not living with their husbands, three-quarters said the reason for the separation was the fistula. Thirty per cent of all the patients said their husbands had taken other wives after they began leaking.

Nearly a third of the patients came alone to the hospital, not accompanied by a husband or other relative. Approximately one fifth of the women were visited by their mothers, and a quarter by their husbands. BMC nurses and members of the Project Team were often the only people who provided company on the ward. In many cases, the women said their friends and family were afraid to be made financially responsible for the treatment, and so chose to stay away from the hospital.

Of the women who came to BMC for repair, only 18 per cent reported becoming pregnant again after acquiring VVF; studies from other countries indicate that many women experience lack of menstruation following fistula.[27,28] This intensifies the experience of isolation and shame.

Many of the women who came to BMC in search of a cure said they had lived with VVF for a long period of time (Table 3). Almost a quarter had been living with fistula for a decade or more. Research from India suggests that some women had been living with this condition for over 20 years before it was repaired.[27]

Participants in the study were asked about their experience living with VVF and how their lives had changed since they began leaking and were awaiting repair. Two thirds of the girls and women reported experiences of isolation. One third reported that they were doing different work than before the leaking began and many worked alone rather than around others. Over two-thirds worked inside their homes,

Table 3. Length of time living with fistula (n=48)

Number of years	Number	Per cent
>1	11	22
1-3	15	30
4-6	5	10
7-9	6	12
10+	11	22

and a similar number said that the VVF made it difficult for them to do work at all.

While most of the study participants said that their families and friends treated them the same as they had before the leaking began, nearly 90 per cent said they felt ashamed of themselves. Over three-quarters said the leaking caused them to feel differently about going out of their homes or socialising, having sexual relations or working, or going out to pray (Table 4).

When asked if they would like to marry again, over a third of the patients said no, and when asked about having children, over half said they did not want to try again. Staff of the Addis Ababa Fistula Hospital report that patients there also felt extreme anxiety about attempting childbirth again, given the risk of repeated fistula and the shame it brings.[29]

When counselled to refrain from sexual relations for six months after repair in order to heal fully, one patient in the study said firmly that she would make sure she didn't have sexual relations for a year. BMC staff and patients have expressed concern, however, that women who have been repaired will quickly be pressured to resume sexual relations and face another pregnancy that leads to another fistula. One BMC patient was cured of fistula but was left with severe stenosis of the vagina, making sexual relations difficult if not impossible; she refused any procedure to open the vagina as she feared the leaking would again begin.

Table 4. Changes in how women feel about their lives with VVF (n=50)

Negative feelings about:	Number	Per cent
Wanting to go outside of home	40	80
Having sexual relations	40	80
Working to earn money	39	78
Talking and sitting with others	34	68
Having visitors	31	62
Going to pray	30	60

At the same time, many patients who were cured demonstrated outward optimism and confidence in the future. The Addis Ababa Fistula Hospital specialists told BMC staff that the surest sign of a cured patient is when she begins to braid her hair again.[6] And indeed, BMC staff often saw girls and women who had been cured sitting on the hospital balcony braiding each other's hair before being discharged.

Discussion and recommendations for action

Health workers in Africa working in the field of VVF state emphatically that poverty is a key factor putting girls and women at risk of VVF. The BMC study reinforces this view and suggests that limited personal finances may heighten women's risk of inadequate care during delivery and constrain their ability to seek VVF repair once injured. In the BMC study, large numbers of patients came from subsistence backgrounds and had lived with VVF for many years. Many reported that they worked alone and had trouble earning cash income, and this social exclusion may well limit economic opportunity further. Evidence of patients' limited access to cash, coupled with the costs of treatment and transport, suggests that VVF care is likely to be out of reach for many who are living with the condition. Given that repeated visits to a hospital are required for many patients, treatment and care becomes even more elusive.

VVF is also a reflection of inadequate provision at the health sector level. System-wide deficiencies are seen in the large percentage of study participants who went through childbirth alone, delivered without trained assistance, and laboured for long periods of time before reaching a health facility. Because VVF repair is done in very few hospitals, the distance women had to travel for repair was often even longer than to a service delivery point that could assist with childbirth.

Data from the BMC study and other research point clearly to the severe impact of VVF on the lives of those who have the condition. Only half of the study participants who were married were still living with their husbands; in other studies, abandonment of women with VVF was even more common. Stigma associated with the inability to bear further children is likely to be part of this problem. Most study participants reported significant deterioration in their sense of self after beginning to leak. Over three-quarters felt differently about walking out of their homes.

Prevention of prolonged, obstructed labour is needed to reduce the incidence of VVF. Thus, attention to VVF should be mainstreamed into a larger reproductive health and rights agenda that can address broader aspects of women's lives. Mainstreaming may bring greater attention and resources to a specific issue such as VVF, and make initiatives to address the condition more sustainable.

Because thousands of women are already living with VVF and the condition is likely to persist for a long time to come, more and better services should be established that are accessible and affordable to women, including those unable to pay.

Hands-on training for doctors and nurses in surgical and post-operative nursing care is needed, with doctors conducting repairs alongside skilled surgeons. Post-operative care is essential to successful VVF repairs, and as such, training for nurses should focus on the specific protocol required. Training for both doctors and nurses should include the psycho-social support needed by patients before, during and after repair.

Potentially difficult decisions may be called for to assure that training is provided to professionals who are committed to VVF care. Training is a popular activity and medical professionals are unlikely to decline an opportunity to learn new skills. Doctors and nurses who participate in VVF training should be willing to provide treatment afterwards with the full recognition that VVF care typically pays poorly and holds little status in the medical community. At the same time, the health care facilities where those doctors and nurses are employed need to ensure adequate supplies and equipment for VVF care so their staff can conduct repairs after they have been trained.

Given the highly stigmatised nature of VVF, special clinics within established health facilities are an excellent opportunity to ensure appropriate and timely care for women in a safe and respectful way. Financial resources are critical if VVF clinics are to provide free treatment to those who could otherwise not afford care. Religious institutions and women's rights advocates might be particularly good partners in raising funds for VVF care.

Averting future cases of VVF and treating those girls and women who already have it requires sustained investment in peripheral level health facilities, affordable health care for the poor, and reduced fees for VVF treatment. The capacity to prevent and treat VVF is likely to be constrained sharply by local budgets, and the fact that cost-sharing programmes may be making health care less accessible for the poor and less utilised.[30-32]

VVF needs to be leveraged onto health agendas in Africa and internationally in order to increase human capacity and funding to address the problem. Advocacy on VVF should address global development issues that undermine the provision of health care in countries such as Tanzania, where insufficient government allocations to health care and the burden of debt servicing[33] threaten the capacity of the health system to manage obstetric emergencies along with other health conditions. In Tanzania, where the government spends nine times more on debt repayments than on basic health,[34] it is not surprising that investment in primary health is insufficient.

Conclusion

Programmes focusing on safe motherhood seek to increase the capacity of health facilities to reduce maternal mortality. This is extremely important, but where there is obstructed labour leading to maternal mortality, there is also likely to be significant morbidity,[35] including VVF. Decreasing maternal morbidity is often perceived as even more difficult than decreasing maternal mortality. Nonetheless, it is imperative that reproductive health initiatives increase attention to the quality of life of women who survive after complications of childbirth, and who live many years with the often devastating consequences.

Acknowledgements

Sincere thanks to Blandina Lwamenzi for excellent help with interviews and answers to questionnaires; Celestina Solo for early help with interviews; Rebecca Balira, Genoveva Kalaye and Frola Gabone for assistance with data entry and analysis. We appreciate feedback of staff and colleagues of the Bugando Medical Centre VVF Project who participated in the workshop on the research findings; including Drs Kimaro and Ng'walida; and Nurses Gondwe, Bakari, Leonard, Ziota, Bushiri, Mach and the late Ms. George. Thanks to Rakesh Rajani for support in developing the data collection instrument and comments on this article. The BMC VVF Project was funded by the Royal Netherlands Embassy, Alliances, kuleana centre for children's rights, Maryknoll Fathers and Brothers, individual contributors in the United States and BMC.

Correspondence

Maggie Bangser, Women's Dignity Project, 118 Highland Road, #1, Somerville, MA 02144 USA. Fax: 1-617-625-7784. E-mail: mbangser@hotmail.com

References

1. *Obstetric Fistulae: A Review of Available Information.* WHO/MCH/MSM/91.5, World Health Organization, Geneva, 1991.
2. Harrison KA, 1989. Obstetric Fistulae. Paper prepared for a Technical Working Group of the World Health Organization. Unpublished.
3. Mustafa AZ, Rushwan HME, 1971. Acquired genito-urinary fistulae in the Sudan. *Journal of Obstetrics and Gynaecology of the British Commonwealth.* 78:1039-43.
4. Harrison KA, 1985. Childbearing, health and social priorities: a survey of 22,774 consecutive hospital births in Zaria, Northern Nigeria. *British Journal of Obstetrics and Gynaecology.* Supplement 5: 119.
5. Kelly J. Personal communication, January 1998.
6. Wolde AM. Personal communication. 1997.
7. Leonard D. Personal communication. 1997, 1998.
8. Hamlin C. Personal communication, July 1996.
9. Murphy M, 1981. Social consequences of vesico-vaginal fistula in northern Nigeria. *Journal of Biosocial Sciences.* 13:139-50.
10. Muhammad H, 1998. Obstetric fistulae as seen at Dodoma Regional Hospital, Tanzania. Paper presented at workshop: Maternal Health in sub-Saharan Africa. Dar es Salaam, June.
11. *The Prevention and Treatment of Obstetric Fistulae. Report of a Technical Working Group.* WHO/FHE/89.5, World Health Organization, Geneva, April 1989.
12. Kimaro E. Personal communication, December, 1998.
13. Lawson J, 1989. Tropical obstetrics and gynaecology: vesico-vaginal fistula – a tropical disease. *Transactions of the Royal Society of Tropical Medicine and Hygiene.* 83:454-56.
14. Kelly J, 1979. Vesicovaginal fistulae. *British Journal of Urology.* 51:208-10.
15. *Demographic and Health Survey 1996.* Republic of Tanzania Bureau of Statistics Planning Commission and Macro International Inc. 1997.
16. *The Girl Child in Tanzania: A Research Report.* UNICEF, Dar es Salaam, 1995.
17. Kelly J, Kwast BE, 1993. Epidemiologic study of vesicovaginal fistulas in Ethiopia. *International Urogynecology Journal.* 4:278-81.
18. *The State of the World's Children.* UNICEF, New York, 1998.
19. Ampofo K, 1990. Epidemiology of vesico-vaginal fistulae in Northern Nigeria. *West African Journal of Medicine.* 9(2):98-102.
20. Hanif H. Personal communication, 1989. See ref [1].
21. Arrowsmith S, Hamlin EC, Wall LL, 1996. Obstructed labour injury complex: obstetric fistula formation and the multifaceted morbidity of maternal birth trauma in the developing world. obstetrical and gynecological survey. *CME Review Article.* 51(9):568-74.
22. Tahzib F, 1983. Epidemiological determinants of vesicovaginal fistulas. *British Journal of Obstetrics and Gynaecology.* 90:387-91.
23. Haile A, 1983. Fistula – a socio-medical problem. *Ethiopian Medical Journal.* 21(2):71-78.
24. Shah KP, 1989. Enquiry on the epidemiology and surgical repair of obstetric related fistula in South-East Asia. Paper prepared for a Technical Working Group for the World Health Organization. (Unpublished)
25. Aziz FA, 1965. Urinary fistulae from obstetrical trauma. *Journal of Obstetrics and Gynaecology of the British Commonwealth.* 72:765-68.
26. Kelly J, 1992. Vesico-vaginal and recto-vaginal fistulae. *Journal of the Royal Society of Medicine.* 85:257-58.
27. Bhasker Rao K, 1972. Vesico-vaginal fistula – a study of 269 cases. *Journal of Obstetrics and Gynaecology of India.* 22(5):536-41.

28. Evoh NJ, Akinia O, 1978. Reproductive performance after the repair of obstetric vesico-vaginal fistulae. *Annals of Clinical Research*. 10:303-06.
29. Befekadu, A. Personal communication, August 1997.
30. Hussein AK, Mujijna PGM, 1997. The impact of user charges in government health facilities in Tanzania. *East African Journal of Medicine*. 74(12):752-53.
31. Mmbuji PDL, Ilomo PA, Nswilla AL, 1996. *Implementation of Health Services User Fees in Tanzania: An Evaluation of Progress and Potential Impact.* United Republic of Tanzania Ministry of Health. Dar es Salaam.
32. Moses S, Manji F, Bradley J et al, 1992. Impact of user fees on attendance at a referral centre for sexually transmitted diseases in Kenya. *Lancet*. 340:463-66.
33. Lawson A, 1997. *Tanzania: Public Expenditure Review – Budgeting Priorities in the Social Sectors.* Oxford Policy Management.
34. *Debt Relief for Tanzania: An Opportunity for a Better Future.* Oxfam International, April 1998.
35. Maternal morbidities affect tens of millions. *Network*. 1994; 14(3):8-11.

Women's Experiences of Utero-Vaginal Prolapse: A Qualitative Study from Tamil Nadu, India

TK Sundari Ravindran, R Savitri and A Bhavani

This paper reports on women's experiences of uterine prolapse and their perceptions of its causes, based on interviews and clinical examination. Of 37 rural, poor women in Tamil Nadu, India, who thought they had uterine prolapse and volunteered to be examined by a gynaecologist, clinical examination confirmed the diagnosis in 32 of them. All 32 women worked as agricultural wage labourers. The mean age at which they first developed symptoms of the condition was 26.2. All but two of them had had uncomplicated deliveries, yet 13 of them first experienced symptoms of prolapse after their first or second deliveries and many of the women had suffered from this condition for over ten years. The women considered strenous manual work soon after delivery to be an important factor associated with uterine prolapse, alongside frequent childbearing and trauma to the pelvic floor following surgery. Uterine prolapse seriously compromised the quality of life of those affected by it and had far reaching consequences not only for their physical health, but also for their ability to work and earn a livelihood and their sexual lives. They faced a series of barriers to medical help for uterine prolapse which prevented them from getting successful treatment, ranging from lack of familial support and their own reluctance to mention the problem to a doctor, to long waiting times to be treated, ineffective treatment, and high monetary and opportunity costs. A community-based women's health organisation can offer prevention education and support for affected women and their families and help women to obtain treatment.

PROLAPSE of the uterus is usually described as one of the long-term sequelae of a difficult delivery. It can be caused by damage to the pelvic floor muscles because of bearing down during delivery before complete dilation of the cervix and can sometimes also occur following gynaecological surgery.[1-3]

An early study in India during 1952-54 found that among 5,494 women with gynaecological complaints visiting private clinics in Bengal, Delhi, Punjab and Uttar Pradesh, one in five women examined suffered from uterine prolapse.[1] Another more recent study, conducted in MGM Hospital in Eastern India in 1991, found that genital prolapse constituted 20 per cent of all gynaecological admissions.[2]

There are three degrees of utero-vaginal prolapse. In first-degree prolapse, the cervix appears at the vaginal opening only when the woman bears down. In second-degree prolapse, the cervix descends to the level of the vulva, and in third-degree prolapse, the cervix protrudes outside the vulva. The entire uterus may also protrude outside the vulva, bringing with it the vaginal wall.

Prolapse which causes discomfort is most commonly treated surgically by vaginal hysterectomy or by partial amputation of the elongated cervix. Occasionally, a polythene ring pessary may be used to keep the cervix from descending into the vagina.[4]

In India, women with utero-vaginal prolapse are treated by vaginal hysterectomy. Ring pessaries are rarely used because of the associated risk of vaginal infections. Women from low-income groups do not usually opt for surgery, however, either because they are in poor health or because they cannot afford it. Instead, women seeking help from public health facilities are often treated with drugs for secondary infections, ulceration and pain.

A woman with prolapse may complain of a

lump in the vagina or a feeling that 'something is coming down', back-ache, a bearing-down sensation, abdominal pain, vaginal discharge, disturbances of micturition, frequent urination and dysuria, stress incontinence, difficulty in defecation, profuse menstrual periods, irregular vaginal bleeding or bleeding due to a protruding prolapse becoming ulcerated. With the more serious forms of prolapse, the external swelling may affect the woman's ability to walk and to carry out her every day duties.[5]

Most published studies to date on uterine prolapse are hospital-based and clinical, and examine aspects such as numbers of women with the condition, characteristics of those diagnosed with the condition and prognosis following surgical repair.[6-10]

This paper reports on a community-based study of women's perceptions of the causes of uterine prolapse and the problems they experienced from it, carried out among women suffering from this condition in several villages in Tamil Nadu, India. The data are based on information collected from 37 rural, poor women who volunteered to have a clinical examination by a gynaecologist. Although the data come from a small, self-selected sample of women, the relevance lies in the focus on women's perceptions of the causes of uterine prolapse and the impact of this condition on their daily lives.

Background and methodology

The women whose perceptions and experiences are reported in this paper come from the villages surrounding Chengalpattu town in Tamil Nadu, India. As part a community health project, the Rural Women's Social Education Centre (RUWSEC), a grassroots women's organisation working in these villages who also run a small non-profit hospital, learned from a baseline survey that 106 of the 4,117 women between 15 and 50 years of age in the villages covered by the project were suffering from second- or third-degree uterine prolapse (according to the women's own self-reports). Following this finding, there was a demand from the community for a clinical check-up.[11]

The clinical examination was organised in a community hall in Tirukkazhukundram town, located centrally and well-connected by public buses to the villages from which the women came. The women were compensated for the bus fare, and the clinical examination was carried out free of cost. Drugs for vaginal infections and to treat ulceration and pain were also dispensed free of cost following the clinical examination.

The day's events consisted of a workshop in the morning on utero-vaginal prolapse and its management and treatment. The workshop session had built in a lot of discussion – time for women to ask questions and clarify their doubts. This was followed in the afternoon by the clinical examination of the women by a senior gynaecologist.

Information on women's perceptions and experiences on uterine prolapse was collected by RUWSEC's senior community workers in one of the rooms, with the help of a check-list, at the same time as the gynaecologist performed the clinical examinations in another room. The interviews were carried out in privacy and with the informed consent of the women. The primary purpose of the data collection was to help RUWSEC with suitable follow-up activities.

Characteristics of the women and extent of uterine prolapse

All 37 women who volunteered for the clinical examination and attended the workshop were from landless, agricultural labouring households, and belonged to the Scheduled Castes. All of them worked as manual wage labourers in agriculture. Nearly all of them (34 out of 37) were illiterate.

Thirty-two of the 37 women (87 per cent) were found to be suffering from utero-vaginal prolapse on clinical examination, while five did not have any apparent gynaecological problem. The high level of correspondence between the women's self-reports and the medical diagnosis in this instance is noteworthy. The mean age of those with prolapse at the time of the examination was 37.5.[12] However, the mean age at which the women had first developed symptoms of the condition was 26.2 years. Indeed, many had been suffering from the condition for more than ten years (mean 12.3 years).

Ten of the women said they had developed symptoms of uterine prolapse after their very first delivery, three after their second delivery, 11 after their third delivery, nine after their fourth to sixth deliveries and two after their ninth delivery.

Thirty-five of the women had experienced only normal deliveries; one had had a forceps-

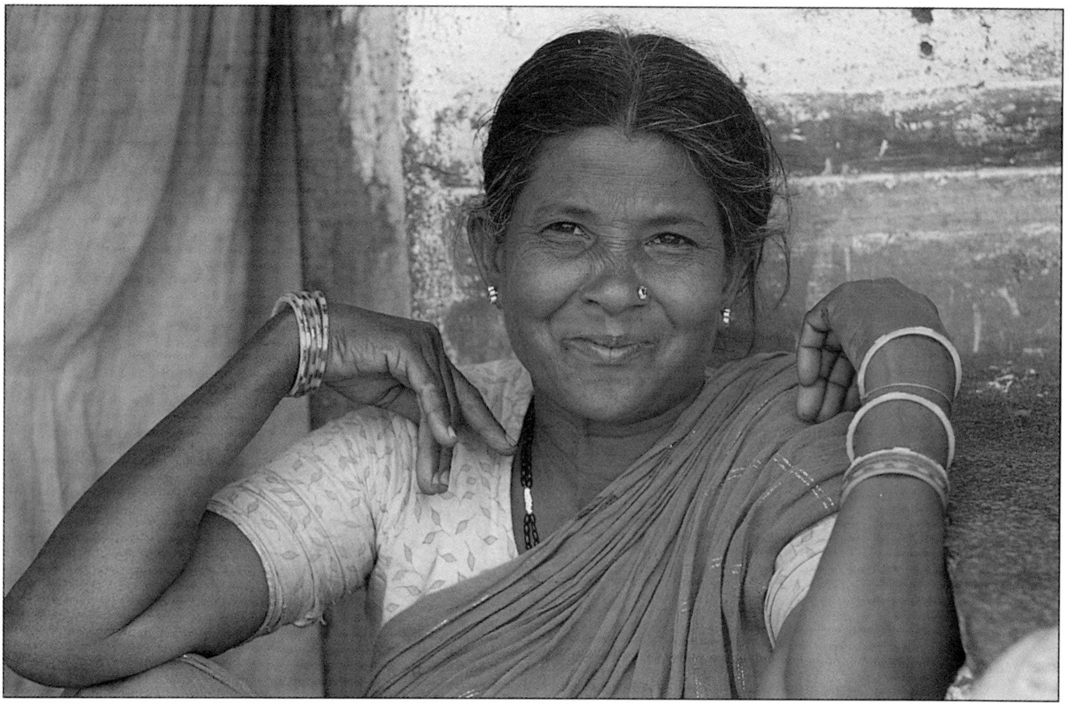

VICTOR LAMONT / HUTCHISON LIBRARY

assisted delivery and one a stillbirth. Thirteen of the 32 women (40 per cent) had delivered all their babies at home, while nine (28 per cent) had had all their deliveries in a public hospital, and the remaining ten had delivered some babies at home and some – usually their first and last – in hospital. Twenty-two of the 32 women had undergone tubal ligation in hospital – the 19 who had had hospital deliveries and three others.

The profile of those with prolapse in this instance appears to vary from that commonly found in medical textbooks. For example, one text book describes the typical patient who complains of prolapse as a 'woman aged about 50 years, who has given birth to several children and who usually gives the history of a difficult confinement or of the birth of large children'.[5] Studies from industrialised countries have also reported that the woman's age, parity and weight are significantly associated with the risk of uterine prolapse.[7,9]

However, according to some developing country studies, uterine prolapse may also occur in a relatively young population. Although rural women delivering in hospital may not be representative of the population of childbearing women as a whole, a study in two hospitals in Kenya in the period 1989-1993 found 156 women in one hospital and 195 women in the other with uterine prolapse, in both cases from among a mainly rural, relatively young population.[13] In another study in Dakar of 104 cases of genital prolapse, the average age of the women was 30, and 64 per cent were between the ages of 20 and 39.[14] A 1951-1954 study in India of 214 women admitted to the gynaecological ward of the Osmania Hospital, Hyderabad, also observed that uterine prolapse was not necessarily the outcome of repeated childbirth but often followed damage to the pelvic floor as early as after the very first delivery.[15]

Perceived causes

When the women were asked what they thought had caused the uterine prolapse, 18 of the 32 women mentioned heavy manual labour within a week to a fortnight following delivery as the cause. The stories of these 18 women were very similar – of having lifted up water pots or the heavy instrument for pounding rice or millet – and sensing a protrusion soon after.

'I delivered my first child in my husband's home, because my mother was too poor to bring me home for delivery. I had no rest even for a week. One day, I had to carry a huge basket of cow dung. As I bent down and lifted it up from the floor to put it on my head, I felt something give way inside.' (30-year-old woman with 3 children)

'After my third delivery, I had to do all the household work from the very next day. I had to boil the paddy to dehusk it (to make rice). After sitting next to the fire for many hours, when I lifted the large vessel up to drain the water, I blacked out and fainted. Since this, I have had the prolapse.' (42-year-old woman with 3 children)

'We are very poor. My husband and I were both bonded labourers in those days. It was soon after my first delivery, I had to carry a heavy bundle of firewood on my head. That's when it happened.' (45-year-old woman with 9 children)

All but three of the women who developed prolapse after their first or second deliveries (10 of 13 women) reported such incidents. Of the other three, two thought that a difficult first delivery had caused the prolapse. In the case of one woman, her child had been stillborn following her first pregnancy. She was returning home to her village from hospital afterwards, travelling by three-wheeler taxi (auto rickshaw). The vehicle met with an accident and she was flung out. She suffered serious injury and dates her uterine prolapse from that time.

Of the remaining 11 women who mentioned other causes, four women mentioned first birth at a young age (between 15 and 18 years of age) followed by frequent childbearing as responsible for their uterine prolapse. There are few methods of contraception available from the family planning programme in India for spacing births, except for IUDS, which women tend to avoid, mainly because of reproductive tract infections and excessive bleeding.

Five others said that the prolapse had followed surgery – sterilisation in three cases, induced abortion in one case and surgery for fibroids in one case. Another had developed symptoms of uterine prolapse following a miscarriage.

One woman reported violence on the part of her husband as the time when her experience of the problem began. This woman had had to return to hospital for a resuturing of her tubectomy incision. Her husband was very angry that she had gone away yet again, leaving him to manage everything at home. Finding her lying down after her return from hospital, he physically assaulted her.

Particularly heartrending was the history of one 26-year-old woman, whose two babies had both died in infancy. She had a second-degree prolapse and was afraid of another birth, but she also badly wanted to have a baby because her husband was contemplating remarriage.

Associated health problems

Sixteen of the 32 women (50 per cent) had been living with uterine prolapse for more than ten years, while six had been suffering from it for six to ten years and ten had developed it within the previous five years. Those who had had the condition for many years reported that the degree of severity of the prolapse had been increasing over time, and that it was becoming more and more difficult to live with it.

The women were suffering from a number of health problems associated with uterine prolapse. The problems mentioned most often were difficulty in standing and sitting because of the prolapse, an obstructed and blocking feeling (16 women) and backache (14 women). Obstruction while passing urine and bowel motion (seven women) was the next most common problem. Four women had acute lower abdominal pain, and six others complained of profuse and smelly or itchy white discharge. Other problems included recurrent episodes of urinary tract infection (four women) and heavy menstrual bleeding (three women). Some women suffered from more than one of these problems.

Three women with third-degree uterine prolapse said they had ulcers on the 'protruding part' and five women (including these three) complained of their protrusion 'getting caught' in their sarees when they worked, often causing ulceration with blood oozing out.

'The saree gets caught when I get up, and water starts oozing out of the wound. I have heavy bleeding during periods.'

'The pain in my genital region is unbearable.'

'I am unable to do any work and feel very depressed. Very often I get acute pain and a burning sensation during urination. There is also a profuse and smelly white discharge on many days.'

While only eight women reported problems related to ulceration, 16 women were found to have cervical erosion and/or ulcerated cervix on clinical examination, and were referred for a biopsy for cervical cancer.

Difficulties with housework and labouring

Living with uterine prolapse is far more than a health problem for poor women dependent on heavy manual labour to earn their livelihood. Twenty-one of the 32 women talked about the problems they faced because of their 'inability to lift heavy objects' (seven women) and 'difficulty in working in the farm' (14 women).

'I have been unable to go for harvesting for the past two years, because I am not able to carry the bundles of harvested paddy or remove the chaff from the grain (which involves lifting up the basket of grain and chaff above one's head)... And you know that the highest wages are earned during the harvest.'

All the women with third-degree prolapse and ten of the 13 with second-degree prolapse said that as they grew older, they were finding it increasingly difficult to do even routine domestic tasks such as fetching water, carrying firewood or lifting pots up from the fire while cooking.

'When I carry something heavy, it comes down more. I can hardly walk then.'

'Squatting down to wash clothes and vessels is becoming excruciating.'

Problems with sexual relations

Relations with spouses were strained because of the problems women had during sexual intercourse. Twenty-two women said that they tried to avoid sex, and that this was a source of constant friction between themselves and their husbands. In the case of 12 women, sexual intercourse was an ordeal to be endured, at most once in two weeks and for others even less frequently, once in several months. The remaining ten said that their husbands regularly forced themselves on them, despite it being not at all enjoyable and indeed, often extremely painful for the women. Violence and battering associated with forced sexual intercourse were reported by eight of these ten.

'My husband beats me daily as I am neither able to go to the fields to work nor willing to sleep with him.'

'He refuses to believe that I am in pain. He says, "What's wrong with you, you look healthy and robust, who are you waiting for, if not me?"'

'When he is drunk, there is no reasoning with him. If he is sober, he is considerate.'

Barriers to medical help

Twenty of the 32 women had not sought any medical help for their condition. Most of them (15) did not give any reasons why when asked. The five women who did give reasons mentioned fear of surgery (2), lack of time (1) and not being permitted by their husband to seek medical help for this condition (1).

Four women had sought treatment and had been on medication for some time, but could not give details as to whether these were meant to treat associated infections or were painkillers. They said they had received no information from the doctors or other health workers who attended them on the course of action required for this condition. Because they felt no better, they had stopped taking the medications.

'I went to the hospital more than ten years ago. They said I would get better with drugs and that no surgery was required. I did not get any better. So I stopped taking the drugs, and did not go again.'

One woman said, however, that although she had gone to the hospital several times, she had never been able to tell the doctor that the prolapse was the actual reason for her visit. Instead, she had complained of breathlessness, difficulty walking, aches and pains, and had hoped the doctor would probe further. This had never happened, and so she was usually given pills for 'strength'.

Another woman had gone to the hospital several only to be told to come back after a month or two for admission for surgery, because there was a long waiting list for gynaecological surgeries. She had given up after four such visits.

Six women had been admitted to hospital for tests and surgery, but had left without any treatment, for a variety of reasons. Two others had left hospital because of emergencies at home – in one case the death of her father-in-law, and in the other case the death of her infant daughter. The woman whose infant daughter had died, who was 50 years old with five children and who thought she had developed prolapse after aborting her sixth pregnancy, said she had had no free time to go back. Two others had stayed in the government hospital for over a month waiting for surgery; they had left against medical advice, because they could not stay away any longer. Two others had been refused surgery after admission because they were acutely anaemic and were considered a surgical risk.

Twenty-nine of the women interviewed requested medical help from RUWSEC. Five were shown how to do pelvic floor exercises and recommended to try these for a period of six months, and then return for another check-up. All the rest of the women, for whom surgical correction (11) or biopsy (16) was recommended, were keen on going through with the procedures. However, the costs were a major worry for all of them. Although treatment provided at RUWSEC's hospital is subsidised to the extent of 50 per cent of the total cost, the women were not in a position to afford even this much and asked to be charged a flat rate of Rs 500/- (US$ 12.50) This represented 80 per cent of their monthly earnings, but it would have covered only 10 per cent of the costs incurred by the hospital.[16]

Removal of the cost barrier alone would not have made treatment accessible for all the women. Four of them were afraid that their husbands would not permit them to go in for the surgery even at the reduced cost of Rs 500/- because there would be other expenses involved, e.g. costs for visiting and for food for a companion who would stay with them in hospital. Moreover, the women's absence from home would be an inconvenience for their husbands. Two women worried about lack of support for taking care of their children while they were away in hospital, and also to help them with domestic tasks after the surgery.

Conclusions

The literature on obstetric morbidities such as uterine prolapse rarely gives a glimpse of what it means to women to live with this condition for years on end without support from their husbands, and without access to appropriate medical help in the way that has been described here.

The women in this group thought that strenous manual work soon after delivery was an important factor associated with uterine prolapse, alongside frequent childbearing and trauma to the pelvic floor following surgery. For many of them, symptoms begin to appear at an early age, after their first or second deliveries.

Uterine prolapse seriously compromised the quality of life of the women affected, with far-reaching consequences not only for their physical health, but also for their sexual lives and their ability to work and earn a livelihood. They faced a series of barriers to medical help for uterine prolapse, ranging from their own reluctance to mention it to a doctor and husbands unwilling to allow them to seek treatment, ineffective treatment and high monetary and opportunity costs, especially long waiting times for surgery in hospital.

The level of correspondence between the women's self-reports and medical diagnosis of uterine prolapse (86.5 per cent) was high. A study in Istanbul reported a similarly high level of specificity – 95.7 per cent when women's reporting of pelvic relaxation was compared to medical diagnosis.[17] This suggests that community-based surveys with well-constructed questionnaires could be a reliable means of identifying women suffering from utero-vaginal prolapse. The perceptions of the women in this present study of the possible causes of prolapse were also notable in that they were medically valid and plausible causes.

Some degree of relaxation of pelvic muscles, and a consequent mild degree of genital prolapse may not be totally preventable, especially as women grow older. However, severe forms of early uterine prolapse, such as those described in this study, are avoidable, even in poor, rural communities. Community-based organisations like RUWSEC who are working in the area of women's health, could initiate interventions that would help to alleviate the needless suffering of poor women with this condition, including to:

- carry out community education on limiting women's exposure to the risk of uterine prolapse from an early age, e.g. that pregnant women should avoid bearing down during delivery before the cervix has dilated completely; after delivery, women should avoid strenuous work for a period of at least six weeks and should do pelvic-floor exercises in the post-partum period;
- make a wider choice of temporary contraceptives available to women for spacing births;
- suggest ways to minimise and alleviate problems in day-to-day life faced by women affected, e.g. counselling women, their husbands and families, to help them appreciate the nature of the problem and ways in which they could be supportive of affected women;
- organise support networks for affected women, e.g. to accompany them to hospital and help them with domestic tasks; and
- find ways to make appropriate medical help more accessible to women, e.g. arranging for subsidised treatment, including surgery.

Correspondence

TK Sundari Ravindran, Rural Women's Social Education Centre, Nehru Nagar, Vallam Post, Chengalpattu-603 002, Tamil Nadu, India. Tel/Fax: 91-4114-30682.

References and Notes

1. Satur DM, Chakraverti J, 1955. A statistical survey of prolapse of the uterus with respect to age and parity. *Journal of Obstetrics and Gynaecology of India.* 6:147-50.
2. Kamini Naik, Ahuja M, Kaduskar N et al, 1993. Are the trends in genital prolapse changing? *Journal of Obstetrics and Gynaecology of India.* 1:426-31.
3. Gynecological examinations and managing common gynecological problems: Training Course in Women's Health, Module 4, 1993. Institute for Development Training, New York.
4. Chamberlain G (ed), 1996. *Gynaecology by Ten Teachers.* 16th edition. Elbs, London.
5. Padubiri VG, Daftary SN (eds), 1994. *Shaw's Textbook of Gynaecology.* Hawkins and Bourne. (11th edition).
6. Dutta DK, Dutta B, 1994. Surgical management of genital prolapse in an industrial hospital. *Journal of Indian Medical Association.* 92(11):366-67.
7. Virtanen HS, Makinen JI, 1993. Retrospective analysis of 711 patients operated on for pelvic relaxation in 1983-89. *International Journal of Obstetrics and Gynecology.* 42(2):109-15.
8. Allahbadia GN, 1992. Reproductive performance following sleeve excision anastomosis operation for genital prolapse. *Australia New Zealand Journal of Obstetrics and Gynaecology.* 32(2):149-53.
9. Mant J, Painter R, Vessey M, 1997. Epidemiology of genital prolapse: observations from the Oxford Family Planning Association Study. *British Journal of Obstetrics and Gynaecology.* 104(5):579-85.
10. Banu LF, 1997. Synthetic sling for genital prolapse in young women. *International Journal of Obstetrics and Gynecology.* 57(1):57-64.
11. Report of the baseline survey on women's health, 1996-97. Chengalpattu (India), Rural Women's Social Education Centre, Unpublished monograph, May 1998.
12. A comparison of the characteristics of the 37 women who volunteered for the clinical examination with that of the 106 women who had reported suffering from utero-vaginal prolapse in the baseline survey shows that the latter were a much younger group (mean age 31.9 years). This is possibly a reflection on the women's health-seeking behaviour – they wait till the problem becomes very difficult to cope with. Nearly 60 per cent of them had delivered their first babies in a hospital, and 50 per cent of all deliveries had taken place in hospital. Ninety-eight per cent of the deliveries were normal and full-term, and about one per cent each were pre-term and forceps deliveries respectively.
13. Lukman Y, 1995. Utero-vaginal prolapse: a rural disability of the young. *East African Medical Journal.* 72(1):2-9.
14. Dia A, Toure CT, Diop MB et al, 1991. Les prolapsus genitaux a Dakar. *Dakar Medicale.* 36(1):39-46.
15. Ramachandran AS, 1955. A statistical survey of prolapse of the uterus in relation to parity and age. *Journal of Obstetrics and Gynaecology of India.* 6:162-65.
16. RUWSEC decided to raise funds to make treatment available at a price affordable to the women, and even to perform surgeries free of cost to those who could not afford to pay at all.
17. Filippi V, Marshall T, Bulut A et al, 1997. Asking questions about women's reproductive health: validity and reliability of survey findings from Istanbul. *Tropical Medicine and International Health.* 2(1):47-56.

Preventing maternal deaths through effective policies and programmes

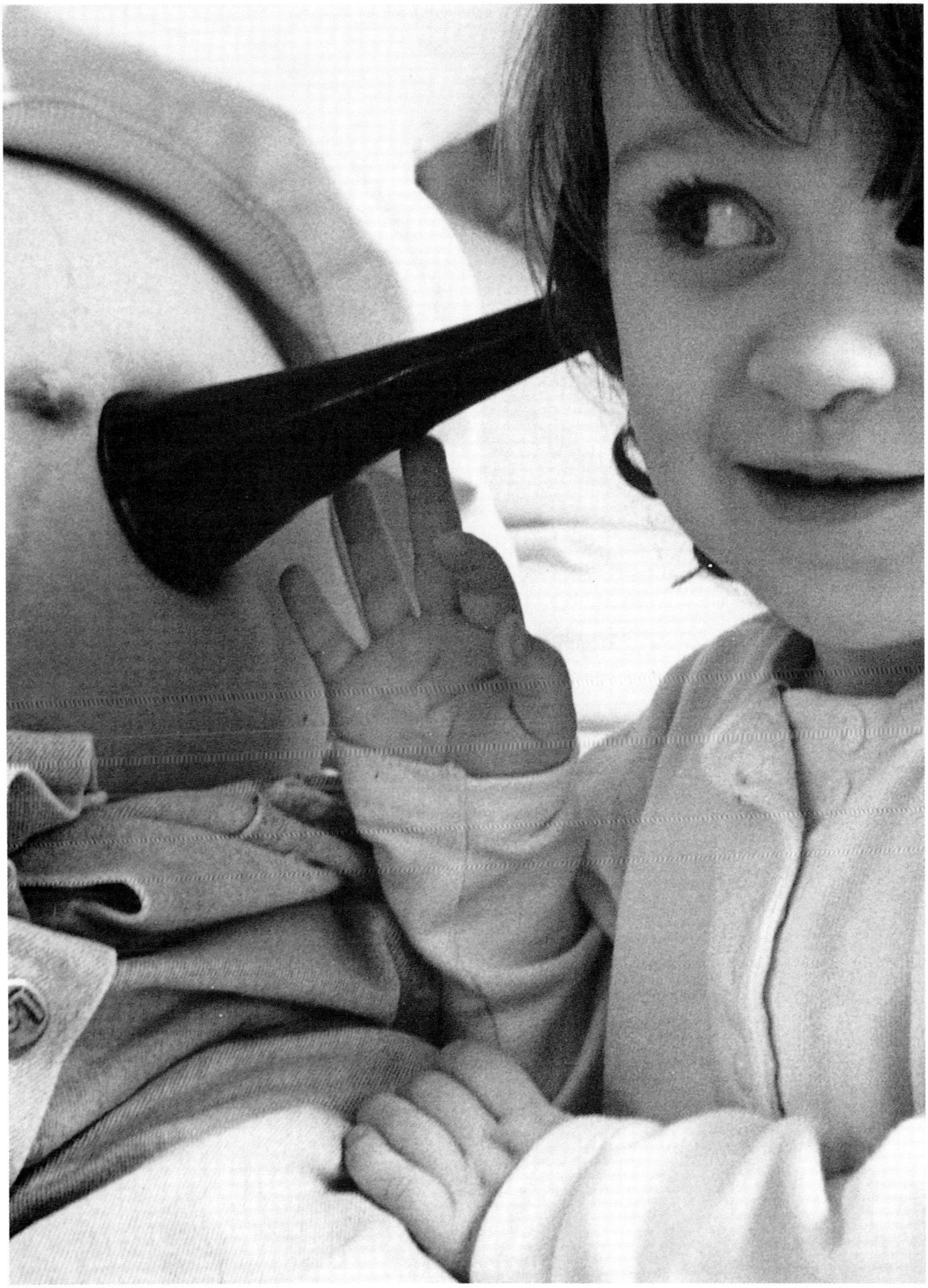

NANCY DURRELL McKENNA / HUTCHISON LIBRARY

What's So Special About Maternal Mortality?

Deborah Maine

The Safe Motherhood Initiative has not accomplished as much as expected during its first decade. There are relatively few large programmes specifically directed at preventing deaths among women who develop obstetric complications, even though effective treatments have been available for half a century. On the other hand, there is much more clarity now about the actions needed to prevent such deaths, especially the central role of emergency obstetric care. Now, we must build strong, effective programmes on this new understanding. Such programmes will not address all the problems that women face, or even all their reproductive health problems. But they will prevent the deaths of millions of women who die in agony and terror. We have had enough advocacy, enough meetings, enough manuals. Now we need programmes that reach the women who will otherwise suffer and die.

"A deep, dark continuous stream of mortality... how long is this sacrifice to go on?"
William Farr, 1838[1]

SINCE the Safe Motherhood Initiative began, more than a decade ago, there have been a number of important developments in the international women's health field. Perhaps the most important of these is the growing emphasis on reproductive and sexual health, so clearly voiced at the Cairo and Beijing conferences,[2,3] which viewed women's reproductive health as a whole, rather than just a collection of diseases or states (e.g. pregnancy). Why, then, does it still make sense, at the very end of the 20th century, to devote an entire book to maternal mortality? What makes maternal mortality so special?

There are at least three ways in which maternal mortality is special: first, its magnitude; second, its epidemiologic nature; and third, its programmatic requirements.

The magnitude of maternal mortality

The facts about maternal deaths are often repeated – more than half a million deaths each year (or more than one a minute), 99 per cent of which are in developing countries.[4] Of all the health indicators monitored by the United Nations, the biggest discrepancy between developed and developing countries is in maternal mortality. While impressive, such facts can be numbing, or fail to convey the true magnitude and horror. In terms of magnitude, the sheer numbers can be staggering. For example, there are an estimated 33,000 maternal deaths each year in Bangladesh, but less than 500 in the United States, although the US population is roughly twice as large as that of Bangladesh. Sadly, William Farr's question about maternal deaths in England in 1838 (quoted above) is still relevant today in many countries.

One of the crucial characteristics of maternal death is that women run this risk every time they become pregnant, and this risk adds up over their lifetime. Many developing countries have both high maternal mortality ratios (average risk of death per pregnancy) and high fertility rates (average number of births per woman). The result is astoundingly high cumulative or 'lifetime' risks faced by women in many areas. For example, an estimated 1 in 12 women die of maternal causes in West Africa, compared to 1 in 4,000 in Northern Europe.[2]

As for the horror, we have all had our hearts wrenched by photographs of starving children. But how many people have imagined what it means to be in labour for five days, in pain, exhausted, knowing that your baby is already dead and you will die soon because the hospital where a caesarean section could be done is out of reach, either physically, financially or socially?

The nature of maternal mortality

There is little mystery about the complications that kill pregnant women, and surprisingly little difference in causes between developed and developing countries. Table 1 shows remarkable similarities between the main causes of maternal death in the world and in the United States.[2,5,6] The WHO estimates for the world are, in effect, the causes in developing countries, since nearly all of the maternal deaths in the world occur in these areas. The similarities are found in haemorrhage, sepsis and hypertensive disorders of pregnancy (such as eclampsia).

Table 1. Obstetric deaths by cause: global estimates (1993) and United States (1987-90)[4-6]

Cause of death	World: 1993 estimates (%)	United States: 1987-90 (%)
Haemorrhage	25	29
Sepsis	15	13
Hypertensive disorders	12	18
Unsafe abortion	13	*
Obstructed labour	8	*
Embolism	*	20
Cardiomyopathy	*	6
Anaesthesia	*	2
Other direct causes	8	*
Indirect causes	20	*
Unspecified	*	13
Total	100	100
Deaths per 100,000 live births	430	9

** = negligible*

There are telling differences as well as similarities, however. Unsafe abortion accounts for 13 per cent and obstructed labour for an estimated 8 per cent of maternal deaths in developing countries, but each of these conditions accounts for less than 1 per cent of maternal deaths in the United States. Deaths from induced abortion have been virtually eliminated in countries where safe, legal abortion is widely available,[4] while deaths from obstructed labour are now almost unknown in developed countries due to the use of caesarean section.

If we are to reduce maternal mortality in developing countries we need to base our actions on knowledge. By 'knowledge' I do not mean the precise level of maternal mortality in a given country at a given time. As other articles in this book demonstrate, that information is costly and difficult (if not impossible) to obtain[7] and not useful for designing and monitoring programmes.[8] The knowledge that we need in order to design effective programmes is knowledge of how maternal mortality 'works'. For example, a recently published article reported that close spacing of births, which has a powerful effect on infant survival, was not found to increase maternal mortality.[9] This finding has been greeted with consternation and disbelief, even though it is not a new finding.[10] The consternation is, I believe, due to a continuing misunderstanding of how maternal mortality works – i.e. the causal model.

The causal model for infant mortality in developing countries is an additive model: if a child's health sustains various insults (e.g. measles, diarrhoea, malnutrition, respiratory infections) and if enough of these add up, then the child will die. A similar model has been assumed to apply to maternal mortality: the woman's health sustains various insults (such as poor nutrition, hard physical labour and repeated childbearing) and these add up to death.

Yet the literature indicates that an additive model is not appropriate for maternal mortality. Instead, a binomial model seems more appropriate (one where there are only two possible outcomes, as when flipping a coin): a pregnant woman either does or does not develop a serious obstetric complication (the coin comes up head or tails). If the woman does develop a life-threatening complication, then her survival depends on getting prompt, adequate emergency obstetric care.

Using a binomial model, it is not surprising that birth spacing does not have an effect on maternal mortality. The idea that short intervals between births increases the likelihood of maternal death is based on the assumption that short intervals will weaken the woman and reduce her ability to withstand complications of pregnancy. But this assumption is not supported by history. During the 19th century, living conditions (nutrition, sanitation, etc.) in Europe and North America improved, and this resulted in sustained and impressive declines in infant mortality, and in deaths from infectious diseases among adults (e.g. tuberculosis), well before medical technology to fight these was developed.

During this period, however, maternal mortality remained high.[11] For example, from 1840 (when the first maternal mortality statistics were available in Britain) to the mid-1930s, maternal mortality remained as high in Britain as it is in many developing countries today. Then, after nearly a century of stagnation, maternal mortality declined so sharply that within 15 years it was no longer a major public health problem. Why? Because the technology to treat obstetric complications became available, including antibiotics (first sulfa drugs and then penicillin), banked blood and safer surgical techniques. In 1934, there were 441 maternal deaths per 100,000 births in England and Wales. By 1950, there were 87, and in 1960 there were 39. Similar patterns obtained in other European countries and in the United States (although data were not available in the USA until much later).

In other words, it was not that women were less likely to develop obstetric complications, or more likely to survive complications in the absence of medical care, that led to low levels of maternal mortality in developed countries. Rather, it was the fact that women had access to treatment for complications.

Despite the historical evidence, for decades the focus of maternal health programmes was on antenatal care, screening of pregnant women, and training of traditional birth attendants to do clean deliveries. These activities were based on the assumption that most life-threatening obstetric complications can either be prevented or predicted. Since they have occupied such important places in maternal health programmes for such a long time, these activities will each be briefly discussed.

Antenatal care

The first antenatal clinics, which were introduced between 1910 and 1915 in Australia, Scotland and the United States, represented a new concept of care for pregnant women – the monitoring of apparently healthy women for signs of illness. It was generally believed (by clinicians, policymakers and the general public) that widespread use of antenatal care would reduce maternal deaths. But this did not happen. By the early 1930s, a huge amount of resources had been devoted to antenatal care (e.g. more than 1,200 clinics were opened in the United Kingdom alone)[12] and most women in Western countries received such care. Maternal mortality, however, did not decline, and there was a fierce debate over the value of antenatal care in leading medical journals.[13]

The problem was (and still is) that the major causes of maternal death cannot be detected and averted during pregnancy.[14] Post-partum haemorrhage, the leading cause of maternal deaths, can be caused by a number of events, such as a small piece of placenta being retained in the uterus, or the woman being exhausted after delivery. These problems cannot be predicted, even late in pregnancy, because they only happen during labour and delivery, or the post-partum period. Prolonged labour can be managed by medical intervention, such as use of drugs or caesarean section, but it cannot be prevented. And certainly, unsafe abortion complications cannot be prevented by antenatal care, though they can be prevented by adequate, accessible abortion services.

While some cases of infection will be prevented through clean delivery techniques, other cases of infection will still occur because infection can arise without being introduced from outside the woman's body. For example, in the event of prolonged labour or prolonged rupture of the membranes without delivery, infection often arises from the damaged tissue itself.

In discussions of the possible benefits of antenatal care, pre-eclampsia is often mentioned as the best example of how early signs of complications may be detected (e.g. through blood pressure and urine testing) and managed. Yet the fatal form of this complication (eclampsia, which is marked by convulsions) often arises suddenly during delivery, including in developed countries.[15] Again, what is crucial is to have the facilities to treat the complication once it has arisen.

When the limitations of antenatal care are pointed out, people often raise the possibility of benefits other than predicting or preventing obstetric complications. Suggested components include tetanus immunisation, iron/folate supplementation, and health education concerning danger signs during pregnancy and delivery, and informing women about where to seek help. Certainly these elements may support women's health and can be part of antenatal care, especially if they do not take place otherwise.

However, as programme planners, we should ask whether antenatal care is the best or only place where these activities should be carried out. For example, in some countries the policy is to immunise all women of reproductive age against tetanus, rather than waiting until they are pregnant. Similarly, if anaemia is a problem among women in general, why only try to help those who are pregnant? Furthermore, pregnancy is a time when the side effects of iron (such as nausea and constipation) can be particularly troublesome. And why should information about danger signs and seeking help be targeted only at pregnant women? Would it not be better to make sure that as many people in the community as possible possess this information, especially people who make decisions about medical care, such as family heads and mothers-in-law? Finally, it cannot be said too often that it is unethical to inform people about danger signs when treatment of complications is not accessible.

Thus, the question about antenatal care is not whether to provide it or not, but how, under what circumstances and comprising which elements – and, most important of all, whether it deserves the almost exclusive priority it has been given up to now.

Screening

Screening does not work – it does not identify most of the women who will develop complications during labour and delivery. In fact, screening cannot work for purely mathematical reasons that have nothing to do with the quality of care provided or the skill of the personnel.

There are two major mathematical reasons why screening of pregnant women cannot predict obstetric complications. One reason is that very accurate screening tools do not exist.[17] Even if we had better screening tools, however, prediction would still be very poor, because the incidence of *specific* complications is fairly low. Of course, taking all serious complications together, the incidence is not low – an estimated 15 per cent of pregnant women will develop a serious complication.[2] But the risk factors for haemorrhage (older age of the woman, high parity), are different from those for eclampsia (young age, first birth). Therefore, in assessing the possible efficacy of a screening test, we need to consider the value of screening for the major complications individually.

The more common the condition, the more accurate screening is. Haemorrhage is the most common of the serious obstetric complications; the WHO estimates that haemorrhage occurs in 10 per cent of pregnancies.[3] Hence, haemorrhage can be used to illustrate the problem. Suppose that there was a screening test that allowed us to identify accurately 75 per cent of pregnant women who would haemorrhage (sensitivity = 75 per cent) and 90 per cent of those who would not haemorrhage (specificity = 90 per cent). In fact, this is much more accurate than the currently available screening tests.[15,18] Given an incidence of 10 per cent, using this test only 45 per cent of the women that we identified as being at high risk of haemorrhage would actually develop this complication. Conversely, 55 per cent of the women identified as high risk would be 'false positives', that is, women who would be told that they were at high risk of having this serious complication, but who would not haemorrhage.

For complications with an incidence of 5 per cent (i.e. obstructed labour, pre-eclampsia and eclampsia), the results of using such a test would be even worse: the positive predictive value = 28 per cent; false positives = 72 per cent.

Women's reported 'poor compliance' with advice to come to the hospital for delivery because they are 'high risk' is sometimes interpreted as evidence that they prefer to deliver at home. However, I wonder how much of women's reluctance to follow this advice comes from their understanding that the results of antenatal screening are more often wrong than right. In addition, women are also aware that many health facilities, including hospitals, are not able to treat serious complications, for a variety of reasons – the physician is not there, there is no blood or anaesthesia, etc. So why go to the trouble and expense of going to the hospital at all?

Screening does not, cannot work. This statement still seems like heresy, although it is much more widely accepted than it was a few years ago, as shown, for example, by this statement from the official Safe Motherhood Website:

'Every pregnancy faces risk.'[16]

The text continues:

'During pregnancy, any woman can develop serious, life-threatening complications that require medical care. Because there is no reliable way to predict which women will develop these complications, it is essential that all pregnant women have access to high quality obstetric care...'[16]

Training TBAs

The training of traditional birth attendants (TBAs) is meant to reduce post-partum infection by encouraging cleanliness and discouraging dangerous practices. While such training may reduce these particular problems, labour and delivery will still be complicated in a certain number of cases. TBAs have neither the skills nor the equipment to treat life-threatening complications. A clear distinction should be made between TBAs and midwives who have been formally trained in the 'execution of emergency measures',[5] who can treat a variety of complications and are a valuable part of programmes to reduce maternal deaths.

It has also been said that TBAs can be trained to recognise obstetric complications and refer women with complications to a nearby health facility for treatment. There are two weaknesses in this plan. First of all, the signs and symptoms of serious obstetric complications are not subtle: any bleeding during pregnancy, excessive bleeding during or after delivery; convulsions; fever, chills and foul vaginal discharge; headaches in combination with swollen hands, face and feet; labour for more than 12 hours.[8] Everyone should be taught to recognise these few danger signs, not just TBAs or pregnant women.

The more difficult problem with training TBAs to refer women with complications is that there is often no feasible referral option. In fact, it is precisely in circumstances where medical treatment is least available that training TBAs is usually proposed as a solution.

Programme requirements for reducing maternal deaths

For women who do not wish to be pregnant, family planning and safe abortion programmes make an important contribution to Safe Motherhood. A woman cannot die a maternal death if she is not pregnant, so family planning can directly and substantially reduce maternal deaths by helping women to avoid unwanted pregnancies. Since even the best contraceptive methods fail, even with an exemplary family planning programme there will be unintended pregnancies. Therefore, access to safe, legal termination of pregnancy is of crucial importance to reducing maternal mortality, as experience in Western countries has demonstrated.

As regards preventing deaths from obstetric complications among women who are pregnant and who wish to be pregnant, the thinking about maternal mortality is undergoing a paradigm shift. There are a variety of ways to express this shift, such as changing from an additive to a binomial model, or changing from a focus on risk screening to accepting that 'every pregnancy faces risk'. We are, in my estimation, mid-way through this paradigm shift. Some ideas that were heresy 10 years ago have now become mainstream, as the quotes from the Safe Motherhood Website above show.

Programme strategies, however, have generally not caught up with this revised understanding of the nature of the problem. For example, in lists of priorities, it is still common to see antenatal care listed before treatment of obstetric complications. For example, in WHO's newly issued *Safe Motherhood Needs Assessment*, the section on 'Policy Assessment' contains suggestions for evaluating (in this order):

'...policy on antenatal care services...policy on clean and safe delivery...policy on postpartum care for mother and newborn....policy on essential obstetric care...'

The last item in this list includes the treatment of major complications.[19] Why is 'essential' obstetric care (EOC) listed fourth? Why are the interventions which have been proven to save women's lives listed after those whose value is questionable? Putting essential obstetric care last on the list, repeatedly, sends a message – that it has lower priority or can be done after the other things.

In addition to putting EOC last, this kind of list implies that governments or agencies need to do all these things, when that is not necessarily the case. Consider recently published data from the Matlab research area in Bangladesh, which showed that maternal mortality declined as much in the southern part of the Comparison Area as in the Intervention Area during the study (1987-89).[9] During this period, a number of interventions were carried out in the Intervention Area (including posting trained midwives in the community, and arranging 24-hour transport for women with obstetric complications), while in the Comparison Area there were no such interventions. However, women living in the southern part of the Comparison Area had much better access to comprehensive EOC at the district hospital. This indicates that just improving services at the district hospital would help to save the lives of women living nearby.

Making programmes more effective by re-ordering priorities

So, what would a programme look like if it were based on our accumulated knowledge about maternal mortality? The absolutely first priority would be to get district hospitals functioning. These facilities are fairly well distributed within countries and are supposed to be able to provide comprehensive emergency obstetric care, including caesarean section and blood transfusion. But this is not the case in many developing countries.

Information on whether health facilities provide care for women with obstetric emergencies is just beginning to be gathered. What often has to be used as a proxy measure is the number of caesarean sections performed in hospitals. Caesarean sections are done too frequently in some countries, such as the United States and Brazil (where in 1990, 23 and 26 per cent of deliveries, respectively, were caesarean section).[20] However, an even more serious problem (in terms of mortality and morbidity) is that a substantial proportion of women in developing countries do not have access to this life-saving surgery. In *Guidelines for Monitoring the Availability and Use of Obstetric Services*, issued by UNICEF, WHO and UNFPA in 1997, the minimum acceptable level of caesarean section is set at 5 per cent of births in the population (not births in the hospital). Because of the danger of overuse of caesarean sections, a maximum acceptable level was also set, at 15 per cent of births, which is less than the current US level.

Various studies show that the actual level of caesarean sections in some countries is shockingly low:

- A study in 10 districts in India in 1992-3 showed that half of the districts had a caesarean section rate of less than 1 per cent of births, two districts had rates of 2-4 per cent, while only three had rates of 5-6 per cent – barely meeting the minimum acceptable level set by the UN agencies.[21]
- A study in Bangladesh in 1993 gathered data from district hospitals in 20 districts.[22] Six of these hospitals performed no caesarean sections at all during the previous year, and the rest performed caesareans equal to less than 1 per cent of births in the population.
- An earlier study in East Africa found that less than 1 per cent of births were being done by caesarean section in 1979-81.[23] Given the deteriorating economic and political conditions in many sub-Saharan African countries, the situation may actually be worse now.
- In June 1998, there was no obstetrician at one-third of the provincial hospitals in Morocco, and general practice physicians are not allowed to perform caesarean sections.[24]

A concern that is often raised regarding EOC and hospitals is their cost. True, a district hospital is more expensive than a health centre, and an obstetrician is more expensive than a midwife. However, there are relatively few district hospitals as compared to health centres. Furthermore, in terms of cost-effectiveness, it appears that well-functioning district hospitals may be the most economical way to reduce maternal deaths.[8] Finally, it is important to remember that in most countries these hospitals already exist, and many of them are staffed, although the staff may need better training and supervision. In many cases, only modest improvements in equipment and facilities are needed, as experience in West Africa has shown.[26]

Once district hospitals are functioning, there are several other activities that should be done next. One is community mobilisation. Making sure that people know the danger signs during pregnancy, delivery and the post-partum period may help speed up the process by which the family decides to take the woman for medical care. But often the barriers to care are not so much traditional beliefs or lack of knowledge; rather, they are more concrete problems such as the long distance that must be travelled, and the high cost of travel, services and drugs (either at the hospital or in the town if the hospital is out of stock). Communities can take a number of steps to overcome these barriers, including enlisting local vehicle owners and starting emergency fund societies.[26]

It is crucial, however, to remember that it is extremely unwise (if not unethical) to mobilise the community unless and until EOC services are functioning.

At the same time, extending services out from a district hospital to health centres would be helpful. Clearly, if the peripheral health facilities (i.e. health centres) are not providing EOC, then the difficulty and costs associated with travel are multiplied. Trained midwives, nurses and medical assistants can treat a number of life-threatening complications with what is known as 'Basic Essential Obstetric Care'.[2] (*see box*)

Midwives and other specially-trained, paramedical personnel can and do successfully perform Basic EOC functions in many countries, though in some countries legal restrictions limit their activities (and usefulness) unnecessarily. In addition, it would be helpful if general practice physicians were trained to provide at least Basic EOC, which many are not at present.

Conclusion

There is a pervasive sense that the Safe Motherhood Initiative has not accomplished as much as expected during its first decade. There is some basis for this impression. There are relatively few large programmes specifically directed at preventing deaths among women who develop the age-old complications of haemorrhage, infection, induced abortion, eclampsia and obstructed labour. That is the bad news.

The good news is that there is much more clarity now about the actions needed to prevent such deaths, especially the central role of treatment of complications. This is a major shift in thinking, and it has not been easy. Now, we must build strong, sharply-focused, effective programmes based on this new understanding. Such programmes will not address all the problems that women face, or even all their reproductive health problems. But they will prevent the deaths of millions of women who die in agony and terror. We still have the opportunity to accomplish this. We have had enough advocacy, enough meetings, enough manuals. Now we need programmes that reach the women who will otherwise suffer and die.

Correspondence

Deborah Maine, Professor of Clinical Public Health, Center for Population and Family Health, Columbia University, 60 Haven Avenue, New York, NY, 10032 USA. Fax: 1-212-544-1933. E-mail: dpm1@columbia.edu

Essential Obstetric Care (EOC): Key Functions

Basic EOC

- Parenteral (intravenous or intramuscular) antibiotics
- Parenteral oxytocics (drugs which make the uterus contract to stop bleeding)
- Parenteral sedatives or anticonvulsants (for eclampsia)
- Manual removal of the placenta (to stop haemorrhage)
- Removal of retained products of conception (to prevent bleeding and infection)
- Assisted vaginal delivery (to alleviate prolonged labour)

Comprehensive EOC

Basic EOC plus

- Surgery (caesarean section)
- Blood transfusion

References

1. Farr W, 1838. *Annual Report of the Registrar General of England and Wales.*
2. United Nations, 1995. *Population and Development,* Vol. 1: Programme of Action adopted at the International Conference on Population and Development: Cairo: 5-13 September 1994. (Sales no. E.95.XIII.7)
3. United Nations, 1996. *The Beijing Declaration and the Platform for Action: Fourth World Conference on Women: Beijing, China: 4-15 September 1995* (DPI/1766/Wom). New York: Department of Public Information.
4. World Health Organization/ UNICEF, 1996. *Revised 1990 Estimates of Maternal Mortality.* Geneva. April.
5. World Health Organization, 1994. *Mother-Baby Package: A Road Map for Implementation in Countries.* Geneva: Division of Family Health.
6. Berg CJ, Atrash HK, Koonin LM, Tucker M, 1996. Pregnancy-related mortality in the United States, 1987-1990. *Obstetrics and Gynecology* 88:161-67.
7. Campbell OMR, 1999. Measuring progress in Safe Motherhood programmes: uses and limitations of health outcome indicators. *Safe Motherhood Initiatives: Critical Issues.* M Berer, TKS Ravindran (eds). Reproductive Health Matters, London.
8. Wardlaw T, Maine D, 1999. Process indicators for maternal mortality programmes. (In this book)
9. Ronsmans C, Vanneste AM, Chakraborty J et al, 1997. Decline in maternal mortality in Matlab, Bangladesh: a cautionary tale, *Lancet.* 350:1810-14.
10. Maine D, 1991. *Safe Motherhood Programs: Options and Issues.* Columbia University, Center for Population and Family Health, New York.
11. Loudon I, 1992. *Death in Childbirth: An International Study of Maternal Care and Maternal Mortality 1800-1950.* Oxford: Clarendon Press.
12. Wrigley AJ, 1934. A criticism of ante-natal work. *British Medical Journal.* May: 891-94.
13. Browne FJ, 1932. Antenatal care and maternal mortality. *Lancet.* 2 July:1-4.
14. Rooney C, 1992. *Antenatal Care and Maternal Health: How Effective Is It?* WHO, Geneva.
15. Hall M, Chng P, MacGillivray I, 1980. Is routine antenatal care worthwhile? *Lancet.* 12 July:78-80.
16. Internet: www.safemotherhood.org/action_messages.htm, October 1998.
17. The Kasongo Project Team, 1984. Antenatal screening for fetopelvic dystocias: a cost-effectiveness approach to the choice of simple indicators for use by auxiliary personnel. *Journal of Tropical Medicine and Hygiene.* 87:173-83.
18. Selwyn BJ, 1990. The epidemiology of reproductive risk screening: degree of accuracy and inherent limitations. In: *A Reassessment of the Concept of Reproductive Risk in Maternity Care and Family Planning Services.* J Rooks, B Winikoff (eds). New York, Population Council.
19. World Health Organization, 1998. *Safe Motherhood Needs Assessment.* Geneva, Family and Reproductive Health, p. 30-1.
20. Notzon FC, 1990. International differences in the use of obstetric interventions. *Journal of American Medical Association.* 263:3286-91.
21. Nirupam S, Yuster EA, 1995. Emergency obstetric care: measuring availability and monitoring progress. *International Journal of Gynecology and Obstetrics.* 50(Suppl. 2):S79-S88.
22. Haque YA, Mostafa GA, 1993. Review of the Emergency Obstetric Care Functions of Selected Facilities in Bangladesh. UNICEF, Dhaka, September.
23. Nordberg EM, 1984. Incidence and estimated need of caesarean section, inguinal hernia repair, and operation for strangulated hernia in rural Africa. *British Medical Journal.* 289:92-93.
24. Personal communication, Ministry of Public Health, Rabat, June 1998.
25. Leigh B, Kandeh HBS, Kanu MS et al, 1997. Improving emergency obstetric care at a district hospital, Makeni, Sierra Leone. *International Journal of Gynecology and Obstetrics.* 59 (Suppl. 2):S55-S66.
26. Prevention of Maternal Mortality Network, 1997. *International Journal of Gynecology and Obstetrics.* 59(Suppl. 2):S1-S271. (whole issue)

When Pregnancy Is Over: Preventing Post-Partum Deaths and Morbidity

Carla AbouZahr, Marge Berer

Pregnancy is a process, with each stage critically influenced by what preceded it. This is especially true of intra-partum care and immediate post-partum care, a time when complications and the need for treatment are closely linked. In developed countries, post-partum care is an integral part of delivery care, but it is almost non-existent in developing countries, often with fatal consequences. The poor coverage of the post-partum period is reflected in the limited data available at global level. Less than one developing country in three reports national data on post-partum care, and in others, levels of coverage can be as low as five per cent. Yet the great majority of maternal deaths take place during or after birth, and the events which lead to those deaths mostly arise during delivery. Similarly, deaths from unsafe abortion occur in the hours and days afterwards. Thus, women in developing countries are not getting the care they need at the times they most need it. What is usually called post-partum care, provided in the months after birth, tends to be curative, promotive and preventive in nature, rather than life-saving. The biggest challenge is to develop programmes that are able to provide emergency care during and just after delivery, to reduce the greatest number of maternal deaths.

IT is common practice to divide care for pregnant women into three stages:

- **the ante-partum period**, from the establishment of pregnancy until the onset of labour;
- **the intra-partum period**, from the start of labour until the end of third stage of labour (expulsion of placenta and membranes); and
- **the post-partum period**, from completion of the third stage of labour to 42 days thereafter.

The use of these distinct stages has a number of advantages, particularly in relation to the rather different types of problems that can arise at each stage, e.g. the complications of early pregnancy are manifestly different from those that occur during childbirth or in the period afterwards.

However, such neat distinctions have an important disadvantage. They tend to obscure the fact that pregnancy is a process, with each stage being critically influenced by what preceded it. This is particularly true with regard to the artificial distinction that is commonly drawn between intra-partum care and immediate post-partum care, which tends to make the need for immediate post-partum care invisible, and mix it up with the value and meaning of late post-partum care. This has unfortunate and even fatal consequences for the way that post-pregnancy care is organised and offered to women, particularly in the developing world.

Maternity care in developed countries: last 100 years

Since modern care for pregnancy and childbirth became the norm in developed countries, delivery care has consisted of a relatively long period of supervision by a specialist, either a midwife or a doctor, generally, though by no means exclusively, in an institutional setting. Among comfortably-off women in Europe, North America and Japan during the early years of the 20th century, standard maternity care consisted of a home delivery with regular, frequent visits by the specialist.[1] The arrival of modern obstetric care during the late 1930s did not alter this practice, but gradually moved the whole process to an institutional setting.[2] Women with uncomplicated deliveries were kept in hospital for a period up to ten days; those with complications considerably longer.

Change came about gradually during the 1970s and 1980s as a result of two developments:

one was increasing sensitivity to the costs of keeping essentially healthy women and their infants in hospitals for longer than was necessary; the other was women's own desire to be at home. These became the basis for campaigns to change childbirth, spearheaded by midwives and women's health activists, campaigns which are still evolving and active in many developed countries today.[3]

Today, although the move back to home births has largely not succeeded in most developed countries, and many women with normal, uncomplicated deliveries still have their babies in hospital, they are now discharged within one-two days or even hours after delivery. This does not mean, however, that they no longer receive medical care when they have left hospital. Discharge is contingent upon a system of post-partum follow-up and care by skilled health care providers, generally midwives, nurses or health visitors, and also by doctors, who make regular visits to check on the progress of mother and baby.[3-5]

Thus, pregnant women in most developed countries get an integrated package of delivery and post-partum care, even though their institutional stay is relatively short and even if recent cost-cutting trends have eroded the community-based care that previously existed in some places.[6] This package has been available since the early years of the 20th century – even though its contents, in terms of management of delivery and availability of drugs and technologies, have changed significantly over the years. Antenatal care was a relatively late arrival on the scene, becoming generally available only following the second World War.[7]

A very different path in developing countries

Maternal health care services in developing countries, by contrast, have followed a very different path. Generally speaking, antenatal care is the first intervention to receive resources and be implemented in a widespread fashion within maternal health programmes. Delivery care (whether institutional-based or at home) tends to be a later addition,[8] while systematic and regular post-partum follow-up and care is hardly available at all.

Even where women do have access to a skilled health professional at the time of delivery or actually deliver in a health care facility, they are often discharged within a matter of hours and are not seen again by a health professional until some considerable time afterwards, usually when they bring their babies for a check-up and immunisation.[9] Even then, their own condition and health needs may be ignored. One country, which shall remain unnamed, indicated in their statistics on maternity coverage that their post-partum coverage was nearly 100 per cent. Upon investigation, however, it turned out that this care consisted entirely of monitoring and immunisation of infants, and this is probably not an isolated case.

The poor coverage of the post-partum period is reflected in the limited data available at global level. Less than one developing country in three reports national data on post-partum care, and even in countries with data, levels of coverage are often as low as 5 per cent. Estimates based on the limited data available indicate overall use of post-partum care below 30 per cent for developing countries.[10] By contrast, just over 50 per cent of all pregnant women in developing countries give birth in the care of a health care professional and 65 per cent of pregnant women have at least one antenatal visit (Table 1).

This finding is particularly worrying given what is known about the timing of maternal deaths. Community studies from around the world have found that most maternal deaths take place during delivery or in the immediate post-partum period (Table 2).[11] Almost half of post-partum deaths take place within one day of delivery and some 70 per cent occur within the first week. In other words, there is a mismatch between women's need for maternal health care and the current patterns of provision and utilisation of care in developing countries where

Table 1. Declining coverage from antenatal to post-partum care[10]

	More developed regions	Less developed regions
% of women with at least one antenatal visit	97%	65%
% of women delivering with a skilled attendant	99%	53%
% of women receiving at least one post-partum care visit	90%	30%

Table 2. Percentage of maternal deaths by timing of death, developing countries[11]

Timing of death	Per cent
Ante-partum	23.9%
Intra-partum	15.5%
Post-partum	60.6%

women are not, in fact, getting the care they need at the times they most need it.

A recent study in Nepal provides striking evidence of how quickly most maternal deaths occur. Of 30 women who died in hospital, 66 per cent died within 24 hours of admission. Of the 82 women who gave birth and died in the community, 50 per cent died within 24 hours of delivery, and the proportion was even higher in the subset who died due to retained placenta. Most of the deaths were from post-partum haemorrhage, which was fatal within six hours, not surprising among highly anaemic women such as those in Nepal. Those with obstructed labour died within 2-3 days, while those with sepsis died some 15 days after delivery.[12]

The period of time from the onset of a complication to the woman dying will vary between countries and groups of women, dependent on a number of factors. However, in every case these deaths happen very quickly indeed. Table 3 shows the average time to death from the most frequent causes of maternal deaths in developing countries, as estimated in 1990.[13]

Table 3. Estimated average interval from onset of complication to death for major obstetric complications[13]

Complication	Average hours to death	Average days to death
Ante-partum haemorrhage	12 hours	
Post-partum haemorrhage	2 hours	
Ruptured uterus		1 day
Eclampsia		2 days
Obstructed labour		3 days
Puerperal sepsis		6 days

Main causes of maternal deaths, when they arise and why

The common pre-disposing factors for maternal deaths are mostly pre-existing when pregnancy begins, such as anaemia, poor nutritional status, HIV or malaria. The main causes of maternal deaths can be divided according to when they arise and why:[14]

- those which occur very early in pregnancy, such as ectopic pregnancy;
- those which arise from the complications of abortion, i.e. retained products of conception, haemorrhage, sepsis and perforated uterus, mostly due to the use of unsafe or outdated procedures;[15]
- those which arise mostly during late pregnancy, such as hypertensive disorders of pregnancy leading to eclampsia;
- those which arise during labour and delivery, including prolonged or obstructed labour, retained placenta, vaginal or cervical lacerations, uterine rupture or inversion, which often arise due to poor or inadequate care;
- those which arise from events in labour and delivery but which manifest in the first hours, days or weeks post-partum, including haemorrhage[16] and sepsis, which are often the result of poor or inadequate care; and
- those which are true post-partum complications, such as thrombo-embolic disease.

Post-partum haemorrhage is the single most important cause of maternal death worldwide. The majority of deaths are the consequence of events in the third stage of labour, often as a result of poor management or mismanagement. Bleeding usually occurs in the transition between labour and the post-partum period, and less commonly in the days following birth or even in the second week (secondary haemorrhage). Anaemia is a common pre-disposing factor. Causes of haemorrhage include retained placenta, uterine atony, vaginal or cervical lacerations, and occasionally uterine rupture or inversion.[14,16,17]

The second most important cause of maternal deaths is sepsis following untreated genital tract infection. Symptoms are lower abdominal pain, high fever and foul discharge. Pre-disposing factors include: prolonged labour, premature rupture of membranes, frequent vaginal examination, vaginal electronic fetal monitoring, and especially caesarean section. Use of non-sterilised instruments and unsafe procedures for abortions, carried out by untrained providers,[15] and poorly observed rules of cleanliness on the part of TBAs and others attending births, including lack of gloves, clean water, soap, etc. are also important factors.[14,17] In Egypt, 10-20 per cent of women in one study reported one or more symptoms of genital infection.[18]

Hypertensive disorders of pregnancy may start after about 20 weeks of pregnancy. Eclampsia, the end point of the evolution of pregnancy hypertension or pre-eclampsia, is the third most important cause of maternal deaths worldwide. The typical convulsions most frequently occur during late pregnancy or labour, but some 30 per cent of cases manifest in the first days post-partum.[14] Of the post-partum eclamptic fits recorded in a recent study, more than half presented three or more days post-partum.[19]

The fact is that preventive care at primary level and timely and appropriate care by competent providers, including those trained in emergency obstetric care, would reduce or prevent most complications from developing at all or becoming fatal if they do develop. Delay or failure in dealing with one complication properly can lead to other complication(s), resulting in multiple problems and often death, e.g. prolonged and obstructed labour may lead to ruptured uterus.

Thus, for example, in one hospital in Ethiopia,[20] of 245 women presenting with ruptured uterus, duration of labour (mean 29+ hours) was the most common associated factor. Almost all the women were attended in labour by an untrained relative and mean time to reach the hospital was seven hours. Rupture was complete in all but five women, and bladder rupture also occurred in eight women. Six women had to have a hysterectomy, 238 had the rupture repaired, one was too ill for either. Thirteen of the women died.

Maternal morbidity reported in the months after delivery

The number of health problems reported by women in the first months after delivery is high, ranging from 23 per cent of women indicating problems in India[21] to 47 per cent reporting at least one symptom in England.[22] Some may resolve within weeks or months; others can become chronic. Problems range from:[14] anaemia and nutritional depletion exacerbated by serious blood loss and breastfeeding,[23] backache,[24] urinary incontinence,[25] frequent headaches, mastitis and other breast problems, haemorrhoids, constipation, depression and anxiety (and rarely puerperal psychosis), pain in the perineum and vulva following from poor repair of episiotomy and perineal tears (often having an adverse effect on sexual relations),[26] or disabling conditions such as pelvic arthropathy of pregnancy,[27] unrepaired fistula or uterine prolapse, which in turn may lead to other forms of morbidity, such as constant irritation of tissue and genital infections. Secondary infertility following from untreated genital infection which has ascended to the upper reproductive tract is also not uncommon, especially after more than one episode.

Needs and responses

Given women's needs for essential and sometimes emergency obstetric care during labour, delivery and the post-partum period, and then primary level care in the months afterwards, what are the implications for health care planners and providers? While there is relatively little evidence on the precise mix of interventions likely to be most effective in preventing and managing post-partum complications,[28] specific interventions that have been shown to be effective need to be put in place.

These include prophylactic oxytocic drugs in the third stage of labour, to reduce the volume and the incidence of post-partum haemorrhage;[29,30] magnesium sulphate for treatment of eclampsia;[31] manual removal of retained placenta and removal of retained products of conception;[32] surgical repair of perineal and cervical lacerations; and prophylactic administration of antibiotics in cases of caesarean section, prolonged rupture of membranes or retained products of conception.[14] Early mobility after childbirth has clearly been shown to contribute to the drop in the incidence of post-partum thrombo-embolic disease in developed countries.[33]

Finally, guidelines exist for managing abortion complications,[34] and programmes are being developed in some hospitals to treat these complications.[35] However, if unsafe and outdated procedures were not still being used to

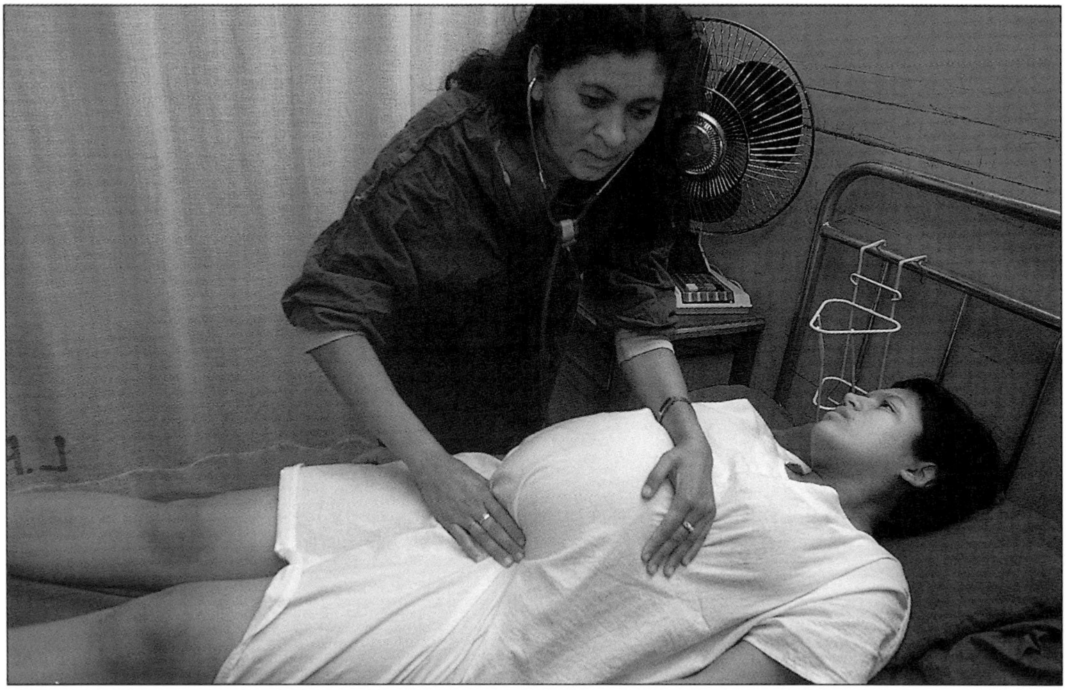

JENNY MATTHEWS / NETWORK

carry out abortions in the first place, the incidence of complications would be very low and rarely serious, let alone fatal, as has been shown in every country where safe abortion is provided.

A striking feature of the post-partum interventions described above is that the most effective ones, in terms of prevention of maternal deaths, are those that are administered close to the time of delivery, and which should really be treated as part of delivery care. The longer the time since delivery, the less likely it is that an intervention will be life-saving. While there are still risks of secondary post-partum haemorrhage, eclampsia, sepsis and thrombo-embolic conditions for some time after delivery, the risks of these complications progressively diminishes over time.

It is only after this critical stage of the early post-partum period, that what is usually understood as post-partum care, such as support for infant feeding and nutrition, as well as detection and treatment of the problems of post-partum morbidity, whether perineal pain, prolapse, fistula, urinary incontinence or mastitis, become predominant. In general, these and other interventions intended to be delivered six weeks or more after pregnancy ends,[36] such as family planning and health check-ups, are curative, promotive and preventive in nature, rather than life-saving.

Providing a service

Given the importance of interventions during birth and the immediate post-partum period, the question that immediately arises is how to ensure access to post-partum care? The fact is that in developing countries, most women deliver at home, yet the presence of a skilled health worker is needed for such interventions. The real challenge is to develop intra-partum and post-partum care programmes able to deliver these interventions at the right times. Few successful examples present themselves to date.

Training in certain types of life-saving skills for those with midwifery skills working at community level is one possibility. As part of Indonesia's community midwifery training programme, for example, for some 54,000 midwives based at village level, training in life-saving skills such as manual removal of the placenta, and preventive measures such as oxytocic drugs to prevent haemorrhage in the third stage of labour, were included in the curriculum.[37]

In Nepal, the fact that post-partum haemorrhage is the leading cause of maternal death led the Ministry of Health to look for innovative ways of improving access to delivery and post-partum care. Clearly, given the terrain and the low levels of delivery coverage (only some 10 per cent of all births take place in a health facility), it would not be feasible or appropriate to consider an approach that depends on trained health care professionals. Instead, the Nepali authorities adopted a dual strategy consisting of large-scale information campaigns and community mobilisation around signs and symptoms of complications, coupled with decentralisation of obstetric first aid to peripheral health centres and to the homes of community midwives. Each community midwife is being equipped with a first aid box containing essential items such as oxytocic drugs for the management of haemorrhage.[12]

A watching brief on these efforts, to determine whether they have an impact, and further action-research will be needed to develop approaches like these and evaluate their feasibility, costs and effectiveness. Such programmes represent forward-looking efforts to provide treatment and care to women in the period of time when most maternal deaths occur; they deserve much more attention and support.

Acknowledgements

Thanks to Erica Royston for help conceptualising the issues, and especially to Anne Thompson for discussion, clarifying points and help with references. The views expressed in this article are those of the authors and do not necessarily represent those of the World Health Organization.

Correspondence

Carla AbouZahr, Department of Reproductive Health and Research, World Health Organization, 1211 Geneva 27, Switzerland. Fax: 41-22-791-4189. E-mail: abouzahrc@who.ch

References and Notes

1. Loudon I, 1992. *Death in Childbirth*. Clarendon Press, Oxford.
2. Campbell R, Macfarlane A, 1994. *Where to be Born: The Debate and the Evidence*. National Perinatal Epidemiology Unit. Oxford.
3. *Changing Childbirth: Report of the Expert Maternity Group*. Department of Health. London 1993. This UK-focused report proposed sweeping changes in the handling of childbirth based on principles and evidence-based practice, prepared by midwifery experts and advocates for women-centred birthing practices.
4. – Evans CJ, 1995. Postpartum home care in the United States. *JOGNN*. 15:401-05.
   – Glazener CMA et al, 1993. Postnatal care: time to change. *Contemporary Review of Obstetrics and Gynecology*. 5:130-36.
   – Garcia J, Renfrew M, Marchant S, 1994. Postnatal home visits by midwives. *Midwifery*. 10:40-43.
   – Marchant S, 1995. What are we doing in the postnatal check? *British Journal of Midwifery*. 3:34-38.
   – Yelland J et al, 1998. Support, sensitivity and satisfaction: Filipino, Turkish and Vietnamese women's experience of postnatal hospital stay. *Midwifery*. 14:144-54.
   – Young D, 1995. Changing Childbirth: for better, for worse. *Birth*. 22:189-90.
5. – Berner LS, 1995. Early discharge rules for mothers and newborns: penny wise and 8 pounds, 2 ounces foolish. *Journal of Women's Health*. 4:479-81.
   – Carty EM, Bradley CF, 1990. A randomized, controlled evaluation of early postpartum hospital discharge. *Birth*. 17:199-204.
   – Margolis LH, Kotelchuck M, 1996. Midwives, physicians, and the timing of maternal postpartum discharge. *Journal of Nurse-Midwifery*. 41:29-35.
6. Thompson A, 1999. Personal communication.
7. Macfarlane A, Mugford M, 1984. *Birth Counts: Statistics of Pregnancy and Childbirth*. HMSO, London.
8. *The World's Women, 1995: Trends and Statistics*. Social Statistics and Indicators. Series K, No.12. United Nations, New York.
9. Ransjö-Arvidson AB et al,1998. Maternal and infant health problems after normal childbirth: a randomised controlled study in Zambia. *Journal of Epidemiology & Child Health*. 52:385-91.
10. World Health Organization, 1997. *Coverage of Maternity Care: A Listing of Available Information*. 4th edition. WHO/RHT/ MSM/96.28.
11. Li XF et al, 1996. The post-partum period: the key to maternal mortality. *International Journal of Gynecology and Obstetrics*. 54:1-10.
12. Government of Nepal, Family Health Division, Department of Health Services, Ministry of Health, *Maternal Mortality and Morbidity Study*, 1998.

13. Maine D, 1990. *Safe Motherhood Programs: Options and Issues*. Center for Population and Family Health, Columbia University, New York.
14. World Health Organization, 1998. *Postpartum Care of the Mother and Newborn: A Practical Guide*. WHO/RHT/MSM/98.3
15. World Health Organization, 1993. *Abortion: A Tabulation of Available Data on the Frequency and Mortality of Unsafe Abortion*. 2nd edition. WHO, Geneva.
– Alan Guttmacher Institute, 1994. *Clandestine Abortion: A Latin American Reality*. AGI, New York.
– Kinoti SN et al, 1996. *Monograph on Complications of Unsafe Abortion in Africa*. Commonwealth Regional Health Community Secretariat for East, Central and Southern Africa, Arusha.
16. Kwast B, 1991. Postpartum haemorrhage: its contribution to maternal mortality. *Midwifery*. 7:64-70.
17. World Health Organization, 1996. *Care in Normal Birth. A Practical Guide*. WHO, Geneva. WHO/FRH/MSM/96.24.
18. Egyptian Fertility Care Society, 1995. Study of the prevalence and perception of maternal morbidity in Menoufeya governate, Egypt. Cairo 1995.
– See also: El-Mouelhy MT, El-Helw M, Younis N et al, 1994. Women's understanding of pregnancy-related morbidity in rural Egypt. *Reproductive Health Matters*. 2(4):27-34.
19. Lubarsky SL, Barton JR, Friedman SA et al, 1994. Late postpartum eclampsia revisited. *Obstetrics and Gynecology*. 83:502-05.
20. Fekadu S, Kelly J, Lancashire R et al, 1997. Ruptured uterus in Ethiopia. *Lancet*. 349(March 1):622.
21. Bathia JC, Cleland J, 1996. Obstetric morbidity in south India: results from a community survey. *Social Science and Medicine*. 43:1507-16.
– See also: Bathia JC, 1995. Levels and determinants of maternal morbidity: results from a community-based study in southern India. *International Journal of Gynecology and Obstetrics*. 50(Suppl 2):S153-S163.
22. Glazener CMA, Abdalla M, Stroud P et al, 1995. Postnatal maternal morbidity: extent, causes, prevention and treatment. *British Journal of Obstetrics & Gynaecology*. 102:282-87.
23. Kusin JA, Kardjati S (eds.), 1994. *Maternal and Child Nutrition in Madura, Indonesia*. KIT, Amsterdam.
24. Russell R, Groves PH, Taub N et al, 1993. Assessing long term backache after childbirth. *BMJ*. 306:1299-1303.
25. Winberg J, Wilson PD, Herbison RM et al, 1996. Obstetric practice and the prevalence of urinary incontinence three months after delivery. *British Journal of Obstetrics & Gynaecology*. 103:154-61.
26. Glazener CMA, 1997. Sexual function after childbirth: women's experiences, persistent morbidity and lack of professional recognition. *British Journal of Obstetrics & Gynaecology*. 104:330-35.
27. Schrader E, 1996. Disability and reproductive rights: complications after regional anaesthesia. *Reproductive Health Matters*. 4(7):135-43.
28. Enkin M, Keirse MJNC, Renfrew M et al, 1995. *A Guide to Effective Care in Pregnancy and Childbirth*. 2nd edition. Oxford University Press, Oxford.
29. Nordström L et al, 1997. Routine oxytocin in the third stage of labour: a placebo-controlled, randomised trial. *British Journal of Obstetrics & Gynaecology*. 104:781-86.
30. World Health Organization, 1990. *The Prevention and Management of Postpartum Haemorrhage*. WHO, Geneva.
31. Eclampsia Trial Collaborative Group, 1995. Which anticonvulsant for women with eclampsia? Evidence from the Collaborative Eclampsia Trial. *Lancet*. 345:1455-63.
– Magee LA, Ornstein MO, von Dadelszen P, 1999. Management of hypertension in pregnancy. *BMJ*. 318:1332-36.
32. World Health Organization, 1995. *The Prevention and Management of Puerperal Infections*. WHO, Geneva. WHO/FHE/MSM/96.24.
33. Swarbreck AB, 1950. Early rising for puerperal women. *BMJ*. 936-38.
– Treffers PE, Huidekoper BL, Weenink GH et al, 1983. Epidemiological observations of thrombo-embolic disease during pregnancy and in the puerperium in 56022 women. *International Journal of Gynecology and Obstetrics*. 21:327-31.
34. World Health Organization, 1994. *Clinical Management of Abortion Complications: A Practical Guide*. WHO, Geneva.
35. Langer A, García-Barrios C, Heimburger A et al, 1997. Improving post abortion care in a public hospital in Oaxaca, Mexico. *Reproductive Health Matters*. 5(9):20-28.
36. Coeytaux F, Winikoff B, 1989. *Celebrating Mother and Child on the 40th day: The Sfax, Tunisia Postpartum Programme*. Quality/Calidad/Qualité Series No. 1. Population Council, New York.
– Brady M, Winikoff B (eds.), 1993. *Rethinking Postpartum Care*. Robert H Ebert Program, Population Council, New York.
37. Muchtar W, 1998. Implementing a program to place midwives in the community. Report for the Government of Indonesia, Ministry of Health.

Efforts to Reduce Abortion-Related Mortality in South Africa

Kim Dickson-Tetteh, Helen Rees

After South Africa's first democratic elections in 1994, a unique environment existed in which to alter a range of legislation which had systematically denied rights and services to the most disadvantaged in the country. Under the new Constitution, which recognises gender and reproductive rights, it became possible for abortion law reform to be implemented. The Choice on Termination of Pregnancy Act came into force in South Africa in February 1997. Before the law was passed, some 425 women died in hospital each year from complications of unsafe, clandestine abortions and some 14,000 or more per year attended hospitals for treatment of complications. Considered one of the most liberal abortion laws in the world, the new Act permits the termination of pregnancy upon the request of the woman up to 12 weeks of pregnancy, and on certain defined grounds after 13 weeks of pregnancy. This paper describes the requirements of the Act as regards service provision, its implementation through a National Abortion Care Programme, and the details of a national curriculum and training programme for physicians and especially midwives who are gradually setting up services. A combination of values clarification workshops for health service providers, and a nationally coordinated and localled-controlled implementation plan are ensuring that this legislation is translated into widely accessible services at provincial level and reducing the incidence of abortion-related mortality and morbidity.

THE South African Constitution states that all people should have a right to health care, including access to reproductive health care, and the government has begun a process of transforming legislation that denied rights and services to the most disadvantaged.

The inequity of race and class has been clearly demonstrated in South Africa in relation to women's access to safe abortion. Before the change of government, access to safe, legal abortions was limited to a few wealthy women who could afford to pay a willing gynaecologist to guide them through the bureaucracy required by the State before a pregnancy could be terminated. Of a total of 868 legal (reported) abortions in 1988, 69 per cent of the women were white women (whites were just over 12 per cent of the South African population at that time). Most of those abortions were performed on the grounds of 'threat to the woman's mental health'.[1]

The campaign to liberalise abortion laws was not only grounded in liberation politics, but also supported on public health grounds by national data which showed that approximately 425 women died each year in public hospitals as a result of clandestine, unsafe abortion procedures. The national research also estimated that of the 44,686 women admitted to South Africa's public hospitals each year with incomplete abortions, at least one third had medical complications that indicated their abortions were induced using unsafe procedures.[2] A significant number of women are also likely to have died unreported in the community or suffered acute and chronic morbidity as a result of such procedures.

Complications of unsafe abortion are a leading cause of maternal deaths worldwide, causing an estimated 14 per cent of pregnancy-related deaths.[3] These deaths are almost all entirely preventable. They occur in developing countries which have not liberalised their abortion legislation, a necessary first step towards ensuring access to safe abortion services, particularly for the most disadvantaged women.

There have been some notable exceptions; Zambia has had a liberal abortion law since the 1970s[4] and Guyana introduced a liberal law in 1995.[5] In both instances, however, implementation has been plagued by infrastructural, attitudinal and resource problems. Advocates who may have thought that with the changing of the law their job was nearly complete, have found that putting the law into practice provides its own challenges. With the recent revision of the South African abortion law, the lessons learnt from these countries were carefully noted.

Prior to 1975, abortion was illegal in South Africa under any circumstances, unless the life of the woman was at risk. The Abortion and Sterilisation Act of 1975 permitted abortion in cases where childbirth presented a serious threat to the woman's physical health, or danger of permanent damage to her mental health, or where the woman was mentally handicapped, or rape or incest had occurred, or the child would be born with a mental or physical handicap.[6] The provisions of this Act remained restricted, and legal abortions in South Africa continued to be inaccessible.

The procedure to obtain an abortion under this Act included: finding a doctor to recommend the procedure, then finding two other doctors to claim in good faith that the abortion was indicated. At least one of the doctors should have been practising for at least four years, and neither could participate in the procedure. Further, the termination had to take place in a state-controlled health facility, or one specifically intended to provide abortions. As a result of such stringent conditions, the great majority of women could not obtain legal abortions and only about 40 per cent of applications for a legal termination each year were approved. Women therefore continued to resort to illegal and often dangerous abortions instead.[7]

The Choice on Termination of Pregnancy Act 1997

In February 1997, the Choice on Termination of Pregnancy Act came into force in South Africa. The mandate given to those who formulated the Act, as part of an effort to address the problem of abortion-related mortality, was to create a framework in which safe abortion could be made accessible to the most vulnerable groups, including rural women and teenagers. The new Act promotes reproductive rights and extends freedom of choice by affording every woman the right to choose whether to have an early safe and legal termination of pregnancy (TOP), according to her individual beliefs.

The Choice on Termination of Pregnancy Act permits termination of pregnancy upon the request of the woman up to and including 12 weeks of pregnancy, under certain defined circumstances from the 13th to the 20th week of gestation, and in more limited circumstances after the 20th week of pregnancy. In the case of young women and girls under the age of 18, the law does not require the signature of a parent or guardian; the decision relies solely on the consent, after counselling, of the young woman herself.[8] The Act is now considered to be one of the most progressive pieces of legislation to be implemented anywhere in the world.

However, even a liberal abortion law alone cannot guarantee that services are widely available and accessible, especially in the early phases of implementation. The initial experience in South Africa was that many women were still compelled to resort to unsafe abortions due to the lack of services. The main aim in implementing the Act was to provide abortions free of cost at the appropriate level of care, depending on the number of weeks of pregnancy (i.e. first trimester procedures at primary care facilities). The provision of free services at the primary care level ensures that even the poorest and most disadvantaged women, who also had the highest risk of complications due to their inability to pay for safe procedures, will be able to access services. To ensure that services could be made widely available, the Act facilitates the decentralisation of services by allowing registered nurse-midwives to perform first trimester abortions, as well as doctors. Since nurses run most South African clinics, nurse-midwives were identified as being critical in the provision of abortion services.

While the Act allows for conscientious objection on the part of health care providers, the legislation also clearly states that if a woman requests a termination of pregnancy, she also has rights under the Act. If the health care provider cannot, or will not, provide an abortion, he/she is obliged to refer the woman to a health professional who is prepared to provide the service. According to the Act, preventing a lawful termination of pregnancy or obstructing access to a facility for the termination of pregnancy is a punishable offence. Conviction could result in a fine, or imprisonment not exceeding ten years.

The first year under the Choice on Termination of Pregnancy Act

Implementation of the new Act posed a major problem to South Africa's national and provincial health authorities. In the first year, as expected, there was a surge in the number of legal abortions requested and performed, which indirectly reflected a reduction in unsafe abortions and associated mortality and morbidity. However, access remained restricted and unequal. Of the total of 31,312 legal abortions performed in the first year, almost all were carried out in tertiary centres in urban areas.[9] Indeed in the first three months after the Act was passed, 60 per cent of all legal abortions were performed in urban Gauteng Province, home to the cities of Johannesburg and Pretoria.[10] A year later only one-third of the hospitals and clinics that were designated to provide abortions were actually providing services.[11]

Health care providers had not been prepared to implement the new Act; they lacked the necessary skills and were also ignorant of the terms of the Act. Many health providers were also resistant to providing termination of pregnancy services. As a result, in the first year the Planned Parenthood Association of South Africa (PPASA), the Reproductive Health Research Unit (RHRU) and the Reproductive Rights Alliance (RRA) conducted values clarification workshops across the country.[12] These workshops aimed to:

- give service providers the time and space to reflect on their feelings and thoughts on termination of pregnancy,
- educate them on the provisions of the new Act and the need for services,
- encourage them to view termination of pregnancy in a non-judgemental way and to treat women seeking abortion with dignity and respect, irrespective of their own views.

Many providers were actually forced to attend these workshops, and some had no idea what they were for before they arrived. In one such workshop, some of the doctors actually walked out. The doctors tended to be more resistant than the nurses, but on the whole, they would sit and listen.

Various exercises were conducted at the workshops. For example, one exercise was 'The last abortion scenario' in which the provider could provide one last abortion to only one woman. S/he had to choose which woman from among several, all of whom had a particularly urgent problem, e.g. a woman dying of AIDS, a girl who had been raped, a woman with eight children, and so on. Each workshop participant had to say which woman s/he would choose and defend the decision. Most people argued their case quite strongly. Another type of exercise was where a sentence would be read out, such as: 'Most women who have abortions do not seriously consider the consequences' or 'Teenage girls should be made to get permission from their parents before being allowed to have an abortion'. Participants would be asked to say whether they strongly agreed or disagreed with the statement and why.

The goal set for the facilitators was to get providers to see that there was always more than one way of looking at these issues, but that it was the woman whose choice had to be respected in the end. It became clear that it was important not to mix different groups or levels of providers, as some people would not get the chance to voice their opinions.

Over 4,000 providers attended these workshops, which were quite successful in helping to change the attitudes of many providers. A pilot study done by PPASA in Cape Town showed that nearly 70 per cent of workshop participants felt that the workshop had helped them deal with abortion patients 'quite a bit' or 'a lot' better than before the workshop.

Attitudes of some providers remain a problem, however. In September 1998 a schoolgirl seeking an abortion was turned away by nurses in Mpulaneng Hospital in Bushbuckridge. The girl went to a male nurse who did an illegal abortion in his room. The girl died and the nurse dumped her body a few meters away from the residential quarters.[13]

Public knowledge of the Act was also limited; over 30 per cent of abortions performed in the first year were second trimester terminations.[14]

Many women were also requesting terminations for pregnancies beyond the 20-week cut-off point (except for abortions on limited health-related grounds) specified in the legislation. Organisations such as the RRA and the National Progressive Primary Health Care Network began community awareness-raising efforts; however, these were not extensive, as services were still limited.

The Reproductive Rights Alliance also undertook to act as a 'watchdog' with regard to implementation of the Act, through ensuring balanced media reporting and publication of the *Barometer*, a quarterly publication that reports on TOP statistics, analyses the status of implementation, and collates information to help coordinate the work of NGOs, government and other key decision-makers.

Six months after the Act was passed, three anti-abortion groups challenged its constitutionality in court on the grounds that the Act violated the rights of the fetus. The government argued that the Constitution does not protect the fetus as a bearer of rights and that the plaintiffs therefore did not have a case. They further argued that 'it would be disastrous for the State to prohibit women from accessing abortion under safe, controlled conditions' and subject them once again to the indignity of having to seek unsafe, illegal abortions. The court ruled in favour of the Act in July 1998.[14]

A National TOP Advisory Group was set up to coordinate and monitor implementation of the Act. This group consisted of National and Provincial health service managers, representatives from the country's eight medical schools, academics and specialists, the South African Nursing Council, researchers and the non-governmental sector. The group meets every four to six months, monitors provincial progress in the implementation of the Act, and makes recommendations to government on relevant critical issues.

Although there were ongoing activities to facilitate the implementation of the Act and to decentralise services, a co-ordinated strategy was identified as necessary. By the end of the first year, efforts had begun to set up a nationally co-ordinated programme to ensure that abortion services were set up throughout the country. The training of midwives in the simple, cost-efficient manual vacuum aspiration (MVA) technique was to be a key activity of this programme, with the National TOP Advisory Group to oversee and review its activities.

The National Abortion Care Programme

The National Abortion Care Programme was officially started in April 1998 with donor funding. The programme is a partnership between the Maternal, Child and Women's Health Directorate (MCWH) of the Department of Health, the Reproductive Health Research Unit (RHRU), the provincial health departments and academic institutions, co-ordinated by RHRU. Ipas, an NGO with extensive experience training health care providers in the manual vacuum aspiration technique, provide technical assistance to the Programme.

The National Abortion Care Programme was designed to reduce maternal mortality from unsafe abortions by developing the capacity to provide safe, efficient and accessible abortion services in public sector hospitals and clinics. The aim is to introduce abortion services, particularly at the primary and secondary care levels, bringing services closer to the community and making them more accessible. These services include techniques for the termination of pregnancy and to manage incomplete abortions and the complications of unsafe abortions appropriately. The programme also focuses on ensuring that all services provide adequate post-abortion family planning counselling and methods, to contribute to the reduction of unwanted pregnancy, and ensuring that abortion services are linked with other, related reproductive health services.

The key elements of the National Abortion Care Programme are:

- training of physicians in cost-efficient techniques to manage abortions,
- midwifery training in carrying out abortions, including training in the MVA technique to provide first trimester abortions and to manage incomplete abortions; and
- midwifery training in post-abortion family planning counselling.

The programme has been designed to run for three years. In its first few months, the national co-ordinators worked with all nine provinces in South Africa to develop provincial plans. Each province is to work in collaboration with a medical school or a nominated tertiary training hospital. Work also began to develop training for midwives.

In November 1998, two national training-of-trainers workshops were held for physicians and midwives, to which each province sent two or more physicians and midwives. Twenty physicians were designated as provincial trainers; they were to be responsible for the training of other physicians and midwives in their provinces. They were also to be responsible for establishing and monitoring abortion services in their provinces.

Nurse-midwives are the major providers of health services at the primary care level; hence, the training of nurse-midwife trainers in the MVA technique was a particularly significant part of this programme's aim to decentralise service provision and make services accessible. Twenty-five nurse-midwives were also trained as trainers in post-abortion family planning counselling. They were to work with the physicians to ensure that all abortion services to be set up would have nurse-midwives on site who could provide adequate counselling pre- and post-abortion.

The Midwifery Training Programme

The Choice on Termination of Pregnancy Act provides that 'a registered midwife who has completed the prescribed training course' as well as a medical practitioner may perform a termination of pregnancy of less than 12 weeks gestation. The training course was to be 'prescribed' by the South African Nursing Council (SANC). When the Act was introduced, no such course had as yet been formulated or approved. In July 1997, the South African Nursing Council, with technical support from the RHRU, produced comprehensive guidelines for the formulation of a short course for the training of registered midwives in the termination of pregnancy and related reproductive health matters.

The guidelines prescribed a 160-hour course combining theory and practicals for midwives. The theoretical part of the course could be offered through attendance of a class or in the form of self-directed study with the aid of a learning package. Clinical practicals under supervision were a compulsory component of the course. Midwives could only be certified to provide abortions after they had successfully completed both the theory and the practicals. The Council required that a registered nurse-midwife or a medical practitioner be involved in both the theoretical and the practical teaching.

In October 1997, the RHRU was mandated by the National Termination of Pregnancy Advisory Group to develop a national core curriculum for training registered midwives in abortion care, which could then be modified to meet provincial needs as required. A draft curriculum and training manual were put together and circulated to major stakeholders for comment, including representatives of the SANC, midwifery training institutions, medical schools, national and provincial reproductive health departments, practising midwives and reproductive health and rights organisations. A national workshop brought all the major stakeholders together to discuss the draft. By the end of October 1998 the training manual had been revised and was ready for training the first batch of midwives.

The curriculum[15] endorses the principle of safe, sustainable and cost-effective abortion care in South Africa, and reflects an holistic approach to the termination of pregnancy as part of comprehensive reproductive health services, in line with the National Abortion Care Programme. The curriculum includes an overview of the Choice on Termination of Pregnancy Act and the problem of unsafe abortion, professional practice and ethics, communication skills and counselling techniques, patient assessment and preparation, pharmacology, the MVA technique, infection control, management of abortion complications, post-abortion family planning, emergency contraception, identification and treatment of sexually transmitted infections (STIs) and strategies for dual protection against unwanted pregnancy and STIs. (see Box)

Before any training could be initiated, dedicated midwives who wanted to be trained and skilled physicians willing to train them had to be identified. Primary and secondary level health care facilities with appropriate referral centres also had to be identified. A long-term plan for the provinces to incorporate the training into the basic training curriculum of midwives is still being developed. These steps would ensure not only the initiation of the programme, but also the sustainability of the programme and services.

Many South African midwives have shown great interest in the training programme. In the first six months, the National Abortion Care Programme received 148 requests for training, from whom 83 midwives had already been trained as of this writing. The first group, 22 midwives, attended a two-week national training workshop in November 1998 using the new curriculum. The participants were practising, registered midwives working in reproductive health services. After completion of the theoretical component, they were given a period of three months to complete the two-week clinical training successfully at an accredited institution within their province.

These midwives have now gone back with the aim of setting up services in their provinces. This has been a slow process, however, since the provinces have said they first want to strengthen their secondary and tertiary services before offering abortions at primary level. Only three midwives are actually already providing abortion services at primary level at this writing. One midwife left the public health service after being trained but has gone on to work for an NGO providing women's health services, where hopefully she will be able to use her training. Another was reallocated to different duties.

However, two further national training workshops have since been held and a further 61 midwives have been trained. The provincial reproductive health co-ordinators have requests from many more midwives who would like to be trained, and the provinces will soon start their own training. The practice of the trained midwives is being monitored and supported by the provincial physician trainers and the National Abortion Care Programme coordinators.

One problem that has arisen due to the slowness in getting primary level services up and running to meet the rapidly increasing demand, is burnout among the few hospital-based physicians providing abortions and the nurses who are working with them. Their numbers are so limited in some places that rotation of staff, an important practice, has not been possible. In the absence of support systems for these providers, which there has barely been time to set up, burn-out is becoming an issue.

Problems are also emerging with untrained providers who were working illegally. For example, one midwife who was performing abortions in a private clinic without having done the prescribed training course is currently facing criminal and professional charges. Cases like these are perhaps the inevitable but temporary sorts of problems which emerge when dangerous, illegal abortion services are replaced by legal ones.

Curriculum for training registered midwives in the termination of pregnancy[15]

The objectives of the curriculum are such that the trained midwife should be able to perform a TOP or manage an incomplete abortion patient with a normal, under-12-weeks pregnancy. The midwife should also be able to stabilise and refer a patient with an under-12-weeks pregnancy with complications, or a pregnancy of over 12 weeks. By the end of the course, the registered midwife should be able to:

- Assess clients and establish the length of pregnancy
- Assess the woman for reproductive tract infection
- Provide pre- and post-TOP counselling using appropriate communication skills
- Perform essential pre-TOP investigations, e.g. a pregnancy test
- Perform a manual vacuum aspiration to terminate a pregnancy and manage incomplete abortion (for the under-12-weeks pregnancy)
- Administer medication responsibly during the management of the abortion within the midwife's scope of practice
- Institute emergency treatment in the event of an untoward reaction or complication during the management of an abortion
- Make appropriate referral to other agencies
- Provide contraceptive methods following medical eligibility criteria for post-TOP family planning
- Implement comprehensive patient education with regard to contraception, sexually transmitted diseases, HIV/AIDS and safer sexual practices.

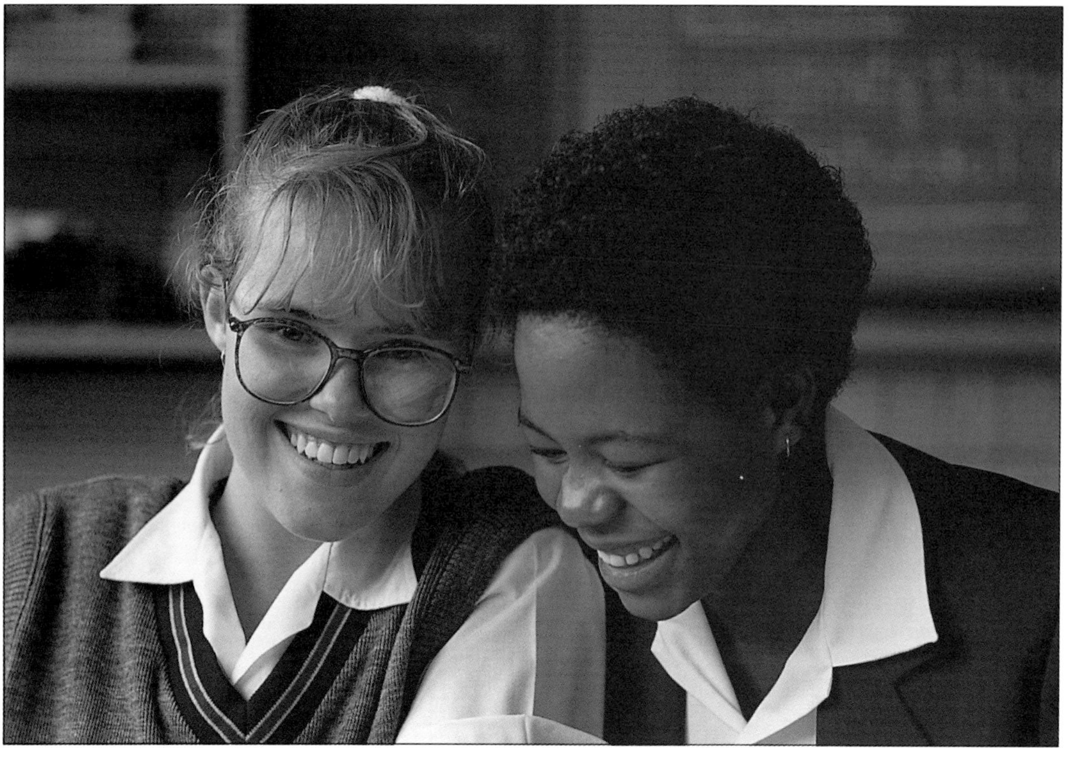
INGRID HUDSON / HUTCHISON LIBRARY

Conclusion

The National Abortion Care Programme shows commitment on the part of the government of South Africa to reduce abortion-related mortality. The training of registered midwives in MVA will ensure broad-based provision of abortion services in South Africa and promote access for those who most need these services. Even though it is still too early to measure the impact of the programme on maternal mortality and morbidity, there are some examples of places where the provision of safe and legal abortion services has brought about a reduction in the number of women seeking treatment for abortion complications.

At the Kalafong Academic Hospital in Pretoria, in the first year of the new Act, there was a significant decrease in both the total and relative number of patients admitted with complications of abortion. The complication rate decreased from 50.7 per cent in 1996 to 29.4 per cent the following year. Conversely, when the same hospital stopped doing second trimester terminations, the rate of complications rose again from 25.9 per cent to 35.3 per cent, another indication of the importance of access to safe services for women.[16]

National Guidelines for Contraceptive Services are currently being drawn up to help improve contraceptive service delivery within the country. Along with these, the Choice on Termination of Pregnancy Act is part of the government's commitment to promoting an holistic approach to reproductive health care, reducing maternal mortality and the number of unwanted pregnancies, promoting reproductive choice and sustaining and improving the quality of women's lives. The long-term aim, which is beginning to be realised, is to make reproductive choice a reality for all South African women, without fear of death, through safe, legal and high quality services.

Acknowledgements

The National Abortion Care Programme is supported by grants from the Henry J Kaiser Family Foundation, USA, and Department for International Development (DFID), UK. We would like to acknowledge Ipas for technical support to the National Abortion Care Programme and Mrs Mosotho Gabriel for dedicated assistance in the preparation of the midwifery training curriculum and the co-ordination of the National Abortion Care Programme.

Correspondence

Dr Kim Dickson-Tetteh, Reproductive Health Research Unit, Department of Obstetrics and Gynaecology, Chris Hani Baragwanath Hospital, P. O. Bertsham 2013, Johannesburg, South Africa. Fax: 27-11-933-1227. E-mail: kimdt@obs.co.za

References and Notes

1. Rogers B. 1972. *Population dynamics and migrant labour in South Africa. South Africa the Bantu Homelands,* London International Defence and Aid, Cited in Edmunds M, 1981.
2. Rees H, Katzenellenbogen J et al, 1997. The epidemiology of incomplete abortion in South Africa. *South African Medical Journal* 87(4):432-37.
3. Division of Family Health, World Health Organisation, Abortion 1994. *A Tabulation of Available Data on the Frequency and Mortality of Unsafe Abortion.* Geneva: WHO.
4. Zambia: Termination of Pregnancy Act 1972. Act 26. *International Digest of Health Legislation,* 1973. 24:448-49.
5. Nunes F, Delph Y, 1997. Making abortion law reform work: steps and slips in Guyana. *Reproductive Health Matters.* 9:66-75.
6. Abortion and Sterilisation Act 1975. Act 2. Capetown: South African Government Gazette.
7. Rees H, 1991. The abortion debate in South Africa. *Women's Global Network for Reproductive Rights Newsletter.* 36:32-35.
8. Choice on Termination of Pregnancy Act 1996. Act 96. Capetown: *South African Government Gazette.* For a summary of the main clauses of the Act, see *Reproductive Health Matters* 5(9):116-18.
9. Department of Health, Republic of South Africa, 1998. *Epidemiological comments. Termination of Pregnancy.* 24(3):2.
10. Reproductive Rights Alliance, 1998. Directory of designated hospitals. *Barometer* 2(1): 30-31.
11. Reproductive Rights Alliance, 1998. Editorial. *Barometer* 2(1):1.
12. The Reproductive Health Research Unit is an academic center of excellence devoted to policy and programme development, research and training within the new reproductive health paradigm, and was formed in 1994 to help develop and improve reproductive health services in South Africa. The Reproductive Rights Alliance is an umbrella organisation of 30 women's groups and other organisations committed to promoting reproductive rights and freedom of choice for women, through its member organisations.
13. *Sunday Times of Johannesburg,* September 1998.
14. Reproductive Rights Alliance, 1998. Legal update. *Barometer* 2(2):20.
15. Dickson-Tetteh KE, Gabriel M, Gringle R et al, 1998. *Abortion Care Manual: A guide for the training of registered midwives in termination of pregnancy, the management of incomplete abortions and related reproductive health matters.* Reproductive Health Research Unit/ Ipas, South Africa.
16. De Jonge ETM, Pattinson RC, Mantel GD. Termination of pregnancy (TOP) in South Africa in its first year: is TOP getting on top of the problem of unsafe abortion? (Submitted for publication 1999)

HIV/AIDS, Pregnancy and Maternal Mortality and Morbidity: Implications for Care

Marge Berer

Most developing countries in which HIV is prevalent in women of childbearing age are also countries in which the risks of maternal mortality and morbidity are high, creating a serious threat to safe motherhood. This paper discusses the limited but growing evidence from developing countries that: (1) complications of pregnancy, delivery and induced abortion are more frequent and more severe in HIV positive than HIV negative women, especially those who are symptomatic, (2) pregnancy may contribute to HIV disease progression, immune deficiency and AIDS, in pregnant as compared to non-pregnant women, and (3) AIDS is an underlying factor in direct maternal deaths, contributes to indirect deaths from other causes and is an indirect cause of maternal death in itself. The presence of HIV in a large proportion of an antenatal population has serious implications for antenatal, delivery and post-partum care, emergency obstetric care and abortion provision, as well as the training of health care workers providing these services. These services, along with focused prevention efforts, need to be strengthened, not only to reduce maternal and infant mortality and morbidity, but also to take account of the needs and problems of pregnant women with HIV and AIDS.

AN estimated two million HIV positive women worldwide were expected to give birth in 1998,[1] while well over half a million women were expected to die from complications of pregnancy, childbirth and abortion.[2] There is a significant though unquantified overlap between these two groups of women in sub-Saharan Africa and other developing countries where rates of HIV among women and maternal mortality and morbidity are high.

Women cannot easily protect themselves from HIV infection when they are trying to get pregnant, or during pregnancy, or when they resume sexual relations after the post-partum period. Many women only learn they are HIV positive from an antenatal HIV test, which in developing countries often means in the second or third trimester of pregnancy, or only when their infants become ill. Women who start to protect themselves during or after pregnancy may be too late, as they may already have been infected with HIV.[3,4]

Prevention efforts to date have failed to reduce the incidence of HIV infection or maternal mortality and morbidity in women of childbearing age, particularly in developing countries. These efforts have been further hampered because maternal mortality and HIV/AIDS are usually addressed separately, in spite of how inter-related they are. A more integrated approach is long overdue.

This paper discusses the limited but growing evidence from developing countries that: (1) complications of pregnancy, delivery and induced abortion, and complications arising from certain life-saving interventions such as caesarean section, may be more frequent and more severe in HIV positive than HIV negative women, especially in women who are symptomatic, (2) pregnancy may contribute to HIV disease progression, immune deficiency and AIDS, in pregnant as compared to non-pregnant women, and (3) AIDS is an underlying factor in direct maternal deaths, contributes to indirect deaths from other causes and is an indirect cause of maternal death in itself.

A Medline search was done using the key words 'pregnancy', 'HIV' and the major direct and indirect causes of maternal deaths. The data summarised in this paper came from three systematic reviews, studies reported in journals in the past five years on maternal mortality and morbidity and HIV/AIDS in women, and abstracts from the most recent World AIDS Conference in Geneva, July 1998. This is not an exhaustive review. Existing data are limited; they come from disparate settings, based on disparate study designs and sometimes very small sample sizes, and only rarely control for confounding factors. This is further complicated by the need to compare HIV positive and HIV negative pregnant women for some associations, and pregnant and non-pregnant HIV positive women for others.

Although limited, however, the existing data suggest that poor women with HIV infection in developing countries may be at greater risk of maternal death and yet receive little or no sustained care or support. More thorough study, using more rigorous research protocols, would clarify the association between HIV/AIDS, pregnancy and the risk of maternal mortality. In the meantime, there is a clear need for national health programmes to take account of the risks faced by women with HIV and AIDS who are pregnant, within wider efforts to reduce maternal mortality and morbidity.

Extent of HIV in pregnant women

Internationally, half of all new HIV infections in women reported globally in 1998 were in the 15-24 age group,[5] and sentinel surveillance throughout the past decade has shown that growing numbers of women attending antenatal clinics are HIV positive.[6,7] Figures range from less than one percent in low HIV prevalence settings (e.g. in western Europe) to as high as 30-40 per cent and more in some parts of sub-Saharan Africa. Table 1 gives data reported to UNAIDS through

Table 1. Median HIV Prevalence in Women Attending Antenatal Clinics in Major Urban Areas and among Sex Workers,[7] Selected Countries*

Country	Year	Antenatal clinic attenders – HIV positive (%)	Year	Sex workers – HIV positive (%)
Bahamas	1993	3.6	–	–
Botswana	1997	38.5	–	–
Brazil	1996	5.1	1994	6.3
Burkina Faso	1996	9.6	1994	57.2
Cambodia	1997	0.8	1997	39.3
Cameroon	1996	4.5	1995	16.5
Côte d'Ivoire	1997	9.1	1995	69.2
Ethiopia	1996	18.2	1991	67.5
Ghana	1996	2.2	1991	37.5
Guyana	1992	6.9	1993	25.0
Haiti	1993	8.4	1989	41.9
Honduras	1996	1.0	1995	20.5
India	1997	4.3	1995	27.3 (range 4.6–49.9)
Jamaica	1992	0.4	1995	20.5
Kenya	1997	15.9	1995	55.5
Malawi	1996	30.5	1994	70.0
Nigeria	1994	6.7	1994	29.1
Sierra Leone	1992	2.0	1995	26.7
Sudan	1996	4.5	–	–
Thailand	1997	1.3	1997	13.0
Uganda	1997	14.7	–	–
Zambia	1994	26.5	–	–
Zimbabwe	1995	31.0	1995	86.0

** Reported to end 1997*

the end of 1997 in selected countries, to show the range of prevalences; in some cases, data are not reported annually and figures are from previous years, up to six years out of date. Some 79 countries in all regions, developed and developing, had not reported figures from antenatal clinics at all; these were mostly but not only low HIV prevalence countries.[7]

HIV was reported in more than 20 per cent of antenatal clinic attenders in major urban areas in the following countries: Botswana, Burundi, Lesotho, Malawi, Rwanda, South Africa, Swaziland, Zambia and Zimbabwe.[7] In South Africa, the rate of HIV infection in antenatal clinics nationally rose from 17.04 per cent in 1997 to 22.8 per cent in 1998.[8]

Pregnant women in rural areas, particularly poor women, are even less likely to attend antenatal clinics than women in urban areas, so recorded data from these clinics may not be representative of the population as a whole.

Data for women sex workers in the selected countries are also included in Table 1.[7] Sex workers are often young women and have babies, often as single mothers, and these figures indicate the much greater risk of HIV that exists for women involved in sex work. This epidemic is thriving on the fact that single and married women are at risk from unprotected sex with their partners/husbands who have unprotected sex with other women, including sex workers. This is a major source of risk for both mothers and babies.[9]

Does pregnancy contribute to HIV disease progression?

A growing number of controlled studies in developed countries which have compared disease progression in HIV infected women who have had pregnancies, with HIV infected women who have not had a pregnancy, show that pregnancy appears to have no discernible effect on the early progression of HIV disease in asymptomatic women.[3] In developing countries, the lack of adverse effects is not so clear.

In developed countries the great majority of pregnant women with HIV are asymptomatic. One review[10] of controlled studies, including a French prospective cohort study with 61 months of follow-up,[11] found no difference in the rate of acceleration of HIV disease in pregnant women as compared to non-pregnant women.

A systematic review of studies from 1983 to 1996 with a meta-analysis of data from seven prospective cohort studies,[12] six of which were carried out in developed countries, investigated HIV disease progression and survival in pregnant women as compared to non-pregnant women in relation to: clinical setting (developed or developing countries), methodological quality (high or poor) and whether studies had controlled for potential confounding factors. The risks of an adverse maternal outcome as reported in this review are shown in Table 2.

The authors conclude[12] that HIV disease progression related to pregnancy was significantly more common in the developing as compared to the developed country settings and was detected more accurately in high quality studies than low quality ones. There appeared to be less progression of HIV disease and progression to AIDS in two studies which attempted to control for confounding factors, although this was not statistically significant in either case. The association appeared to be somewhat stronger in the one developing country study, but large-scale, comparable studies with long-term follow-up in more settings would be needed to get more definitive information.

Perhaps most noteworthy is the lack of well-conducted, controlled studies anywhere globally, but particularly in developing countries with high HIV prevalences in women.

Table 2. Risk of adverse maternal outcome related to HIV in pregnant women in seven cohort studies, 6 in developed countries and 1 in a developing country[12]

Outcome	Odds ratio
Death	1.80 (95% CI 0.99-3.3)
HIV disease progression	
– All studies	1.41 (95% CI 0.85-2.33)
– Developing country	3.71 (95% CI 1.82-7.75)
– Developed countries	0.55 (95% CI 0.27-1.11)
– High quality studies	3.71 (95% CI 1.82-7.57)
– Low quality studies	0.55 (95% CI 0.27-1.11)
Progression to an AIDS-defining illness	1.63 (95% CI 1.00-2.67)
Fall of CD4 cell count to below 200x10(6)/L	0.73 (95% CI 0.17-3.06)

The role of HIV/AIDS in complications of pregnancy and childbirth

In some studies of maternal deaths, data on the role of AIDS is now being included. These show that:

- AIDS is an important underlying factor in direct maternal deaths,
- AIDS is an indirect cause of maternal death in itself, and
- AIDS is a contributor to other indirect causes of maternal death.[13]

In South Africa, deaths due to AIDS comprised 13 per cent of all maternal deaths; women who died of AIDS tended to be younger on average and with lower parity than women who died from other causes.[14] In Brazzaville, Congo, from 1993 to 1994, AIDS was a direct cause of maternal death in 4.2 per cent of cases, and was described as both the main indirect cause of death and the primary mortality factor in pregnant women.[15] In 1993 in Bulawayo district of Tanzania, AIDS was the fourth leading cause of maternal death.[16]

Direct and indirect causes of maternal mortality and morbidity may be more severe or debilitating in HIV positive women, especially in those with symptomatic HIV disease or AIDS, than in women who are HIV negative. HIV positive women may also be more susceptible to complications, including from surgical interventions that are meant to be life-saving.

Even five years ago, mostly anecdotal information existed on this subject, based on the personal observations of clinicians, some of which have been confirmed. For example, a clinician in Zimbabwe[17] noted more severe reproductive tract infection, puerperal sepsis and other post-partum complications following caesarean section and tubal ligation in women with HIV, as well as increases in tuberculosis peritonitis and recto-vaginal fistulae.

As early as 1993, caesarean sections and laparotomy were already being avoided in the University Teaching Hospital in Lusaka, Zambia, unless there was no other option, because a large majority (75 per cent) of HIV positive women having caesarean sections were found to experience delayed wound healing and, with both procedures, an increased risk of infection.[18]

A number of studies[10] have found higher rates of ectopic pregnancy, bacterial pneumonia, urinary tract infections and other infections in HIV positive as compared to HIV negative pregnant women. Studies from South Africa and Mozambique show that infectious complications are also more common during the post-partum period in HIV positive women.

One recent review[19] has found evidence of lower fertility rate ratios in HIV positive as compared to HIV negative women in cohort studies in African populations, as have other studies, probably as a consequence of other sexually transmitted infections and impaired immune function.

A Rwanda study[20] found that HIV positive pregnant women had significantly more sexually transmitted infection and were also more likely to experience post-partum haemorrhage than HIV negative pregnant women.

Studies in Italy,[21] Rwanda,[22] Uganda[23] and Germany[24] have found a higher risk of major and minor complications following caesarean section in HIV positive women as compared to HIV negative women. In the Rwanda study,[22] the severity of complications was also greater, with a high number of maternal deaths among women with severe immune deficiency.

When prophylactic penicillin was administered following emergency caesarean section to 477 women in the controlled study in Uganda,[23] 98 women with asymptomatic HIV infection experienced no significantly greater morbidity than HIV negative women. The incidence of maternal morbidity due to pre-operative dehydration, anaemia, labour lasting more than 18 hours and ruptured membranes, and the incidence of post-operative wound sepsis, genital tract infection and duration of stay of over eight days in hospital (30.6 per cent) was high for all the women, though not significantly different between the two groups. However, there were seven maternal deaths, of which two were directly due to AIDS.

The German study[24] found that the risk of both major and minor complications with laparotomy, caesarean section and induced abortion was significantly higher in HIV positive than HIV negative women (18.3 per cent vs 4.2 per cent, $p < 0.0001$). The highest rate occurred with laparotomy (70 per cent vs 20 per cent), followed by caesarean section (42.9 per cent vs 7.1 per cent) and induced abortion (13.0 per cent vs 2.2 per cent). Severe infection was the most frequent complication observed in HIV positive women (42 per cent), followed by secondary

Complications of pregnancy and delivery found among HIV positive (mainly symptomatic) women as compared to HIV negative women, reported in at least one study in developing countries, 1990-99

- More frequent and severe reproductive tract infections
- More severe and more frequent blood loss, sepsis and delayed wound healing after caesarean section, tubal ligation, laparotomy, and induced abortion
- More urinary tract infections
- Lower fertility rate ratios
- Insufficient weight gain in pregnancy
- Higher rates of ectopic pregnancy
- Greater risk of post-partum haemorrhage and post-partum sepsis
- More frequent and severe anaemia and malaria, and possibly tuberculosis
- Complications of AIDS-related conditions, such as bacterial pneumonia
- Maternal deaths from AIDS and AIDS as a contributor to or underlying factor in maternal deaths from other causes, including in the late post-partum period (from 42 days to two years after the end of pregnancy)

surgery (18 per cent), healing impairment (12 per cent), fever (8 per cent) and blood transfusion (6 per cent). Poor immunological status correlated with a greater risk of complications.

Pregnancies may also be complicated by AIDS-related conditions. In one Swiss study,[25] there were 16 cases of severe maternal morbidity in 153 pregnancies: 14 pneumonia, 1 pyelonephritis and 1 cerebral toxoplasmosis. A recent case report[26] described a maternal metastatic malignancy with non-Hodgkin lymphoma of B-cell origin, an AIDS-related cancer. In this case, the malignancy was revealed upon histological examination of the placenta following caesarean section; HIV infection was confirmed afterwards.

AIDS-related conditions caused appreciable maternal morbidity and mortality in a controlled, prospective study[27] of pregnant women with transfusion-dependent beta-thalassaemia major in India from 1990 to 1997. Among 39 women who had AIDS, 31 per cent had a miscarriage by eight weeks of pregnancy and 13 per cent died undelivered by 32 weeks of pregnancy from pneumocystis carinii pneumonia. In contrast, the women with asymptomatic HIV disease remained well throughout pregnancy.

HIV/AIDS and anaemia, malaria and tuberculosis in pregnancy

HIV/AIDS combined with other indirect causes of maternal death and morbidity can have severe consequences. In Malawi, asymptomatic HIV infection was associated with an increased prevalence and severity of anaemia in pregnancy[28] in an antenatal population with a high prevalence of both anaemia (60 per cent) and HIV (30 per cent).

Malaria has serious adverse effects on pregnant women. In a hospital study in Mozambique between 1989 and 1993,[29] 15.5 per cent of 239 pregnancy-related maternal deaths were directly attributable to malaria, mostly associated with severe anaemia, of which 37.8 per cent were in adolescent girls in their first pregnancies. HIV complicates this further. Malaria rates were significantly higher at first antenatal visit in HIV positive women at all gravidities and from earlier in gestation than in HIV negative women in a study in Malawi.[30] In a large group in Kenya, HIV positive women had more and higher density of malaria in all birth orders than HIV negative women.[31] These studies suggest that HIV may reduce pregnant women's ability to control malaria, particularly in higher birth orders.

Tuberculosis (TB) kills more women than any other infectious disease, and women have a higher progression from infection to disease and a higher case-fatality rate than men.[32] TB is the most common opportunistic infection associated with HIV in the developing world;[10] in 1996, HIV was expected to be responsible for 20 per cent of the projected increase in global TB.[33] Evidence of an association between HIV, the development of tuberculosis and recent childbirth was found in 1990 in Nairobi: five in seven HIV positive women who delivered children had active tuberculosis, compared with one in eight HIV negative women.[34] However, a more recent case-control study in Santo Domingo, Dominican Republic found that neither recent pregnancy nor childbirth was associated with an increased risk of developing active tuberculosis in HIV positive or HIV negative women.[35] Further exploratory studies seem to be called for.

Late post-partum mortality from AIDS in sub-Saharan Africa

Women with HIV in several sub-Saharan African countries have been shown to be at greater risk of dying up to two years after pregnancy than HIV negative women. For example, a prospective study of maternal mortality in rural Malawi[36] found that HIV infection and anaemia were strongly associated with death three to ten months after delivery.

Mortality and morbidity requiring hospitalisation during pregnancy were not significantly different among HIV positive and HIV negative pregnant women from the second trimester of pregnancy to two years after delivery in Kampala and Harare (1990-1994).[37] However, HIV positive women in Kampala were 31 times more at risk of dying between 42 days and two years after delivery than HIV negative women and in Harare the relative risk was 18. Causes of death included AIDS, parasitic infections and other illnesses.

Similarly, higher death rates in women with AIDS were found in a three-year study in an obstetric ward and follow-up clinic at a large municipal hospital in Zaire.[38] Overall, families in which the mother was HIV positive experienced a five- to ten-fold higher maternal, paternal and early childhood mortality rate than those in which the mother was HIV negative. HIV positive women who transmitted HIV to their most recently born child had lost a greater number of previously born children (mean 1.5 versus 0.5; $p < 0.05$), were more likely to have had AIDS at delivery (25 per cent versus 12 per cent; $p < 0.01$) and were more likely to die during follow-up (22 per cent versus 9 per cent; $p < 0.01$) than HIV positive women who did not transmit HIV infection to their newborn child.

Women with AIDS-defining illnesses in sub-Saharan Africa may feel compelled to continue to get pregnant due to social and familial pressure to reach an acceptable family size. In a qualitative study among antenatal women in Abidjan, Côte d'Ivoire, most said they were unable to tell anyone of their positive HIV status, and almost all of them felt they had to have four children, in spite of fears for their own health and that of their babies.[39]

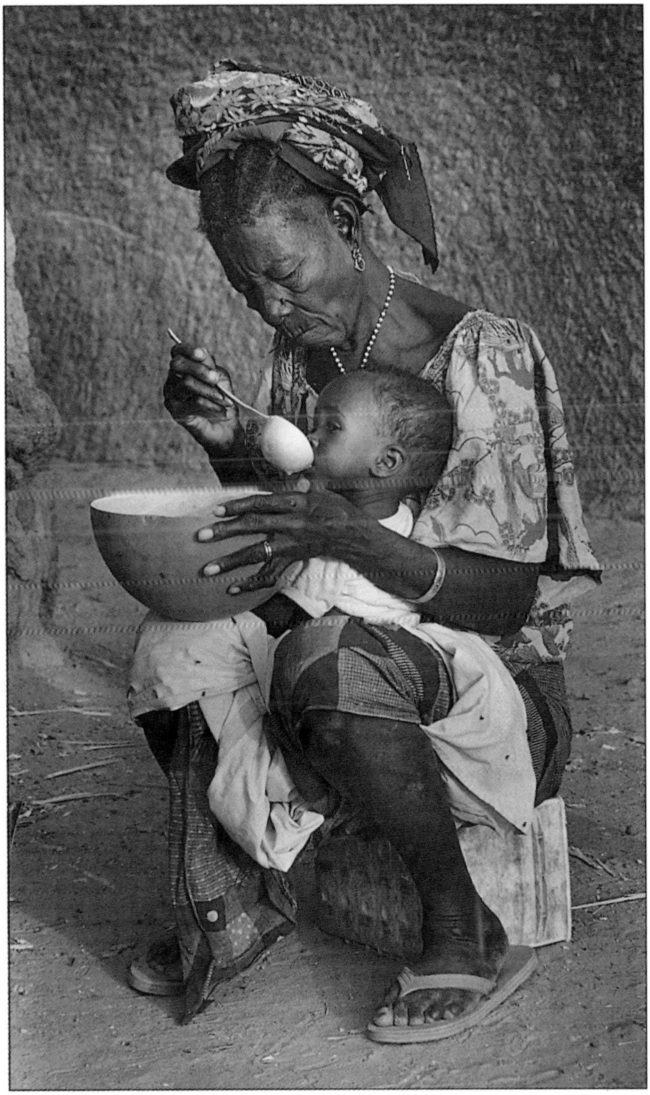

RON GILING / STILL PICTURES

The role of HIV infection in adverse perinatal outcomes

A recent systematic review of the literature and meta-analysis of studies investigating the association between maternal HIV infection and perinatal outcome[40] analysed 31 prospective studies (21 of them from developing countries) of cohorts of HIV positive pregnant women and HIV negative pregnant controls. The summary odds ratio of the risk of adverse perinatal outcomes related to HIV infection is shown in Table 3.

The association between infant mortality and maternal HIV infection was stronger in studies conducted in developing (OR 8.6 95% CI 0.53-141.05) as compared to developed countries (OR 3.72 95% CI 3.05-4.54); studies of higher vs poorer methodological quality; and those which controlled for confounding factors as compared to those which did not.[40]

Only one of the developing country studies included in the review attempted to measure the rate of miscarriage. Nearly all the studies of mortality were carried out in developing countries, and the association between maternal HIV infection and infant mortality in developing countries was strong. There was a statistically significant risk of stillbirth in developing country studies but not developed country ones. The differences in mean birthweight and pre-term delivery were also greater in developing than developed country studies.[40] The limitations on these data arise mainly from the fact that: (1) only two of the studies reported outcomes for asymptomatic and symptomatic women separately, even though this has been shown to make a difference to these outcomes, (2) only two studies attempted to control for confounding factors, e.g. other sexually transmitted infections or injection drug use, and (3) viral load and treatment regimens of the women were rarely described, all of which could have affected outcomes.[40]

Table 3. The association between maternal HIV infection and adverse perinatal outcomes, summary odds ratios from 31 studies (10 in developed countries and 21 in developing countries), 1988-1996[40]

Outcome	Number of studies	Odds ratio
Spontaneous abortion	4	4.05 (95% CI 2.75-5.96)
Stillbirth	11	3.91 (95% CI 2.65-5.77)
Fetal abnormality	7	1.08 (95% CI 0.7-1.66)
Perinatal mortality	6	1.79 (95% CI 0.7-1.66)
Infant mortality	9	3.69 (95% CI 3.03-4.49)
Intrauterine growth retardation	12	1.70 (95% CI 1.43-2.02)
Low birthweight	17	2.09 (95% CI 1.86-2.35)
Pre-term delivery	22	1.83 (95% CI 1.63-2.06)
Neonatal mortality	3	1.10 (95% CI 0.63-1.93)

Other studies have explored some of these issues. A prospective study of transplacental transmission of HIV[41] showed an increased rate of spontaneous fetal death in HIV positive women compared to HIV negative women; HIV was detected in placental and fetal tissues in 7 of 14 losses in 124 pregnancies. Further, women with AIDS more often had fetal loss associated with HIV transmission than did asymptomatic women.

The extent of HIV disease progression and immune suppression are important factors in the increased risk of poor outcomes. In an observational study in 1995-96 in two antenatal care centres in Abidjan, Côte d'Ivoire,[42] the risk of having had at least one miscarriage or stillbirth was significantly higher for HIV positive than HIV negative women, when social and demographic factors were controlled for.

Insufficient weight gain in pregnancy was more frequent in HIV positive women (46.3 per cent) than HIV negative women (30.6 per cent) in São Paulo, Brazil between 1988 and 1996.[43] Those with insufficient weight gain had higher rates of vertical HIV transmission, premature birth and low birthweight than those with normal weight gain, which suggests immune dysfunction was also greater.

Injection drug use can also contribute to poor pregnancy outcomes in association with HIV infection. In the Swiss study mentioned above,[25] 15 per cent of 153 pregnancies in HIV positive women were premature, which was significantly higher for the 100 women using injection drugs (20 per cent) than for those not using drugs (5.6 per cent). Premature labour or rupture of membranes (n=13), maternal illness (n=8) and fetal complications (n=2) were the most frequent reasons for prematurity, and the women tended to have lower CD4 cell counts than those with full-term delivery (29.4 per cent vs 12.0 per cent with CD4<200).

A less noted limitation of such studies is that they do not report the maternal outcomes of pregnancy loss, such as from miscarriage and stillbirth, in any depth or at all. Hence, any resulting morbidity in the women is invisible. Yet the cumulative effects of the number of previous term pregnancies, pregnancy losses, safe or unsafe abortions and their outcomes in terms of maternal morbidity are surely relevant to understanding why women in developing countries are experiencing complications more than those in developed countries.

Furthermore, community-based studies seem to be rare, even though women attending antenatal clinics are not necessary representative of childbearing women most at risk of HIV infection. An additional unknown is whether some women are less likely to attend an antenatal clinic after their first or second pregnancies in some developing countries, because by then they are supposed to 'know what it's all about'. These limitations may also bias the outcomes found.

Discussion and recommendations for service provision

Clearly, HIV and AIDS in women of reproductive age have serious implications for safe motherhood and maternal mortality and morbidity. Women with symptomatic HIV infection in developing country settings where other direct and indirect causes of maternal deaths are prevalent, may be at increased risk of maternal death and more susceptible to and adversely affected by obstetric complications, as compared to HIV negative women, and may progress to AIDS and die more rapidly than non-pregnant women.

The lack of comparable adverse effects in developed countries is at least partly because women are generally in better health (i.e. not malnourished, anaemic or suffering from tropical diseases); maternity care is of a much higher quality, with complications treated rapidly; and HIV positive women have access to prophylactic and curative treatments for opportunistic infections and are more likely to remain asymptomatic longer. Hence, they are less likely to experience many of the problems that women in developing countries go through, who have more and later pregnancies, receive minimal maternity care and inadequate and delayed attention to obstetric and HIV-related complications, and have little or no access to treatment and care for HIV/AIDS-related illnesses.

Where antenatal HIV prevalence is increasing or high, research on maternal mortality and morbidity and safe motherhood programmes must also take the effects of HIV infection into account, and offer concrete recommendations to service providers for appropriate care. This is not yet happening in many instances. For example, a recent study in Uganda among rural pregnant women[44] found that 66 per cent reported having suffered from malaria during their current pregnancy, yet HIV and AIDS were not even mentioned.

Many women with HIV infection are not using maternity services sufficiently, if at all, in spite of the increased risks. Among 615 adolescents (aged 10-19 years) who attended for a first antenatal care visit at two rural hospitals in southern Malawi,[45] the prevalence of anaemia, malaria and HIV infection was high, yet only 41.5 per cent came for a supervised delivery. In many places, this is because delivery services are unavailable or inaccessible to rural women.

The presence of HIV in an antenatal population has wide-ranging implications for public health education and community education. It is important to determine the information needs of women and address these through appropriate channels. Antenatal, delivery and obstetric care, provision of safe abortions, and the training of maternal and child health care workers, midwives and obstetricians are also affected, as well as the availability of drugs such as oxytocin and antibiotics, life-saving procedures and the safety of blood for transfusion.

Provision of adequate women-centred HIV testing and counselling which includes the kind of information contained in this paper, and on prevention of perinatal HIV transmission and the relative benefits and risks of breastfeeding, are also important.[46-48] These should ideally be provided for women considering pregnancy. For those who are already pregnant, it should be early enough in pregnancy to allow a decision on whether to continue the pregnancy. This information should be made available to women in the community and through other accepted channels as well. First, however, the social conditions which encourage women (and their partners) to be tested need to be in place and support for those who are HIV positive needs to be in place as well.

Where there is a high prevalence of antenatal HIV, especially where there is little or no access to or low uptake of HIV testing, assumptions of HIV positivity in all antenatal and birthing women, and use of appropriate universal precautions by health professionals when providing care, are advised.[49] Lack of information, experience and resources for dealing with infected patients will result in fear and poor care. There has been anecdotal evidence that health workers who are not informed about taking these precautions have refused to attend birthing women or have taken a 'space-suit' approach to delivery. Discrimination against those with HIV affects pregnant women too. Doctors have been reported to pressure women to abort wanted pregnancies because of HIV in some settings and in others have refused women abortions for fear of becoming infected themselves. Many refuse women attention for fertility problems. Health care workers also need good information in order to provide appropriate care without discrimination or fear.[50]

HIV positive women have unwanted as well as wanted pregnancies and for some, HIV may be a reason to terminate a pregnancy, use contraception or have a sterilisation. If women are unable to admit to others that they have HIV, accessing these services may be more difficult.

Women with HIV may be at high risk from sepsis, haemorrhage and perforated uterus and their sequelae following unsafe, illegal abortions or attempts to self-abort. No data appear to exist on this because of the continuing illegality of abortion. However, women with HIV infection should qualify for a legal termination of pregnancy in almost all countries. The fact that many physicians in countries with restrictive laws are afraid to provide this service openly (or at all) for fear of repercussions means that outreach is greatly restricted, and young, single women will be particularly disadvantaged.[51]

Guidelines for health care professionals on the provision of antenatal and emergency obstetric care and post-partum follow-up for HIV positive (and untested) women in settings where maternal mortality and morbidity and HIV prevalence are high are also needed. The sorts of improvements needed in service provision include:

- HIV testing and counselling which addresses the information needs of HIV positive pregnant women, including the benefits and risks of breastfeeding and of alternative forms of infant feeding;
- better management of pregnancy, labour and delivery to prevent and treat haemorrhage, anaemia, sepsis, obstructed labour, delayed wound healing and fistulae;
- early and effective treatment of HIV-related disease, malaria and tuberculosis;
- safe abortion services; and
- post-partum and post-abortion contraceptive services.

More specifically, such guidelines would include:

- universal precautions for infection control and to prevent needlestick injuries;
- transfusion of blood and blood products to be reserved for life-threatening complications only;[52]
- pre-operative antibiotic prophylaxis where HIV positive women need surgical or invasive obstetric interventions, in order to reduce the risk of morbidity from blood loss, infection and delayed wound healing;
- more aggressive use of antibiotics for treatment of infectious diseases and complications in HIV positive women;[52]
- awareness that the presence of pneumonia that does not respond rapidly to treatment (i.e. pneumocystis carinii pneumonia, a rapid killer) in young pregnant women may be a sign of HIV infection;[14]
- research on the frequency and timing of malaria treatment in pregnant women, to determine whether the currently recommended course needs to be altered for primi- or multi-gravid women.[30]

Some interventions raise medical-ethical dilemmas which deserve greater attention. Elective caesarean section has been shown to decrease the risk of perinatal HIV transmission in a growing number of studies,[53] including one randomised controlled trial.[54] Such results make the clinical decision whether to perform an elective caesarean on women with symptomatic HIV infection extremely difficult, as the risk of morbidity in the woman must be balanced against preventing HIV in the infant. This is particularly true in resource-poor settings, where prophylactic antibiotic treatment may not be available and where the ability to provide treatment for post-operative complications may be limited. In addition, in areas with high HIV prevalence in the antenatal population and a low caesarean section rate, the caesarean section rate would have to increase several fold to provide the necessary coverage. This would require huge additional resources in terms of qualified medical and midwifery staff, hospital inpatient care, etc .

In general, because an infant is inseparable from its mother until it is born, and mothers are so important for infant and child survival and health, there are important benefits of studying outcomes and complications and the effects of interventions (or their absence) in both mothers and their babies – and in the same study. Six to eight weeks post-partum seems to be an inadequate period of follow-up; given evidence of a high rate of infants deaths and late post-partum deaths in women, a longer period seems to be called for. Only then can life-saving, evidence-based practice, benefiting both women and their babies, be determined and put into practice. Unfortunately, the current research agenda has focussed very much around the prevention of mother-to-child transmission of HIV, a worthy but too narrow focus; women and babies would benefit if a broader range of stakeholders were involved in setting the research and action agenda for the future.

Conclusions

In developed countries the majority of pregnant women have access to effective anti-HIV therapies, including during pregnancy, and a high quality of maternity care. Many of these treatments and services, both preventive and curative, are considered too expensive to provide in the developing world, where the public health need in terms of numbers is the greatest. Treatment for opportunistic infections and combination antiretroviral therapy would help to keep HIV positive women in developing countries healthier longer as well, but these are not available except through private purchase and personal contacts, with the exception of a few countries, most notably Brazil. In some cases, even the cost of essential antibiotics is beyond the capacity of health systems to provide. Greater priority in public health policy to making appropriate therapies available to pregnant HIV positive women in developing countries is called for. Negotiations with pharmaceutical companies to provide these drugs at greatly reduced, affordable public sector prices should be put high on the international health policy agenda by UNAIDS, UNICEF and WHO.

At the same time, interventions that are available and appropriate in developed country settings – where fewer pregnant women with HIV are symptomatic and more are able to live in good health much longer than those in developing countries, and who do not suffer the same risks of maternal mortality and morbidity – cannot simply be recommended for developing countries settings, where the quality of antenatal, delivery and post-partum care, abortion provision and emergency obstetric care, is limited and often inadequate. In these settings, HIV and AIDS make an already difficult situation even more difficult. Needs assessments and priority setting must determine necessary improvements and how and when these can be implemented incrementally.

An integrated approach to women's reproductive health brings into sharp focus the need to address HIV/AIDS in women in the context of Safe Motherhood initiatives and creates a challenge to previously vertical programmes. Practical information and guidance for policy-makers and service providers must be disseminated in accordance with best practice in the prevention of maternal mortality and morbidity and also in the prevention, treatment and care for women with HIV and AIDS.

Correspondence
Marge Berer, Reproductive Health Matters,
E-mail: RHMjournal@compuserve.com

References and Notes

1. Nieburg P, Stanecki KA, 1998. The global burden of mother-to-child transmission of HIV-1. 12th World AIDS Conference. Geneva, July.
2. *Revised 1990 estimates of maternal mortality: a new approach by WHO and UNICEF, 1996.* WHO/FRH/MSM/96.11. The previous estimate of 500,000 deaths per year was changed to 585,000 deaths per year globally.
3. Alger LS, Farley JJ, Robinson BA et al, 1993. Interactions of human immunodeficiency virus infection and pregnancy. *Obstetrics & Gynecology.* 82(5):787-96.
4. Taha TE, Dallabetta GA, Hoover DR, 1998. Trends of HIV-1 and sexually transmitted diseases among pregnant and postpartum women in urban Malawi. *AIDS.* 12(2):197-203.
5. UNAIDS, 1998. New World AIDS Day Report finds global HIV infections increased 10 per cent in 1998. Press release, UNAIDS. Geneva, 24 November.
6. Smith NH, Lu-Yu Hwang, 1996. Risk factors for HIV in pregnant women. *International Journal of STDs & AIDS.* 7(October):388-95. Data reported in this paper are mostly pre-1990 but include a wide range of studies internationally.
7. Annex. HIV/AIDS estimates and indicators, end 1997. *UNAIDS/WHO Report on the Global HIV/AIDS Epidemic.* Joint UN Programme on HIV/AIDS, World Health Organization. Geneva, June 1998.
8. – Whiteside A, 1999. South Africa's 1998 survey results show no let-up. *AIDS Analysis Africa.* 10(1):1/10.
   – See also: Wilkinson D, 1998. Antiretroviral drugs for pregnant women in rural South Africa: cost effectiveness and capacity. 12th World AIDS Conference. Geneva, July. Abstract 23297.
9. See for example: – Ray S, Maposhere C, 1997. Male and female condom use by sex workers in Zimbabwe: Acceptability and obstacles. *Beyond Acceptability: User's Perspectives on Contraception.* Ravindran TKS, Berer M, Cottingham J (eds). Reproductive Health Matters/WHO, London.
   – Meursing K, Sibindi F, 1995. Condoms, family planning and living with HIV in Zimbabwe. *Reproductive Health Matters.* 3(5/May):56-67.
   – Kuntolbutra S, Celentano DD, Suprasert S et al, 1996. Factors related to inconsistent condom use with commercial sex workers in northern Thailand. *AIDS.* 10(5):556-57.
   – Maticka-Tyndale E, Elkins D, Haswell-Elkins M et al, 1997. Contexts and patterns of men's commercial sexual partnerships in northeastern Thailand: implications for AIDS prevention. *Social Science and Medicine.* 44(2):199-213.
   – de Zoysa I, Sweat MD, Denison JA, 1996. Faithful but fearful: reducing HIV transmission in stable relationships. *AIDS.* 10(Suppl A):S197-S203.
10. McIntyre J, 1999. *HIV in Pregnancy: A Review.* WHO/UNAIDS, Geneva.
11. Hocke C, Morlat P, Chene G et al, 1995. Prospective cohort study of the effect of pregnancy in the progression of HIV infection. *Obstetrics & Gynecology.* 86(6):886-91.
12. French R, Brocklehurst P, 1998. The effect of pregnancy on survival in women infected with HIV: a systematic review of the literature and meta-analysis. *British Journal of Obstetrics & Gynaecology.* 105(8):827-35.
13. AbouZahr C, 1998. Maternal mortality overview. In: *Health Dimensions of Sex and Reproduction.* Murray CJL et al (eds). Global Burden of Disease and Injury Volume 3. World Health Organization, Geneva.
14. National Committee on Confidential Enquiries into Maternal Deaths, 1998. *First Interim Report on Confidential Enquiries into Maternal Deaths in South Africa 1997.* Department of Health, South Africa, April.
15. Iloki LH, G'Bala Sapoulou MV, Kpekpede F et al, 1997. Maternal mortality in Brazzaville (1993-1994). *J Gynecol Obstet Biol Reprod.* (Paris). 26(2):163-68.
16. MacLeod J, Rhode R, 1998. Retrospective follow-up of maternal deaths and their associated risk factors in a rural district of Tanzania. *Tropical Medicine & International Health.* 3(2):130-37.
17. Verkuyl DAA, 1995. Practising obstetrics and gynaecology in areas with a high prevalence of HIV infection. *Lancet.* 346(29 July):293-95.
18. Luo NP, Sikazwe C, 1993. Unpublished data, personal communication.
19. Zaba B, 1998. Evidence of impact of HIV on fertility in Africa. 12th World AIDS Conference. Geneva, July. Abstract No. 24196.
   – See also: Gray RH, Wawer MJ, Serwadda D et al, 1998. Population-based study of fertility in women with HIV-1 infection in Uganda. *Lancet.* 351 (10 Jan):98-103.
   – Lee LM, Wortley PM, Gray RH, Fleming PL. Reduced fertility and duration of HIV-1 infection in American women. 12th World AIDS Conference. Geneva, July 1998. Abstract No. 24198.
   – Nicoll A, Stephenson J, Griffoen A et al, 1998. A method of adjusting HIV prevalences derived from pregnant women to allow for the effect of fertility. 12th World AIDS Conference. Geneva, July 1998. Abstract 23459.
20. Leroy V, Ladner J, Nyiraziraje M et al, 1998. Effect of HIV-1 infection on pregnancy outcome

in women in Kigali, Rwanda, 1992-1994. Pregnancy and HIV Study Group. *AIDS*. 12(6):643-50.

21. Semprini AE, Castagna C, Ravizza M et al, 1995. The incidence of complications after caesarean section in 156 HIV-positive women. *AIDS*. 9(8):913-17.
22. Bulterys M et al, 1996. Fatal complications after cesarian section in HIV-infected women. [Letter]. *AIDS*. 10(8):923-24.
23. Kigongo WS, Tamale JAK, Mmiro FA et al, 1998. Maternal morbidity following emergency lower segment caesarean section in asymptomatic HIV-1 infection in Mulago Hospital. 12th World AIDS Conference. Geneva, July. Abstract 32229.
24. In this retrospective study, 141 HIV positive women who underwent 191 obstetric and gynaecological surgical procedures between 1984 and 1997 were compared to matched HIV negative women with the same operations. Dathe O, Lutz-Friedrich R, Grubert T et al, 1998. Post-operative complications following 191 gynecological and obstetrical surgical interventions in HIV-infected women. 12th World Conference on AIDS. Geneva, July. Abstract No 13391.
25. Zurrer M, Biedermann K, Rudin C et al, 1995. [Premature labor in HIV infected women. Swiss HIV and Pregnancy Study Group - article in German]. Z Geburtshilfe Neonatol . 199(2):58-64.
26. Pollack RN, Sklarin NT, Rao S et al, 1993. Metastatic placental lymphoma associated with maternal human immunodeficiency virus infection. *Obstetrics & Gynecology*. 81(5-Pt 2):856-57.
27. Kumar RM, Khuranna A, 1998. Pregnancy outcome in women with beta-thalassaemia major and HIV infection. *European Journal of Obstetrics, Gynecology and Reproductive Biology*. 77(2):163-69.
28. van den Broek NR, White SA, Neilson JP, 1998. The relationship between asymptomatic human immunodeficiency virus infection and the prevalence and severity of anaemia in pregnant Malawian women. *American Journal of Tropical Medicine & Hygiene*. 59(6):1004-07.
29. Granja AC, Machungo F, Gomes A et al, 1998. Malaria-related maternal mortality in urban Mozambique. *Annals of Tropical Medicine and Parasitology*. 92(3):257-63.
30. Verhoeff FH, Brabin BJ, Hart CA et al, 1999. Increased prevalence of malaria in HIV-infected pregnant women and its implications for malaria control. *Tropical Medicine and International Health*. 4(1):5-12.
31. Steketee R, Nahlen B, Ayisi J et al, 1998. Association between placental malaria infection and increased risk of mother-to-infant transmission of HIV-1 in western Kenya. 12th World AIDS Conference. Geneva, July. Abstract No. 13298.
32. Diwan VK, Thorson A, 1999. Sex, gender and tuberculosis. *Lancet*. 353:1000-01.
33. World Health Organization 1995. *Tuberculosis and HIV: Towards Solutions: Results of a WHO Workshop on the Formulation of a New Research Strategy*. WHO Geneva. Referenced in: MacNeil JM, Anderson S, 1998. Beyond the dichotomy: linking HIV prevention with care. *AIDS*. 12(Suppl 2):S19-S26.
34. Gilks CF, Brindle RJ, Otieno LS et al, 1990. Extrapulmonary and disseminated tuberculosis in HIV-1-seropositive patients presenting to the acute medical services in Nairobi. *AIDS*. 4(10):981-85.
35. Espinal MA, Reingold AL, Lavandera M, 1996. Effect of pregnancy on the risk of developing active tuberculosis. *Journal of Infectious Disease*. 173(2): 488-91. See also *Journal of Infectious Disease* 1997; 175(4):1025 for comment.
36. McDermott JM, Slutsker L, Steketee RW et al, 1996. Prospective assessment of mortality among a cohort of pregnant women in rural Malawi. *American Journal of Tropical Medicine & Hygiene*. 55(1-Suppl):66-70.
37. Mmiro FA, 1998. Controlling the spread of HIV. Presentation to Women's Health in Developing Countries, organised by the Royal College of Obstetricians and Gynaecologists, London, 29 June.
38. Ryder RW, Nsuami M, Nsa W et al, 1994. Mortality in HIV-1-seropositive women, their spouses and their newly born children during 36 months of follow-up in Kinshasa, Zaire. *AIDS*. 8(5):667-72.
39. Aka-Dago-Akribi H, Desgrées du Loû A, Msellati P et al, 1999. Issues surrounding reproductive choice for women living with HIV in Abidjan, Côte d'Ivoire. *Reproductive Health Matters* 7(13):20-29.
40. Brocklehurst P, French R, 1998. The association between maternal HIV infection and perinatal outcome: a systematic review of the literature and meta-analysis. *British Journal of Obstetrics & Gynaecology*. 105(Aug):8836-48.
41. Langston C, Lewis DE, Hammill HA et al, 1995. Excess intrauterine fetal demise associated with maternal human immunodeficiency virus infection. *Journal of Infectious Diseases*. 172(6):1451-60.
42. Desgrées du Loû A, Msellati P, Ramon R et al, 1998. HIV-1 infection and reproductive history: a retrospective study among pregnant women, Abidjan, Côte d'Ivoire, 1995-1996. Ditrame Project.

International Journal of STD & AIDS. 9(8):452-56.
43. – Ladner J, Castetbon K, Leroy V et al, 1998. Pregnancy, body weight and human immunodeficiency virus infection in African women: a prospective cohort study in Kigali (Rwanda), 1992-94. *International Journal of Epidemiology.* 27:1072-77.
– Duarte G, Quintana SM, Cavalli RC et al, 1998. Influence of maternal weight gain on vertical transmission and pregnancy outcome among HIV+ women. 12th World AIDS Conference. Geneva, July. Abstract No. 32232.
44. Ndyomugyenyi R, Neema S, Magnussen P, 1998. The use of formal and informal services for antenatal care and malaria treatment in rural Uganda. *Health Policy and Planning.* 13(1):94-102.
45. Brabin L, Verhoeff FH, Kazembe P et al, 1998. Improving antenatal care for pregnant adolescents in southern Malawi. *Acta Obstet Gynecol Scand.* 77(4):402-09.
46. See Berer M. Reducing perinatal HIV transmission in developing countries in the context of antenatal and delivery care, and breastfeeding: supporting infant survival by supporting women's survival. *Bulletin of the WHO.* (Accepted for publication 1999).
47. Graham WJ, Newell M-L, 1999. Seizing the opportunity: collaborative initiatives to reduce HIV and maternal mortality. *Lancet.* 353(6 March):836-39.
48. UNAIDS/UNICEF/WHO, 1998. *HIV and Infant Feeding: Guidelines for Decision-Makers; A Guide for Health Care Managers and Supervisors; A Review of HIV Transmission through Breastfeeding.* UNAIDS/UNICEF/WHO.
49. – World Health Organization, Global Programme on AIDS,1995. *Preventing HIV Transmission in Health Facilities.* Geneva, WHO/GPA/TCO/HCS/ 95.16.
– See also: Dick S, 1993. A London midwife's experience and recommendations for infection control policy for all pregnant women delivering in hospital. *Women and HIV/AIDS: An International Resource Book.* Berer M with Ray S (eds). Pandora Press, London.
50. Berer M, 1993. Safe motherhood and HIV/AIDS: the issues for women. *Women and HIV/AIDS: An International Resource Book.* Berer M with Ray S (eds). Pandora Press, London.
51. Anecdotal information from various sources in Africa via personal communication. For evidence of the marginalisation of young, single women and their lack of access to safe, hospital-based abortion services in a context of continuing illegality of abortion, see: Hardy E, Faúndes A, Bugalho A et al, 1997. Comparisons of women having clandestine and hospital abortions: Maputo, Mozambique. *Reproductive Health Matters.* 5(9):108-15.
52. World Health Organization, 1998. *Post-Partum Care of the Mother and Newborn: A Practical Guide. Report of a Technical Working Group.* WHO/RHT/MSM/98.3.
53. International Perinatal HIV Group, 1999. The mode of delivery and the risk of vertical transmission of HIV-1. A meta-analysis of 15 prospective cohort studies. *New England Journal of Medicine.* 340:977-87.
– See also cautions expressed in the editorial in this same journal issue by Riley LE, Greene MF. Elective cesarean delivery to reduce the transmission of HIV.
– See also: Kind C, Rudin C, Siegrist CA et al, 1998. Prevention of vertical HIV transmission: additive protective effect of elective cesarean section and zidovudine prophylaxis. Swiss Neonatal HIV Study Group. *AIDS.* 12(2):205-10.
54. European Mode of Delivery Collaboration, 1999. Elective caesarean section vs vaginal delivery in prevention of vertical HIV-1 transmission: a randomised clinical trial. *Lancet.* 353:1035-39.

Managing Obstructed Labour: Four Phases of Maternity Care Development

Vivian Taam Wong and Jerker Liljestrand

In cases of advanced obstructed labour, caesarean section is associated with high morbidity and mortality, and also with increased risk of uterine rupture in ensuing pregnancies. In rural areas with poor facilities and transport, certain types of vaginal extraction have proven to be safer than caesarean section, with fewer maternal deaths and less serious complications. Four phases of development in maternity care can be observed. The transition from 'high mortality, high obstruction rate and poor maternity care' to 'low mortality, low obstruction rate and improved maternity care' is associated with a change from the use of vaginal extraction to the use of caesarean section for the management of obstructed labour. Programmes for safe motherhood should be adjusted to correspond to the stage of development in maternity care in order to produce the safest outcome.

OBSTRUCTED labour is one of the main causes of maternal death in developing countries. It has been defined as '... failure of descent of the fetus in the birth canal for mechanical reasons in spite of good uterine contractions'.[1] Its causes are either too narrow a pelvis, often a result of childhood malnutrition, or malpresentation of the fetus. It may also be caused by fetal malformations or soft tissue tumours in the mother. The incidence varies between 1 and 3 per cent.[2] If left untreated, obstructed labour will eventually lead to fetal death. In the mother, it may cause death from uterine rupture, sepsis or haemorrhage. If the mother survives, she is often left with debilitating fistulae, causing lifelong leakage of urine or faeces.[1] In developed societies, such deaths can easily be averted through adequate monitoring of labour and timely use of caesarean section. In developing countries, women with obstructed labour die from lack of access to adequate and timely obstetric care. They may also die from a caesarean section carried out too late, however, in situations where a vaginal procedure would have been more appropriate. This article briefly reviews the use of such alternatives to caesarean section, and the transition in obstetric management which developing countries go through when improving access to obstetric care.

Risks associated with caesarean section

Casarean section is standard procedure when moderate-to-severe obstructed labour is diagnosed in a timely way. However, when a birthing woman reaches a health facility after several days in active labour, she usually has severe dehydration and is very weak or even semiconscious. The fetus is seriously compromised from asphyxia, or is already dead. The membranes have usually been ruptured for several days, and there is commonly a severe intrauterine infection. An abdominal operation implies further risks of spreading the infection. Pre-existing anaemia, malnutrition, malaria, tuberculosis or HIV may have contributed to making the situation worse. The conditions at the receiving district hospital are also often suboptimal. Shortage or lack of essential equipment and drugs are common. If the staff are not fully trained and experienced to deal with such advanced complications, the prognosis will be further aggravated. Evidently, performing a caesarean section under such circumstances involves a considerable operative risk for the woman.[1]

It is thus not surprising that deaths associated with caesarean section under difficult circumstances may occur more frequently than those after vaginal delivery. A study conducted on 7,885 births in five centres in two less developed countries, chosen from an international maternity monitoring network, showed that the maternal mortality ratio from vaginal delivery was 510 and from caesarean section was 3,620 per 100,000, with 1,280 per 100,000 estimated as attributable to the caesarean section operations themselves.[3] The main cause of death among the vaginal births was eclampsia, while sepsis was the reason in caesarean section deaths. Haemorrhage was the second most common cause in both groups. The authors concluded that caesarean section had a markedly higher mortality than vaginal births, that a considerable proportion of the caesarean section deaths were probably attributable to the caesarean section procedure *per se*, and that a large number of caesarean section deaths would have been avoided had the hospitals been better equipped and staffed.

Another risk is that of uterine rupture, via the uterine scar, in ensuing pregnancies. This is particularly true in settings where facilities for monitoring labour and emergency caesarean section are lacking, or where ensuing births may take place at home without skilled attendance. Consequently, caesarean section rates climb steeply after the first one practised, due to the custom of carrying out the same procedure for subsequent pregnancies to avoid the risk of scar rupture. A study from rural Zaire showed that from 1971 to 1992 the incidence of caesarean section rose from 6.2 per cent to 12 per cent, and the fraction of repeat section rose from 17 per cent to 49 per cent.[4] Although the deaths connected to caesarean section decreased from 3.2 per cent to 0.7 per cent, rupture of previous caesarean section scars occurred in 3.5 per cent of the 760 caesarean sections performed. There was no change in perinatal mortality, which was maintained at 20 per 1000. The authors consider that in areas with a poorly supported health system, a high rate of caesarean section is a hazard to maternal health and that there is a need for knowledge about alternative methods of vaginal delivery.

Thus, the total package of maternity care should be considered in the context of available local resources. If many women arrive with neglected obstructed labour, and facilities for the proper management of women with prior caesarean section are not available, service providers have to be cautious in performing a first caesarean section. Previous caesarean section warrants careful and close monitoring of labour and birth by skilled staff. Alternative methods of vaginal delivery cover a range of obstetric interventions such as vacuum extraction, symphysiotomy, podalic version, breech extraction, and (high) forceps delivery when the fetus is alive, and in cases of fetal death, craniotomy and decapitation.[5]

Alternatives when the fetus is alive

Vacuum extraction implies the application with vacuum of a suction cup to the head of the baby, and traction in the cup in synchronisation with the mother's own contractions. It is a safe procedure, easy to learn by staff with midwifery skills. It is very useful in cases of slight disproportion, where the fetus with such traction can still pass through the birth canal.

Forceps delivery is potentially more dangerous, and therefore demands greater skill and experience. In many countries this instrument is reserved for doctors specialised in obstetrics. Applying the obstetric forceps while the baby is still high in the birth canal is particularly exacting, but may be considered by skilled staff where caesarean section is extra risky or has limited immediate availability.

Symphysiotomy implies division of the pubic cartilage under local anaesthesia, and thereafter usually extraction with vacuum extractor. This procedure temporarily widens the birth canal by up to 25 per cent. After birth, the mother rests in bed for up to a week while the pelvis stabilises. It has been reported that subsequent births may also lead to a slight temporary widening of the symphysis, facilitating birth. Permanent pelvic instability is a rare complication. Thirty-one cases of symphysiotomy performed in Mozambique and Botswana, followed up for seven days to six months, showed few complications, and none of them permanent.[6] In rural areas, where caesarean section is not available within a few hours, it is a life-saving operation in cases of moderate disproportion.

Internal podalic version means the turning of the malpositioned fetus via pulling by its foot, with the hand of the birth assistant inserted into the uterus. This is only possible in early stages, before the labour has become impacted. The procedure can be useful, e.g. in cases of twin births where the second fetus after the birth of the first one suddenly positions in a transverse lie. A vigilant attendant can immediately correct the position of the second fetus with this procedure, thus avoiding caesarean section.

Alternatives when the fetus is dead

Destructive operations should be considered where the fetus is dead when the mother arrives in advanced obstructed labour. As indicated above, a caesarean section scar in the uterus increases the maternal risk in subsequent pregnancies, and this, even apart from the mother's condition, should lead to consideration of vaginal extraction when the fetus is dead.

Craniotomy implies perforating the fetal skull with a sharp instrument, emptying it, and thereafter applying forceps to extract the fetus. Once the head has collapsed, the fetus is usually extracted without a great deal of force, and this procedure is thus technically relatively safe. The operation can be performed under mild sedation, is carried out in a matter of minutes, and does not require an operating room. It is particularly essential to inform the woman and her family in advance of such an operation. They should be told that the baby is dead, that the mother is in a life-threatening state, and that this operation will contribute to saving her life. The woman usually recuperates rapidly post partum. The risk of spreading an intra-uterine infection throughout the abdomen, creating peritonitis, and risking scar complications via postoperative infection is thus avoided by preferring craniotomy to caesarean section. While any pelvic constriction will remain, the woman will have no scar in her womb that will make subsequent births extra risky. A special case for using craniotomy is hydrocephalus. Here, the malformed baby is often in the breech presentation, eventually leading to the situation of a dead baby with the body already born, but with the enlarged, liquid-filled head still trapped in the pelvis. A puncture at the base of the neck followed by skillful decompression of the head easily resolves this situation.

The unpleasantness of these and other destructive operations to the staff, including the operator, is appeased by seeing the rapid and uncomplicated recoveries of very ill women. Again, good contact with the woman and her family is both necessary and rewarding.

Decapitation is a more difficult operation, requiring a trained operator, and is best performed in an operating theatre. This implies separation of the head from the body, using a steel wire and delivering the two parts separately. While the interventions mentioned previously are usually carried out in cephalic presentations, decapitation is carried out in cases of neglected transverse lie. Typically, the dead baby is impacted in the pelvis, an arm hanging out of the vagina. Traditional attendants may have pulled on the arm in order to extract the baby, and this may have worsened the situation, as it is not possible for a normal-sized baby to pass through a normal pelvis in the transverse position, shoulder first. The danger comes from the risk of uterine rupture. The womb is contracted around the baby, and any manipulation may cause the uterus to rupture. After having performed the operation, the operator therefore manually checks, via the vagina, that the uterus is intact. If it is not, immediate opening of the abdomen and repairing the uterus is necessary.

Here again, it is essential to give very good information to the woman and family before the operation. On arrival, the family often realise that the baby is dead and therefore cannot be delivered. Avoiding a caesarean section is often also important for cultural beliefs/reasons in many areas.[7] After the operation/birth, the head is sutured back in place, and the baby is draped before the funeral arrangements.

Use of vaginal procedures and destructive operations

A review of the years 1981-91 at a centre in Pondicherry, South India in 1993, showed 6,558 operative vaginal deliveries out of a total of 35,018 deliveries. There were 33 destructive operations (0.094 per cent). Craniotomy was the most common (n=27), the main indications being hydrocephalus, obstructed labour and arrest of the after-coming head. The authors were of the opinion that until socio-economic status, literacy, transport and communication facilities are improved in developing countries, obstetricians and primary health care doctors should be trained to handle any obstetric emergency in rural areas so that a mother's life can be saved by confidently-performed destructive operations, rather than transferring her to a referral institution with the possibility that she might die in transit from a ruptured uterus.[8]

Another study from an Indian hospital compared the use of destructive operations in 56 patients against the use of caesarean section for 27 patients arriving late in labour with a dead fetus and advanced infection. The operations were done for similar indications.[9] There were no maternal deaths and very few complications in those after destructive operations, but in those who had had a caesarean section, one mother died and others had serious complications such as post-partum haemorrhage, post-operative shock and pyrexia. It was felt that in badly infected cases of neglected obstructed labour, with fetal death, destructive operations are safer and thus still have a limited role in developing countries. In Karachi, an evaluation of 32 cases of craniotomy done for hydrocephalus, dead fetus associated with obstructed labour, after-coming head of breech, and failure to progress to the second stage of labour showed maternal morbidity of 12.5 per cent and no maternal deaths.[10] The authors conclude that craniotomy is safe and quicker than caesarean section in selected cases.

Destructive operations, in obstructed labour with dead fetuses, have been found superior to caesarean section in many instances. However, it requires a considerable amount of experience, judgement, skill and competency. Rupture of uterus must be excluded beforehand.

Other reasons for caesarean sections

Caesarean section is used for a variety of maternal and fetal indications, apart from obstructed labour. Prolonged labour can be diagnosed in time using the partograph,[11] and trained staff will resolve the situation with use of, for example, oxytocin or caesarean section. One important indication for performing caesarean section in many situations is fetal distress. A study in two public maternity units in Benin with an overall primary caesarean section rate of 7.5 per cent, showed that fetal distress was the indication for caesarean section in 65.9 per cent.[12] Practitioner experience and fetal distress were the most important factors influencing the decision to perform caesarean section and they differed between the two maternity units. In developed countries, judicious use of electronic fetal monitoring coupled with fetal blood sampling is used to improve the outcome of the babies. Such facilities are beyond the reach of rural centres in most developing countries. A fine balance should be achieved by better training of physicians in anticipating, diagnosing and managing fetal distress to prevent overuse of caesarean section.[13,14]

Four phases of development

Studying the changes in the evolution of maternity care over the decades, one can observe four phases of development, reflected, for example, in the management of obstructed labour. Normally, improvement in maternity care moves in parallel with socio-economic changes that influence improvements in education and family planning, and consequently, in parallel with the transition to lower fertility and mortality. However, there are countries, or parts of countries, where improvement in maternity care has been neglected despite improvements in socio-economic development, with little change in maternal mortality ratios – a policy and operational stagnation that is out of phase with the overall transition.

In Phase I, both maternal and perinatal mortality rates are very high. The standard of maternity care is poor. Many women have no access at all to essential obstetric care, even in cases of severe emergency, and maternal deaths to a large extent occur outside the health care system. The incidence of obstructed labour is high, but most of it is not recorded, because moribund women only rarely reach hospitals. Rates of caesarean section are generally low.

Transition from Phase I to Phase II: the case of North Bengal

Two studies carried out in North Bengal Medical College Hospital between 1965 and 1971, and 1981 to 1987, reported a marginal increase in the obstructed labour rate, from 2.3 per cent to 3 per cent respectively.[15] Over the interval of 15 years, however, destructive operations had begun to be replaced increasingly by caesarean section. The destructive operation rate for obstructed labour fell from 52 per cent to 24 per cent, while the caesarean section rate increased threefold, from 19 per cent to 55 per cent. The maternal mortality rate following obstructed labour rose from 11 per cent to 17 per cent. Although this difference is not statistically significant, it implies that there was no improvement. Among patients with obstructed labour in the 1981-87 series, 12.4 per cent suffered ruptured uterus and 56 per cent had intra-uterine fetal death. The perinatal death rate for patients admitted due to obstructed labour rose from 70 per cent in 1965-71 to 82 per cent in 1981-87. This reflects the poor condition of the patients on arrival at the hospital, after a long period of obstruction.

The above example illustrates the importance of improvement in the standard of maternity care as a package in rural areas. This package must include upgrading the knowledge and experience of the birth attendant as well as the doctor at the first level of referral. It must be supported by improvement in facilities, equipment, supplies, drugs, blood transfusion and referral logistics, including communication and transport. The transition from the use of destructive operations to caesarean section to manage obstructed labour should normally be accompanied by such improvement.

In Phase II, the maternal and perinatal mortality rates are still very high. There is uneven distribution of maternity care with gross inadequacy in rural areas. As the health care system begins to address the issue of maternity care, more mothers shift from traditional to modern methods of care. More mothers are referred to health centres, and often arrive late in a poor general condition. There is an apparent increase of maternal deaths, as deaths hitherto happening at home are now being recorded.

In referral centres, there will be high complication rates and a high risk of perinatal and maternal deaths because of the mother's late arrival at the referral centre in poor condition. In this phase, procedures outlined in this article will often be good options to caesarean section in cases of obstructed labour.

Transition from Phase II to Phase III: the case of rural Zaire

As described earlier, a study in rural Zaire experienced an increase in caesarean section rate with a drop in the overall maternal mortality ratio. All the same, death from caesarean section was still high at 0.7 per cent in 1991-92.[4] It was observed that 93 per cent were emergency caesarean sections, 97 per cent were given spinal anaesthesia and 259 out of the 760 caesarean sections were performed by a nurse or a dentist. This is a unique example of a jump from Phase II to Phase III, using the short-cut of employing non-doctors to perform caesarean sections, and by the provision of skilled attendants at birthing centres.

In Phase III, the transition to lower mortality rates is the result of overall improvement of the maternity care package. In this phase, the number of women with obstructed labour will plateau and eventually go down if birth attendants are taught to detect cephalopelvic disproportion and malpresentation in early labour for urgent referral. The overall caesarean section rate will increase dramatically because of a general reliance on caesarean section to manage most patients with suspected disproportion or prolonged labour. Furthermore, there will be more caesarean sections done for patients with previous caesarean section. The lowering of maternal and perinatal mortality is the result of overall improvement in maternity care, and not the result of caesarean section alone.

Transition from Phase III to Phase IV

In a primary referral hospital in north Jordan, receiving high risk patients from low socio-economic classes, the caesarean section rate was lowered from 15.5 per cent in 1987 to 6.5 per cent in 1990 and 8.7 per cent in 1993 with a persistent fall in perinatal mortality from 52 through 30 to 21 per 1,000 respectively.[16] This success was attributed to active management of labour, trial of labour for previous caesarean section, and vaginal breech delivery in selected women. Another example came from a provincial hospital in Zimbabwe where the introduction of strict guidelines for the management of dystocia, previous caesarean section, fetal distress and breech presentation brought about a drop in the caesarean section rate from 16.8 per cent to 8 per cent over two years.[17] Use of oxytocin increased from 3.4 to 17.4 per cent. The maternal mortality ratio fell from 202 to 57 per 100,000 and the perinatal mortality rate from 71.9 to 56.2 per 1000.

The challenge is in maintaining a low caesarean section rate without compromising the maternal and perinatal outcome. Although there is still room for improvement in the maternal and perinatal mortality in the above examples, the initial formula for success is apparent. Active management of labour with clinical guidelines and proper supervision is essential.

In Phase IV, the low mortality rates would be followed by lower morbidity rates. This phase is reached if and when proper management of labour alleviates uterine dysfunction and those with previous caesarean sections and breech presentations are allowed to try vaginal delivery. Caesarean section rates would fall. The main indications for caesarean section would change from obstructed labour and previous caesarean section to fetal distress and placenta praevia.

Realistic planning

From a review of the literature on the management of obstructed labour in different parts of the world, four phases of development in maternity care are identified. These phases are primarily related to the standard of health care delivery facilities in the district. In planning improvement measures, especially in the training of health care personnel, and provision of equipment and development of guidelines, proper assessment is essential to put together a package that is applicable to the stage of health care development in that locality.

For those who are still at Phase I with a high incidence of obstruction and high mortality rates, it would be sensible to continue training doctors and midwives in the rural areas to perform procedures such as vacuum extraction, craniotomy and symphysiotomy in order to save the lives of mothers. However, it would be essential to seek the funding necessary to upgrade a referral centre to provide essential obstetric care, including capacity for blood transfusion, general anaesthesia, caesarean section and resuscitation of the new-born. This will pave the way to the next phase.

In Phase II, when caesarean section is available, the priority is to train birth attendants or community health care workers in early referral when suspected complications arise. Logistics for referral and transport must be strengthened. The doctors need to acquire the skills in performing both caesarean section and the alternatives to the operation. Furthermore, experience in judging and deciding which is the better alternative is the cornerstone for success.

Once in Phase III, when caesarean section is used to replace many of the vaginal operations, and mortality rates are falling, training and guidelines in the active management of labour, vaginal delivery for previous caesarean section and breech presentation become the priority at the referral centre.

In Phase IV, with improved caesarean section rates, and relatively low perinatal and maternal mortality rates, further improvements in outcome will require continuous developments using a series of interventions for modern perinatal care.

Conclusion

Providing the necessary training in the appropriate management of obstructed labour to maternal health care staff is a considerable challenge. Many urban centres, where training takes place, are in Phase III or IV, while many midwives and doctors will eventually work in rural areas with Phase II-type scenarios. Intermittent training/attachment in peripheral district hospitals, and competent supervision by colleagues with experience in the wider range of management alternatives can remedy this situation. An understanding of the very different situations and needs in under-served areas on the part of the planners is therefore a key requisite. A phased approach, tailor-made for individual areas, could achieve realistic improvement in maternal deaths by addressing immediate deficiencies.

Note

The opinions expressed in this article are those of the authors and do not necessarily reflect the views of the World Health Organization.

Correspondence

Vivian Taam Wong, 401, Administration Block, Queen Mary Hospital, 102, Pokfulam Road, Hong Kong, China. Fax: 852-28185170. E-mail: vcwwong@ha.org.hk

References

1. Philpott RH, 1982, Obstructed labour. *Clinics in Obstetrics and Gynaecology*. 9(3). Dec.
2. World Health Organization/ Harvard School of Public Health/World Bank,1998. *Health Dimensions of Sex and Reproduction. Volume III of the Global Burden of Disease and Injury Series.* Murray CJL, Lopez AD (eds). ISBN 0-674 -38335-4.
3. Chi I-Cheng, Whatley A, Wilkens L et al, 1986. In-hospital maternal mortality risk by caesarean and vaginal deliveries in two less developed countries - a descriptive study. *International Journal of Gynecology and Obstetrics*. Apr; 24(2):121-31.
4. Onsrud L, Onsrud M, 1996. Increasing use of caesarean section, even in developing countries. *Tidsskrift for Norsk for Laegeforen*. Jan 10; 116(1):67-71.
5. Cook J, Sankaran B, Wasunna AEO, 1991. *Surgery at the District Hospital: Obstetrics Section, Gynaecology, Orthopedics Section and Traumatology*. World Health Organization, Geneva.
6. Bergström S, Lublin H, Molin A, 1994. Value of symphyseotomy in obstructed labour management and follow-up of 31 cases. *Gynecologic and Obstetric Investigation*. 38:31-35.
7. Engelkes E, Van Roosmalen J, 1992. The value of symphyseotomy compared with Caesarean section in cases of obstructed labour. Medical and anthropological considerations. *Social Science and Medicine*. 35(6):789-93.
8. Raksha A, Rajaram P, Oumachigui A et al, 1993. Destructive operations in modern obstetrics in a developing country at tertiary level. *British Journal of Obstetrics and Gynaecology*. Oct; 100:967-68.
9. Gupta U, Chitra R, 1994. Destructive operations still have a place in developing countries. *International Journal of Gynecology and Obstetrics*. 44(1):15-19.
10. Tariq TA, Korejo R, 1993. Evaluation of the role of craniotomy in developing countries. *Journal of Pakistani Medical Association*. 43(2):30-32.
11. *Preventing Prolonged Labour: A Practical Guide*, I-IV. World Health Organization, Geneva, 1993.
12. Fourn L, Alihonou E, Seguin L et al, 1994. Incidence and primary caesarean risk factors in Benin (Africa). *Revue d'epidémiologie et de santé publique*. 42(1):5-12.
13. Granja A, Gomes E, Bugalho A et al, 1991 Management of labour following caesarean section in a developing country. *Clinical and Experimental Obstetrics and Gynecology*. 18(1):47-50.
14. De Muylder X, 1998. Vaginal delivery after caesarean section: is it safe in a developing country? *Australia-NewZealand Journal of Obstetrics & Gynaecology*. 28(2):99-102.
15. Konar H, Adhya SA , Chakraborty AB, 1992. Obstetrics - past and present (A comparative review of 210 cases of obstructed labour). *Journal of Indian Medical Association*. 90(1):18-19.
16. Ziadeh SM, Sunna EI, 1995. Decreased caesarean birth rates and improved perinatal outcome: a seven-year study. *Birth*. 22(3):144-47.
17. De Muylder X, Thiery M, 1990. The caesarean delivery rate can be safely reduced in a developing country. *Obstetrics and Gynaecology*. 75(3 Pt I):360-04.

Community Participation and Mobilisation in the Prevention of Maternal Mortality in Kebbi, Northwestern Nigeria

Dora J Shehu

In Maiyama, Kebbi state, in northwestern Nigeria, factors which contributed to maternal deaths included: medical care not promptly sought for any condition; almost all women delivering at home and rarely in a clinic or hospital; delays in seeking and reaching emergency obstetric care due mainly to lack of finance, transport difficulties, absent or unwilling husbands whose permission was required, the cost of hospital deliveries, the unfavourable attitudes of hospital staff and frequent drug shortages. This paper describes a project by the Nigerian team of the Prevention of Maternal Mortality (PMM) Network on mobilising the community to improve maternal outcomes and prevent maternal deaths, using participatory methods. Between 1990 and 1995, following traditional channels, a range of activities was carried out in a collaborative effort between community leaders, local government, community members, and the PMM team. These included a baseline study as a form of social enquiry, analysis of the results, community awareness raising, collaborative design of interventions and their implementation. After five years, local maternity care facilities had been upgraded and expanded, transport for emergency cases had improved thanks to the support of a transport union and subsidised fuel, two income-generating projects were begun, some delays in getting women to hospital for care were reduced and community involvement in preventing women's deaths was greatly increased. The study area presented conditions which were amenable to social change but this required time, patience and persistence. A much longer period of sustained work is needed to ensure permanence in the gains made.

THE Prevention of Maternal Mortality Network (PMM) is an international effort involving multi-disciplinary research teams, comprised of obstetricians, nurses, midwives, community physicians and social scientists, based in universities with teaching hospitals, where women with obstetric complications can be referred which began in 1988. Under the aegis of the Network, these teams have designed specific interventions that could lead to the reduction of maternal deaths in the research locations.

This paper describes a PMM project in Nigeria concerned with community participation and mobilisation to improve maternal health care and prevent maternal deaths, using participatory methods. It was carried out from 1990 to 1995 in the local government area (LGA) of Maiyama, Kebbi State, in northwestern Nigeria, by an operations research team based in Sokoto state, of which I was a member.

The study area

The northwestern Nigerian project was initially located in Sokoto state, in a local government area (LGA) with a fairly rural outlook. In 1991, when a new state was carved out of Sokoto state, the project area was changed to Maiyama in the new state of Kebbi. There are 22 districts in this LGA. The population is about 108,000, living in some 70 villages (1991 census). The ethnic groups are the Hausa and Fulani, many of whom have intermixed.

Infrastructural facilities were few. There was no electricity, though more recently, a few towns have been connected to the national electricity grid. The water supply was through bore holes.

The roads were inadequate; in some communities difficult terrain such as rock outcrops or surface water presented problems in road construction. Communication between the local government offices and the state was limited to a two-way radio link.

Agriculture was the main economic activity of men in the area, with non-farming activities during the dry season. Women processed the harvested products, e.g. grains, groundnut oil and leather ware, and prepared cooked food for sale. The marketing of these products was carried out either by their children or hired help.

Household income varied from about N12,000 to N36,000 (U$180-$400) per annum and fluctuated with the seasons. Socially and politically men took all the decisions affecting the community, within a system of hierarchical authority based on male lineage. Men also decided how household income would be used. The practice of *purdah* or *kulle* (seclusion) was conventional; women, especially those of childbearing age, were required to stay at home. Levels of educational attainment were low. Some 11 per cent of men had completed primary school and 7 per cent of women. School enrolment rates averaged about two girls to every ten boys. Religious instruction and the study of the Koran were a high priority for the people, and participation was nearly 100 per cent.

The project

The importance of involving the community in health care delivery has been widely recognised,[1-3] and participatory research involving the community was relevant for this area, but to do this we had to give consideration to the issue of gender. What strategies could we adopt that would allow the unrestricted involvement of both men and women in the communities, given the nature of the society in the project area? Women could show their power by displaying fortitude during childbirth. In matters of reproduction, especially childbirth, men were firmly excluded. Men were in charge at social, political and household levels. Any strategy for participation had to take cognisance of these nuances of power. To ensure that each group got a fair chance to participate, we decided to follow the traditional hierarchy. The elders were to be mobilised first and, in the role of trainers, would pass information on to the men. The men, as heads of households, would broach these matters with the women in their households. This approach had the appeal of using traditional channels and, we hoped, would make our work easier.[4]

The LGA was divided into four areas, each containing five or six communities. Our activities centred on the largest village, Maiyama, and was then taken to the smaller ones. In order to create a cordial and trusting environment, the mobilisation effort was divided into three phases. The traditional hierarchy recognises distinctions between the *Masu sarauta* (ruling class) and the *tallaka* (the masses) who comprise men, women, and children or youth. Phasing helped to reach all these groups without flouting cultural sensibilities. Each group would have adequate time to interact with the project and reflect on the problem of maternal deaths.

Phase I, the rapport-building phase, was estimated to last about three months – in the event, it took almost a year. Phase II, the collaborative/participatory phase, was envisaged to last 12-15 months; in fact, this stretched to over two years. Phase III was for consolidation, during which we hoped some activities would be implemented and evaluated. By this last stage, some changes in maternal health outcomes should have become apparent, at least as regards increases in the use of health facilities, reduction in delays in seeking care, and an overall improved awareness of maternal health issues.

Building a rapport: Phase I

To gain access to each group in the community, the appropriate channels were used. Introductions and initial contacts were arranged through the local government Primary Health Care officer, who was officially assigned to work with us and who made all our appointments. The PMM team was scheduled to visit the communities each week on either Tuesday or Saturday, while the contact person visited on Fridays on our behalf. He was provided with a motorcycle by the team for this work and we maintained close links with him by radio. The first few months were devoted to acquainting ourselves with the community – the people, their environment and social and cultural organisation. In return, they got to know us, our mission and our aims. This period proved to be the toughest. Following local protocols, we met the elders, explained our mission and eventually asked permission to meet with others in the community, first the married men. After a number of meetings with the men, and at the suggestion of community leaders, we then sought permission to meet their wives and other women. The team learned to give out small gifts – matches, razor blades, cola nut, earrings, bangles, small containers of petroleum jelly and soap – and to accept offers of food and drink in return.

In 1990, after about two months of such visits and with the help of the contact person, we began a baseline study at the hospital, community and household levels, using focus-group discussions and in-depth interviews as a form of social enquiry. The focus-group discussions were with groups of elders (community and religious leaders), married men, married women, youth and traditional birth attendants (TBAs), and the interviews with health professionals and government officials. In each of the four areas, eight or nine group sessions were held, three sessions per group. Altogether 36 sessions were held. The aims were to determine the causes of maternal deaths locally and the underlying social and structural conditions which were contributing to those deaths. From the findings, a community-based agenda was drawn up.

Maternal health care utilisation and services

The study found that knowledge and awareness of reproductive matters and the biology of reproduction were low. It became clear that women delivered at home, rarely in a hospital, except where there was a complication. Medical care was not promptly sought, as a rule, for any condition; this included delays in seeking and reaching emergency obstetric care, due mainly to lack of finance, transport difficulties, absent or unwilling husbands whose permission was required, the cost of hospital deliveries, the unfavourable attitudes of hospital staff, and frequent drug shortages.

The married women said time and again that they were not permitted to go to a hospital to deliver, and that husbands also contributed to delays in cases of complications. The married men frequently said that they did not know when their wives were in labour and they were not informed in good time. It was only when a man realised that his wife had been in labour for a long time that he might find out there was a complication.

A Sisterhood study of maternal deaths in the LGA found that pregnant women had a 1 in 17 chance of dying from pregnancy-related causes in their lifetimes. Causes of maternal deaths were mainly retained placenta (29.4 per cent), obstructed labour (27 per cent), and eclampsia (15 per cent). Haemorrhage, anaemia, ruptured uterus, congestive cardiac failure and malaria in pregnancy added to the numbers of women dying.

There were more than 50 TBAs in the project area, who were largely untrained. Discussions with them revealed that they were not always aware of danger signs, and had their own methods of handling certain conditions.

There was one maternity clinic in Maiyama for the whole LGA, and a Comprehensive Health Centre about 25 km from Maiyama. The nearest teaching hospital offering obstetric services was 50 km from Maiyama, in Birnin Kebbi, the state capital. There was also a private clinic providing general medical care in Maiyama.

It was evident from interviews with health professionals that antenatal care, emergency obstetric care and post-natal care were all limited, and they confirmed that hospital delivery was infrequent. Clinic records for 1992, 1993 and 1994 showed that only 43, 127 and 149 women respectively had had antenatal care, while the numbers of clinic-based deliveries for the same three years were 6, 13 and 28 women.

Antenatal visits: an early intervention

The PMM team began to carry out antenatal visits to pregnant women's compounds during the course of the focus-group discussions. After each session with married men or women, we would ask if there were any pregnant women who would be willing for us to visit. We were able to see about 60 per cent of the women identified in this way. We did routine checks and gave out free drugs – haematinics, folic acid and some daraprin.

This was going well in most communities, but then we faced our first set-back. A local clinic owner who provided ANC to women on a fee-for-service basis felt threatened by the distribution of free tablets, and contrived a story that our real mission was for family planning.[5] This fabrication spread fast to other places. Consequently, our next visits were met with the perfunctory return of the drugs we had given out. To resolve the situation, the Director of Health at local government level held a meeting with the community elders and the clinic owner. However, this created a substantial delay in completing this phase of the project.

Drawing up action plans with the community: Phase II

The second phase of the project began towards the end of 1992. We aimed first to analyse the findings from the baseline study and the problems raised, and through a series of meetings, draw up a plan of activities with community members and engage them in its implementation and evaluation.

Local government officials and community leaders suggested that all district heads should be invited to participate in this phase. Venues and meeting days were agreed upon to take place during the dry season, when farming activities would be slack. The costs of the meetings were to be shared between the local government and the PMM Network. Invitations were sent to all 22 district heads, two TBA leaders and the local government women's affairs co-ordinator. Personnel from the Health Department, the Director of Health and the Co-ordinator of Primary Health Care were also invited.

A chairperson and secretary were selected (the former was a high-standing community leader and the latter the women's co-ordinator). The PMM team members who participated in this exercise were the social scientists, midwife and community physicians. The obstetrician attended twice to inform community leaders about the kinds of complications of pregnancy which they regularly dealt with at the hospital. Minutes were copied to each member. The meetings discussed specific activities which the community could undertake to improve pregnancy outcomes and prevent maternal deaths.

Deliberation on the findings of the baseline study took about three weeks, during which time it became clear that an awareness drive on reproductive health matters was needed, with separate information packets designed for the men, the women and the TBAs, with their own inputs. The PMM team and community leaders worked first on the packet for men. For the women's packet, we worked with the TBA leaders and the women's affairs co-ordinator.

The final segment of the programme, to suggest activities which focused on roles in the community, took about two weeks to design and formed the third information packet.

Information sessions for community leaders

The information to be transferred to all community groups covered: all aspects of reproduction; problems of pregnancy, labour and puerperium; the complications which women may face, including those resulting from delays in getting medical help; the major danger signs to watch out for; and a few basic ways to avert danger and death. The community leaders then turned their attention to spelling out what they thought their role ought to be and to suggest strategies for use when there were obstetric emergencies.

The methods used in meetings with community leaders to provide information included posters and charts, with explanations provided by midwives and physicians, followed by questions and answers. To explain the complications pregnant women face, we used a model pelvis and rag doll as well. Question-and-answer sessions and role-plays also brought out some of the difficulties that women and their families face in the event of an emergency. This led to the compilation of single messages on five common complications of childbirth, which were distributed to everyone with minutes of each meeting. After 16 such meetings over the period of a month, it was decided that the community leaders were ready to conduct similar meetings with the men in their communities. Attendance at these meetings had been 100 per cent, in the sense that where a member could not attend he always sent a representative.

Information sessions for men

It was suggested that Friday afternoons after prayers at the local mosques (most districts had one) be set aside for information and discussion sessions for the men in the communities. All the men attended Friday prayers and used the period afterwards for resting, so the district head literally had a captive audience. The PHC contact person rotated around to these Friday meetings and they were monitored by the Director of Health. PMM team members also carried out occasional checks.

The men were enjoined to ask questions and to inform their wives about what they were learning. Any questions which could not be handled by the contact person were brought the following Tuesday to the meeting of community leaders and officials and the PMM team, where the leaders reported on what had happened in the Friday meetings. This form of information transfer proved interesting and engaged everyone's attention in no small way.

The leaders showed exceptional interest and keenness to participate, as indicated by the high turnout rates. As time went on and they began to understand the biology of reproduction, their propensity to participate actively and ask questions during the sessions increased. They also took their roles as trainers seriously. Indeed, their new role as educators was a boost to their standing.

By the fourth month of these meetings, the PMM team and community leaders had both gained mutual respect and acceptance. In that period of time, the intended information had been transmitted to most of the men in the various communities, and they had begun informing their wives as well. But we wanted to meet with their wives separately too.

Information sessions for women

The community leaders in fact prompted our holding meetings with women; it was a relief for us not to have to ask permission to meet them, since they are generally secluded. The leaders also took it upon themselves to organise the meetings, which always took place in the women's own compounds. Saturdays were their meeting days and PMM members (usually all women – midwives, a social scientist and an obstetrician) met with them, rotating round the villages and attending two groups each Saturday. Unfortunately, the majority of the married women did not turn up every Saturday, and sometimes the meetings were postponed. These meetings therefore took place over a period of seven months. Essentially the same programme was used as with the men's groups but with a different emphasis on pregnancy and childbirth, as well as on the changes they would like to see. The results were equally impressive. As one woman put it: 'Once we were in darkness, but now we've seen light.'

Overall, the phase of participatory information and discussion meetings lasted almost two years. During this period, we were asked to provide several kinds of medical assistance, not only for pregnant women but also investigation of cases of infertility, treatment for sick children, and even income-generating activities in some communities. Greater demands were made on our time, resources and energies than we had been prepared for. On the other hand, the PMM team had gained enough credibility to be accepted everywhere in the area.

Improvements in maternal health services and supporting infrastructure: Phase III

This phase was considered the most fruitful by all partners in the project, as we had all dropped our stereotypical views of each other and begun to consolidate the gains we had made. Importantly, the community leaders' group decided on their own to transform themselves into a local government, safe motherhood committee when the Tuesday meeting was discontinued. We began to meet once every two months with them to review progress and suggest further measures. These joint meetings finally ended in December 1995. Today, this committee takes major decisions regarding women and children for the whole local government area. People in the communities have themselves become more involved and continued to make suggestions for and initiate changes as they identified the barriers to safe motherhood, including:

- The provision of two small facilities for use as maternity centres. In Maiyama, a small dispensary was renovated and refurbished to provide care during labour and delivery. In Mungadi, community members donated a new building and this was refurbished as a maternity centre. Both of these facilities were also utilised by women from other districts for antenatal care and delivery.

  Since then, a new government hospital has

taken over maternity care in Maiyama, the result of successful collaboration between local government, the PMM team and the community. Today, there is also a general primary health care hospital as well as a maternity centre in the Local Government Area.

- The mobilisation of local transport to take women with obstetric emergencies to hospital. The Nigerian Union of Road Transport Workers agreed to assist, and the PMM team provided a day's training programme on how to carry emergency cases to care. Certificates and special stickers for their buses were provided to the drivers who participated (not all did), and a courier system for reaching them on two 12-hour shifts (8am to 8pm) was set up. We also liaised with the local police to cooperate with the drivers.
- The setting up of a safe-motherhood fund for fuel. Fuel shortages were perennial in Nigeria and delays arising from searching for fuel were not uncommon. The PMM Network and some community members provided a small fund for the purchase of fuel at a higher price, which saved time. The money was deposited in the NURTW office at the local government headquarters. Drivers who were contacted to carry an emergency case would call for money there, which was refunded later by the woman's family. When the NURTW office was closed, money for fuel could be borrowed and repaid from the fund later. No provision was made for those who could not pay at all.
- The production of a video docu-drama based on the actual death of a pregnant woman from obstructed labour. This was a tragic case, in which the community leader had to order that the pregnant woman be taken to hospital, but it was too late. The video was produced as a collaborative effort between the community leaders, the PMM team, local government and the specialist hospital, and was shown round all the communities in the area.
- In the Mungadi community, leaders started a campaign for an increase in the enrolment and retention of girls in formal schools. A special fund was subsequently set aside for supporting girls whose parents pledged themselves to keep their daughters in school till they had completed the first six years.

The PMM team also organised a training programme for TBAs, who had requested this during the focus-group discussions. Trained TBAs could then supervise some home deliveries and also liaise with the two clinics and accompany emergency cases to hospital.

Women's need for income

In the mobilisation of community members to take on responsibility for improvements in maternal/pregnancy outcomes, the need for funds cannot be over-emphasised. In our meetings with women, their untenable financial status was stressed and they asked for support for *sana'a* (income-generating activities) such as groundnut oil processing and vegetable growing. Every time we met, they mentioned this. The PMM team therefore obtained some support for these two activities in three communities.[6]

For groundnut oil processing, credit facilities were made available for the purchase of raw groundnuts to be given to the women on credit. Four groups of women could be given credit for three months each at any one time. The credit was for eight to ten 30 kg bags of groundnut. For vegetable growing, two water-pumping machines were obtained for the exclusive use of the women for irrigation. The income generated from these activities ranged from about N3,500 to N6,000 (U$50-$80) per season, and could be used by the women as they pleased.

Outcomes

The effects of these combined activities and efforts were reflected in a number of measurable changes, especially with regard to reducing delays in reaching care, which was crucial in preventing deaths from complications. Using the same questionnaire over the five-year period from 1990 to 1994, women who came for emergency care at the specialist hospital later than they should have come were asked the reasons why. A total of 2,029 cases were recorded. Table 1 shows the causes of delay, ranging from husband being away to lack of transport and money.

Delays caused by a number of factors had appreciably reduced by 1994. For example, it had been agreed in the meetings with men that they would tell their relations to allow their pregnant wives to seek care if the need arose while they

Table 1. Distribution of delay factors in seeking health care in Kebbi State, Nigeria, 1990-1994 (%)

Factors causing delay	Total no. pregnant women (n=2,029)	Overall % of women	% of cases, 1990	% of cases, 1994	% change, 1990-1994
Husband away	225	12.38	5.61	0.73	- 4.44
No permission	320	15.54	4.04	2.71	-1.33
No transport	399	19.38	8.28	0.98	-7.30
No money	88	4.27	0.44	1.67	+1.23
Unaware of severity	858	41.67	23.50	3.64	-19.86
Night time	94	4.57	1.72	0.44	-1.28
Others	45	2.19	0.34	0.34	0

Source: Field work 1990-1996

were away. In 1990, 5.61 per cent of the delays were caused by this factor; by 1994 this had been reduced to 0.73 per cent. Similarly, lack of transport was responsible for 8.28 per cent of the delays to care in 1990; by 1994 this has reduced to 0.98 per cent. Lack of awareness of the severity was a major cause of delay. This reduced from 23.50 per cent to 3.64 per cent. These reductions indicate an improvement in community awareness of obstetric problems.

Transport from the communities to a health care facility also improved. Community surveys carried out from 1990 to 1995 showed that transport workers were indeed carrying more pregnant women (Table 2). From 1990 to 1992 most pregnancy cases were conveyed by commercial buses on a fee-for-service basis; by 1995 the transport scheme supported by NURTW had taken over 13 per cent of the transport requirements.[7] Further, in 1994 and 1995, 29 obstetric emergencies were transported out of 30 calls, and the great majority of outcomes were successful.

The first maternity clinic that the community renovated showed an increased use of antenatal care and some additional deliveries in the clinic between 1992 and 1995 (Table 3).

The costs of all these activities were also tracked and it was found that community collaboration had reduced the costs of providing care, which were shared between the community, local government and the PMM Network. For

Table 2. Mode of transport used by pregnant women in study area, Kebbi state, Nigeria, 1990-1995.

Year	On Foot	Animal	Own car /bus/taxi	Private comm.	Friends /bike	Ambulance /PMM bike	Comm. motor bike	Other	NURTW bus
	% (no.)	% (no.)	% (no.)	% (no.)	% (no.)	% (no.)	% (no.)	% (no.)	% (no.)
1990	3.17	0.29	27.5	47.7	14.4	2.4	4.2	0.3	0
(n=2718)	(86)	(10)	(744)	(1295)	(391)	(66)	(115)	(11)	(0)
1992	2.4	0.11	26.8	50.5	8.2	2.9	8.5	0.3	0
(n=2575)	(63)	(3)	(691)	(1301)	(214)	(77)	(218)	(8)	(0)
1995	2.0	0	20.7	41.6	6.9	3.3	11	0.4	13
(n=2644)	(53)	(0)	(548)	(1101)	(185)	(89)	(311)	(11)	(346)

Source: Field studies 1989-1995

Table 3. Maiyama maternity clinic: antenatal care, deliveries and referrals, Kebbi state, Nigeria, 1992-1995

Year	Attended for antenatal care	Delivered in the clinic	Home delivery attended by trained TBA	Referrals
1992	43	6	nil	18
1993	127	13	163	35
1994	149	28	183	8
1995	252	32	211	4

Source: Maiyama clinic records

example, the costs of providing transport for one emergency case averaged about US $6 instead of the previous US $13, which it had used to cost a woman to seek care. The refurbished maternity care facilities also cost less than they might have, with community contributions.

Lessons learned

Much has been learnt from this project. First, the decision to respect community hierarchies, and to approach and work with community leaders from the first, proved valuable and appropriate, as it helped in articulating the change process throughout.

Maternal deaths in the community are an acknowledged reality of people's lives. At the beginning of this project, these deaths were seen as inevitable and people were generally fatalistic about them; in the course of the project, this perception began to change.

Using local circumstances as the basis for information and discussion can help to move forward a change agenda.[4] The information transfer sessions on reproductive health helped the leaders to become better advocates. Further, the extensive collaboration between local government officials, community people (from the leaders to the grassroots), and the research team, greatly contributed to the success of many activities.

Participatory community mobilisation of this kind requires time, patience and persistence, but the final results can be rewarding. Direct involvement motivated people to start dealing with maternal health problems. For example, community leaders and people from Mungadi visited the Ministry of Health in the state capital to request for a health worker to take charge of the clinic they had renovated. After two years, they finally succeeded. They felt they had a stake in this clinic and were therefore prepared to make the effort to find solutions to their problems. We found that the more successful community people became, the more motivated they were to try out new things.

Though this project ended in December 1995, the communities are continuing many of activities that had been started. Local government has taken over some of the activities, and the PMM Network has recently succeeded in obtaining the services of a volunteer from the Voluntary Services Organisation to assist in Mungadi. Thus, we have shown that there can be a positive outcome to the mobilisation of rural people to play a part in improving maternal health, as an appropriate development objective. The study area presented conditions which were amenable, through a process of social enquiry, to social change. However, a much longer period of sustained work is needed to ensure permanence in the gains made.

Acknowledgements

I wish to acknowledge the contribution of the Prevention of Maternal Mortality team: Dr L Audu, Dr F Tahzib, Dr AA Fadahunsi, Mal M Kuna, Mrs Bello Gunmi, Mrs A Ikeh and Mrs M Hassan. We gratefully acknowledge the Carnegie Corporation, New York, the main funder of the entire Network; the technical support of the Columbia University team and the leadership and support of Deborah Maine and Angela Kamara; and the researchers, local government officials and community members in Sokoto and Kebbi states who have put so much into this work.

Correspondence

Dr Dora J Shehu, Prevention of Maternal Mortality Programme, Usmanu Danfodiyo University, PO Box 4131, Sokoto, Nigeria. Fax: 234-60-230438.

TREVOR PAGE /HUTCHISON LIBRARY

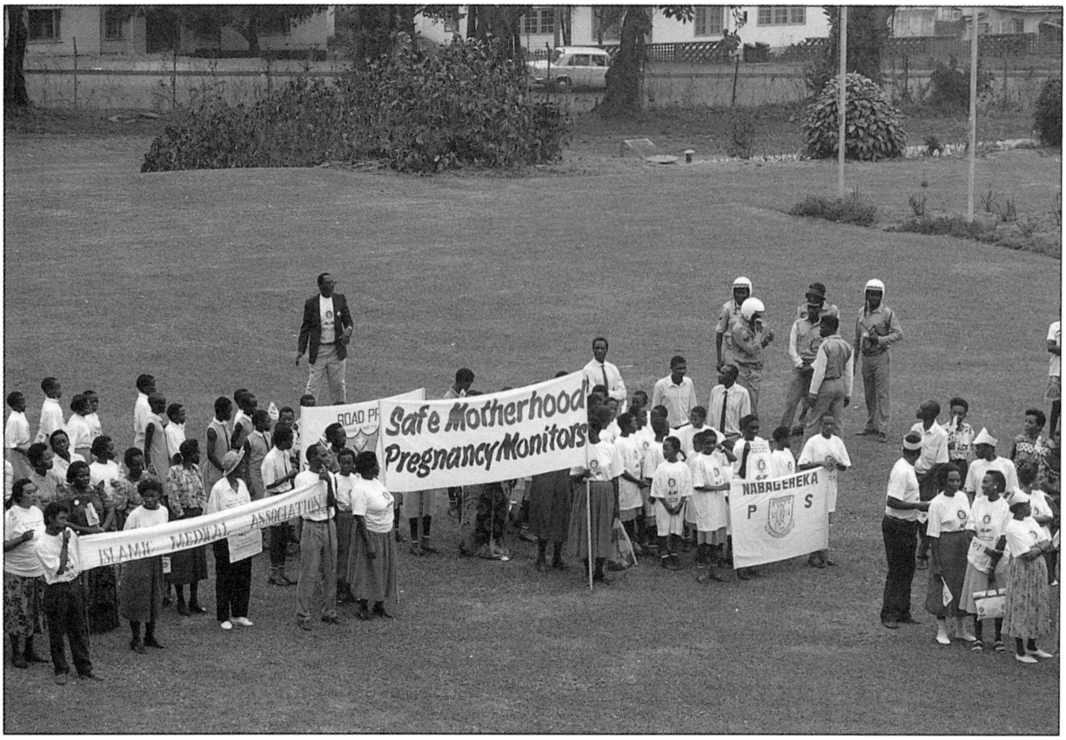

References and Notes

1. Oakley P, 1989. *Community Involvement in Health Development*. WHO Public Health Paper, Geneva.
2. MacCormack C, 1983. Community participation in primary health care. *Tropical Doctor*. 13(2):51-52.
3. Aubel J, Samba-Ndure, 1996. Community participation: lessons on sustainability for community health projects. *WHO Forum*. 17:50-57.
4. Freire P, 1972. *Pedagogy of the Oppressed*. Penguin, London/New York.
5. Family planning is generally regarded with suspicion in northern Nigeria, and there is a general lack of awareness about tablets. Despite our informing them about the use of haematinics and folic acid, the pills were flung back at us.
6. A manufacturer of vegetable oil donated a drum of vegetable oil, which was then sold and the proceeds used for purchasing raw groundnut. The British High Commissioner donated two water-pumping machines. These schemes worked well for about 18 months, after which the agent who assisted with the purchase of the fresh groundnut absconded from the village with the initial capital. The women, through the community leader, agitated for the return of the credit.
7. For details, see Shehu D, Maru I et al, 1997. Mobilising transport for obstetric emergencies in Northwestern Nigeria. *International Journal of Obstetrics and Gynecology*. 59(Suppl 21):S171.

Why Women Need Midwives for Safe Motherhood

Della R Sherratt

The key to safe motherhood in all countries is for the communities to reclaim childbirth as an important and significant event for individual women, families and society. Skilled practitioners, equipped with the appropriate knowledge, skills and attitudes can help achieve this. They do this by working with women, and their families as well as leaders and informers in the community to change attitudes towards childbirth and advocate for social development that benefits women. Safe motherhood is often reduced to discussion of how to prevent maternal mortality. Deaths of women during or around childbirth are only a part of safe motherhood, however. Many women give birth and survive to face the daily reality of a life damaged and hurt, emotionally and or physically, through lack of quality care in pregnancy and birth, within the same scenario as that which leads to other women dying. This paper outlines the essential components of a fitness-for-purpose curriculum for professional training and for defining and evaluating standards of practice, based on the best available evidence, especially in countries where the maternal mortality ratio is high. It uses data and examples from the South East Asian region where I have worked as a midwifery trainer and consultant for many years. It describes a prototype package of standards for practice developed for the South East Asian region. Appropriately educated and skilled midwives are needed to care for women during pregnancy, birth and post-partum. Investing in and strengthening midwifery skills should be seen as an essential component of any social development strategy, health care policy and programme for maternity care.

IN Nepal, every time a woman embarks upon a pregnancy, she faces a 1 in 10 lifetime risk of a maternal death.[1] Compared with the risk faced by women in other countries, such as in the UK, where the calculated lifetime risk is 1 in 5100, or Sweden with 1 in 6000, women in many developing countries are gambling with their lives when they become pregnant.[1]

Although pregnancy is a natural physiological life event, a minority of women and babies will not progress through pregnancy, birth and the puerperium without problems. Some estimates place the number at around 20-30 per cent of all pregnancies.[2] Where a woman lives and where she gives birth, in global terms, makes all the difference between life and death. The only way to ensure that women receive timely and appropriate care is to ensure that they have access to quality maternity care, a major part of which includes access to and support from well-educated practitioners with midwifery skills. As a study in Bangladesh has shown, well-educated practitioners with midwifery skills can do a great deal to reduce maternal mortality and morbidity ratios (MMR).[3]

Access to quality midwifery care is still lacking in many countries, the same countries in which women have low status, few resources and restrictions on mobility and decision-making.[4] Often, however, society and women themselves too readily accept death and disability following childbirth as inevitable. In some instances, women are positively discouraged or forbidden to seek such help, even when it is available. These are the underlying reasons why so more women than necessary are dying of pregnancy-related causes. If reproduction were seen as an essential societal issue, women's gamble with pregnancy would be considered significant and more would be done about it. Many societies consider that other pressing needs, whether income generation or economic reforms, take priority over women's health. Sometimes they believe that tackling economic problems will automatically result in the alleviation of these problems.

Why there are still not enough skilled midwives

Identifying a specific level of care, and the actual skills and competencies of those providing that care, and achieving sufficient numbers of appropriately skilled practitioners, are the major problems facing many developing countries today. Yet the arguments for having someone with 'midwifery skills', who is available to the community, and more specifically to all pregnant women, have been well-rehearsed – most recently at the Technical Consultation on Safe Motherhood in Sri Lanka, October 1997.[5]

One of the reasons why many South East Asian countries are having these problems lies, I believe, in the fact that these countries frequently only have cadres of health workers with a low level of midwifery expertise and skills. Where there are 'trained' midwives, all too frequently there are insufficient numbers of them or they are poorly educated and do not work close to where women give birth. For example, in India, there are only 40 trained midwives for every 100,000 births. In Indonesia, despite an extensive increase in numbers trained in the past decade, there are only on average 16 trained midwives per 100,000 births and in Nepal only 14.[6] With few exceptions those who do work in the community often lack the level of education and/or skills required to be able to offer appropriate, effective and timely care, especially if an emergency or unforeseen problems arise.

Such practitioners are usually not in a position to advocate for changes in societal attitudes and beliefs which would help to unlock the barriers to safe motherhood, as they do not have access to support from the community's elite or to policy-makers. Further, cultural views of women's bodies, especially because of menstruation, which underpin the laws of Purdah, define those who provide care to women in childbirth as being polluted, and therefore are seen as low-grade workers. This is especially the case in Bangladesh and India[7,8] but is also a belief found in the Western Pacific region.[9] Consequently, many families are unhappy to support their children to enter such a low-grade profession, and by the same token, recruitment into non-medical health care positions such as midwifery is aimed at the less academically-able ranks and at lower middle and working class families. As a result, the curriculum is often developed to accommodate the lack of education of the recruits, with little being expected from them and little attention given to their education and training.

All of this may help to explain why so many of the South East Asian countries, especially those with the highest maternal and perinatal mortality rates, have not seen the need to develop appropriate, well-educated midwives. In particular, it helps to explain why they have not concentrated on developing a specialist practitioner to work at the community level who would meet the international definition of a 'midwife', whom they see as a luxury they cannot afford (see Box).

International Definition of a Midwife*

'A person who, having been regularly admitted to a midwifery educational programme, duly recognised in the country in which it is located, has successfully completed the prescribed course of studies and has acquired the requisite qualification to be registered and/or legally licensed to practice midwifery.

'She must be able to give the necessary supervision care and advice to women during pregnancy, labour and postpartum period, to conduct deliveries on her own responsibility and to care for the new-born and the infant. This care includes preventative measures, the detection of abnormal conditions in the mother and child, the procurement of medical assistance and the execution of emergency measures in the absence of medical help. She has an important task in the health counselling and education, not only for the patient, but also within the family and the community. The work should involve ante-natal education and preparation for parenthood and extends to certain areas of gynaecology, family planning and child care. She may practice in hospitals, clinics, health units, domiciliary conditions or any other service.'

**This definition was devised by WHO/ICM/FIGO in 1973-74 and amended in 1976 and 1992.*

Multi-purpose workers cannot achieve safe motherhood

Most South East Asian countries have adopted a model of 'multi-purpose' health worker to provide community care, with the exception of Indonesia and Sri Lanka. In Sri Lanka, over 82 per cent of all births take place in an institutional setting,[10] and even they rely on multi-purpose workers to provide the majority of community-based care in pregnancy, childbirth and the post-natal period.

It is important to differentiate between a 'multi-purpose' and a 'multi-skilled' health worker. Clearly, there are situations where a health worker may have to have additional skills to those usually considered the norm, such as would be required in rural communities with little or no access to specialist centres. 'Multi-skilled' implies that the person has taken extra training and gained additional competencies, as for example a nurse with an additional midwifery qualification. 'Multi-purpose', on the other hand, usually means having a generic training, with the intention that the worker carry out a generic function of health education and promotion, sometimes with limited additional functions such as immunisation and child surveillance.

These multi-purpose workers – whose job titles in the different countries of the region include Lady Health Visitor, Family Welfare Visitor, Community Worker, Multi-purpose Health Worker, Health Assistant – are often overloaded with a multitude of duties and tasks. Frequently, they lack specific skills, especially midwifery skills, as their training has in some instances been very limited. In some countries, the training has also been reduced, e.g. in India the training was reduced in 1978 from two years to 18 months, in an attempt to increase the numbers of women entering other forms of work, as has occurred in Indonesia.

As far back as the mid-1970s in Bangladesh, the government discontinued the training of a cadre of workers who were in effect specialist community midwives, and replaced them with Family Welfare Visitors (FWVs), who were to prioritise the promotion of contraception at the community level.[11] Provision of maternity care suffered. The decision, promoted by large international donors, has been disastrous; it has effectively denied women access to midwifery-trained personnel at community level and this remains the case today. Nurse-midwives in Bangladesh mainly work in institutional settings, where less than five per cent of births take place. Very few work in the community, and the ones who do are usually working in non-governmental organisations (NGOs) or a handful of enterprising practitioners who take private clients.[12]

FWVs in Bangladesh, as with family planning workers in other countries, do not have the necessary component in their training to ensure that they have sufficient midwifery skills. On average, they have only eight weeks' teaching on specific midwifery skills. There is hardly any clinical practice of care during labour and birth in the field, but only simulation in the classroom. Remarkably, it is often they who are charged with training and or supervising traditional birth attendants (TBAs). In addition, it is becoming apparent that excessively heavy workloads, which continue to increase, are having a devastating effect on the quality of the work of FWVs. It may be argued that the heavy workloads contribute to FWVs thinking that maternal and child health (MCH) and maternity care are not priority areas for their work.[11] Even if they did see MCH and maternity care as a priority, their work schedule might well preclude their trying to provide effective care. Thus, FWVs may be considered a barrier to women receiving care in pregnancy in Bangladesh.

Whilst no definitive studies exist to show that multi-purpose workers in other countries face the same problems, anecdotal evidence was reported at a 1995 workshop that throughout the region there was a lack of adequate training in midwifery skills of health workers at the primary care level.[13]

Even today, many at the policy level still believe that with the FWVs, there is no need to have other health workers at community level. Despite evidence to the contrary, there are those in Bangladesh, e.g. the UNICEF in-country office in 1993, who did believe that FWVs could provide that care.[14] There are, however, some signs that with regard to achieving safe motherhood, this opinion may be changing within the government of Bangladesh, as evidenced by recent comments of a senior government official at the Regional Consultation on Standards for Safe Motherhood.[15]

The belief that a cadre of community worker with limited midwifery skills could serve as the main providers of maternity care has had severe consequences for the success of Safe Motherhood programmes in the South East Asia region. These workers do not have the requisite education and skills, and frequently lack the status and power to mobilise communities to bring about appropriate action, including challenging the status quo. Indeed, because they are women, they are prevented from providing effective care by the same barriers that adversely affect the health of women in their countries – lack of mobility, lack of respect, and not being able to address male community leaders. The net result is that woman and the community frequently have little regard for these health practitioners, or their services.

I would argue that multi-purpose workers are not as cost effective as was originally thought, and that it is the development of the multi-purpose worker which has, to a large extent, left many countries facing the new millennium with ambitious but unmet targets for reducing maternal and infant mortality. In some instances, the strategy of developing multi-purpose workers has contributed to the failure of making even small impacts on this major public health and social justice issue.

Why women do not utilise existing services

Possibly as a consequence of the low level of midwifery skills that multi-purpose workers have, there is a low level of expectation among women and families in regard to the type of care and services they expect to receive in pregnancy and childbirth. Evidence is growing of the lack of confidence in the quality of services women would receive if they did seek professional help, particularly in many South East Asian countries, where a large percentage of women only seek assistance from their nearest family relative. In a study to investigate obstetric morbidity in South India, for example, government services, particularly at the sub-centre and primary health care level, were under-utilised. The authors concluded that the community perceived the quality of services at these levels as poor.[16]

Table 1. Different cadres of health worker providing some aspect of maternity care, South East Asia, 1996*

	Nurse-Midwife	Nurse	Midwife	Auxiliary Midwife/ Nurse-Midwife	Health Assistant/ Assistant Nurse	Family Welfare Visitor/ Local Health Visitor	Community Worker	Multi-purpose Worker
Bangladesh	X	X	X			X		
Bhutan	X			X				
India	X			X				X
Nepal	X	X		X		X		
Myanmar	X	X	X	X		X		
Thailand		X		X				
Sri Lanka	X	X	X					
Maldives	X			X	X	X	X	X
DPR Korea		X	X		X			
Indonesia	X	X						

**Source: WHO SEARO survey, 1996*

In many parts of the South East Asia region, anecdotal reports are common of women (or their families or both) who have refused to be taken or transferred to a health facility for specialist care, for fear of the service they will receive, even when their lives or those of their newborn babies is at risk. Unless the community considers that the care given in a health facility is 'good enough', they will not use the service. Often this is not the fault of the individual practitioner, but of weak management, weak policies or weak governance, or the unfair opinions of other health workers.

Equally importantly, the provision of care from pregnancy through birth and post-partum is often the responsibility of many different health practitioners,[17] including many traditional and informal care givers (see Table 1). This militates against quality of care and can result in confusion and chaos. Families want to ensure that women receive proper care for pregnancy and childbirth. Frequently, faced with a myriad of different workers – private, NGO and traditional practitioners, all promoting their own services and often giving conflicting advice – people are left not knowing who to trust or who to turn to for advice and care.

Many reports demonstrate that women do not wish this situation to remain. Women want a healthy life, and safe pregnancy and birth, and they say they would utilise services if the quality were improved and workers were culturally sensitive and effective in aiding them in childbearing.

The need for quality maternity care

In my opinion, it is important to have a named practitioner with knowledge and skills, whom the community can access for maternity care. These practitioners may vary in their level of skills and competency given the exigencies in each country, but they must have a specific and possibly universal core body of knowledge and skills. Adopting a universal name, such as 'midwife', for the person who is equipped and has the appropriate knowledge and skills to assist woman and communities during pregnancy, childbirth and the post-natal period may help to redress this situation. First, it would identify maternity work as special and important for individuals and society.

If these midwives worked as women's advocates and proved they were able to help women, then they might become valued and respected by the community. They would then be able to begin to influence the design and provision of appropriate and sympathetic health care. In time, it may even become possible to change societies' views of childbirth and midwifery care and improve the quality and quantity of skilled midwifery practitioners at the community level.

In South East Asian countries, attempts at improving the quality of maternity care are often reduced to specific interventions. A focus on providing all childbearing women with the appropriate quality care, and the structural changes required to achieve this, are often seen as too complex and difficult to deal with. Without this focus, however, I believe it is unlikely that any of the other interventions will meet with a significant degree of success.

I would argue that, in addition to many of the strategies outlined elsewhere, such as adequate family planning, effective referral systems and Essential Obstetric Care (EOC), it is also important to establish an agreed level or standard of maternity care. These standards must be agreed in consultation with women and the community. Women have the right to expect and to access quality maternity health services; therefore, they also have to right to help to define the kind of care they feel they need.

Given the limited resources facing all developing countries, there is a need to ensure that the resources available are focused on the greatest needs and used to maximum benefit. Therefore, as standards of care and service provision are developed, whilst they may be limited by the available resources, they should always be based on best evidence and proven effectiveness. Strengthening the skills of midwifery-trained personnel working in the community has been endorsed by WHO and the World Bank as a cost-effective strategy in this regard.[18,19]

Evidence suggests that countries which have made the most improvements and invested in the health and care of women in pregnancy, childbirth and the puerperium, are also the ones who have invested in and developed the skilled midwifery-trained practitioners. Some South East Asian countries, e.g. Sri Lanka, Indonesia and the Maldives, have recently embarked on upgrading their midwifery-trained personnel. In the case of

Sri Lanka this, along with other initiatives, has begun to bear fruit, and maternal mortality has declined significantly in recent years.[10] Many argue that this decline can be accounted for by the rise in institutional deliveries, as almost all deliveries now take place in a hospital setting. However, evidence from other parts of the subcontinent shows that hospital-based delivery alone is not always the crucial factor.

The need for standards and other tools to improve quality of care

For quality maternity care to be developed, a sufficient number of educated and skilled midwives is crucial. Investing in and strengthening midwifery skills is not the same, however, as just teaching existing practitioners some additional skills, such as how to give inter-muscular oxytocin for management of the third stage of labour. Strengthening midwifery skills requires a great deal more than this. It means at least setting minimum standards for care during pregnancy, childbirth and the puerperium – and evaluating this care. Setting standards however can be problematic. Faced with low levels of expertise and low levels of expectation from the women and the community, who should be setting the standards in South East Asian countries?

Unfortunately in many of these and other countries, a great deal of the midwifery care offered has been adopted and based on outdated models, methods and concepts, a great deal of which still lacks supporting evidence. It is therefore important that standards are developed following the widest possible consultation with a variety of sources and do not rely on medical practitioners or service providers alone. There is now a body of evidence, documented in the form of technical papers, that demonstrates the need to challenge and change some of these outdated practices. The WHO guidelines on care in normal births[20] is an excellent example.

Standards of maternity care must be based on interventions supported by sound scientific knowledge. They must also be 'women-friendly', by which I mean that they have as a central core the respect and dignity of women and see the individual woman, her baby and family as rightfully at the centre of maternity care. For without careful consultation with women and the community, neither will have the necessary confidence in the standards or utilise the services on offer. A gender perspective is also required, which takes into account both the biological and social contexts of pregnant women.[21] The development of concepts and practical tools to bring about 'quality care' in this way is, I believe, possible in all situations, even in countries where the voices of most women are difficult to hear.

Such an approach must focus on local action, with local communities and health workers, i.e. midwifery-trained personnel, tackling problems and challenges together as partners, not as separate providers and users. However, these local efforts must be supported and underpinned by national systems and national strategies.

Unfortunately, there are few models or frameworks available that have been thoroughly evaluated, on which such an approach can be based. Most of the work to date on frameworks for quality of care have been undertaken in relation to family planning services, the best-known being the Bruce-Jain framework.[22] The International Confederation of Midwives (ICM) in their Triennial Congress in Vancouver 1993[23] and others have developed frameworks for quality assurance (QA) in maternity care, but as yet, evaluation studies are still awaited. Despite the lack of evaluated models, a number of frameworks have been suggested. For example,

Figure 1. Developing standards as a means of improving quality of care

1. Define standard based on best practice (may require a pilot)
   ↓
2. Implement
   ↓
3. Monitor
   ↓
4. Audit
   ↓
5. Develop and implement an action plan to strengthen practice
   ↓
6. Audit again after action plan
   ↓
7. Revise/review standard, based on findings and on new evidence/research and changes in environment
   ↓
8. Start again from the top ↑

Figure 2. Tools to ensure quality of care

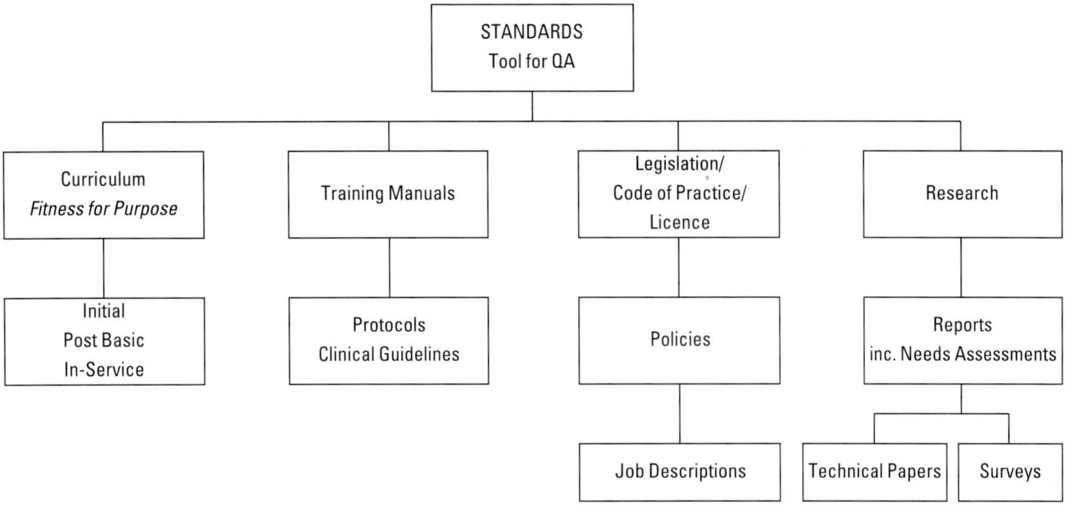

the favoured framework in the UK for QA in midwifery has been the clinical audit tool.[24] Others, however, have suggested linking QA to supervision,[25] while for family planning the Bruce-Jain framework is frequently cited.[22]

There is no short-cut to providing quality maternity care; those who provide the care must be competent and appropriately trained and this training must be based on appropriate standards of midwifery practice. Standards are the key to any improvement in quality of care and should continuously be refined and updated (see Figure 1). Standards are also useful for defining job descriptions and are most important for defining the educational curriculum for midwives (see Figure 2).

Prototype practice standards for WHO South East Asia Region

In an attempt to assist countries in the region and at the request of member States, WHO South East Asia Regional Office has recently developed a package of prototype 'Standards of Midwifery Practice for Safe Motherhood', which have recently been adopted by all the countries in the Region.[26] These standards of practice were developed in consultation with the member countries and were field-tested in four of them, Bhutan, Indonesia, Nepal and Thailand, and are based on the approach described above.

They identify the minimal level of practice required by midwifery-trained personnel in providing essential maternity care, including some essential life-saving interventions appropriate for these countries. We used a 'structure-process-outcome' model for developing them, carried out a review of the available literature and scientific evidence, and included all stakeholders in the process – including policymakers, planners, professional bodies and associations, as well as educationalists, community leaders, women and their families.

The standards define the agreed level of performance, as well as the prerequisites required (structure criteria) for each specific agreed area of practice. In addition, critical tasks (process criteria) required to ensure the standards of practice are achieved are also defined, with full bibliographic references and supporting notes given as appropriate, or requested during field testing. Where there was a suggested change in current practice, full explanations were provided with reference to the research to support this change.

Criteria have been established for each part of the standard and include some expected outcomes as a result of midwifery being practised at the agreed level. These criteria are then used for auditing each standard and developing a series of actions and further checks/audits, to correct deficiencies found and strengthen practice as appropriate.

Outcomes are notoriously difficult to assess[27] and may be influenced by factors outside the control of the midwife or services providers, e.g. floods, natural disasters or civil unrest. Therefore, for the regular monitoring and routine audit of implementation of the standards, attention is concentrated on the structure and process criteria, with the suggestion that outcome criteria form part of a longer-term evaluation.

The audit tool is seen as an essential component of the standard, and it has been suggested that it should form part of the regular supervision and monitoring of the midwives' work. However, to ensure that it is the standard and not the person which is audited, and in an attempt to ensure that the process is not seen as punitive, the audit tool has been developed to ensure multiple data collection, including consultation with women, their families and in some cases the community. Data will be collected from a variety of sources, including direct observations, review of documentation, peer review, information from referral centres and self-assessment.

The approach also allows for some degree of local adaptation and use of local initiatives, but at the same times defines the minimum level of midwifery practice required to achieve Safe Motherhood within an ethical framework. For example, one of the standards for care in labour is that: 'Midwifery-trained practitioners must be able to correctly assess that labour has commenced and provide adequate, culturally sensitive monitoring and care throughout labour that respects the wishes and dignity of women and make referrals as appropriate'.

Using the standards statement it is then possible to identify some outcomes, e.g. mortality and morbidity due to prolonged labour is reduced. It is also possible to identify the essential prerequisites that must be in place to allow this level of practice, i.e.:

- Specify policies/protocols or guidelines required
- Midwifery-trained personnel must be summoned when labour commences
- Specify what training is required
- Specify equipment and drugs required
- Effective referral system must be operational
- Specify what records are required

Defining the critical tasks that must be carried out makes a standard specific. It also allows essential criteria to be identified for the audit. Part of the intention is to remove subjectivity on the part of the auditor and allow flexibility for the midwife to reach the standard, using local adaptations and methods that fit the standard of care defined.

By developing explicit standards of practice and making them available to all stakeholders, it becomes possible to evaluate the effectiveness of maternity care in terms of achieving specific, expected outcomes. The acceptance of the community will be demonstrated through increased utilisation of midwifery-trained practitioners and recorded satisfaction of the recipients of care and those around them.

To date, the results of field-testing these prototype practice standards has been very encouraging. For example, the Indonesian midwives reported an increased uptake of antenatal care during the field-testing period, which resulted in increased earnings for the midwife. All four countries have reported increased satisfaction of the recipients of care. Thailand reported increased confidence among the midwives, who were able to negotiate some changes in routine practice previously dictated by their medical colleagues, such as not undertaking routine shaving and giving routine enemas. They also reported an increase in the number of midwifery-specific research studies, as both they and others began to question why they were undertaking some of the interventions previously considered essential.

Further information on this package will be forthcoming from WHO SEARO, who hope to make it available to the wider community in due course. Work is also underway to see if these standards, or at least the format, can be used to develop a general set of midwifery practice standards that would be helpful for any country developing and strengthening its midwifery-skilled practitioners.

A 'fitness-for-purpose' curriculum for training midwives

In order for the curriculum for midwifery-trained personnel to prepare them to offer quality care, it must be developed on the basis of 'fitness-for-purpose', that is, to produce

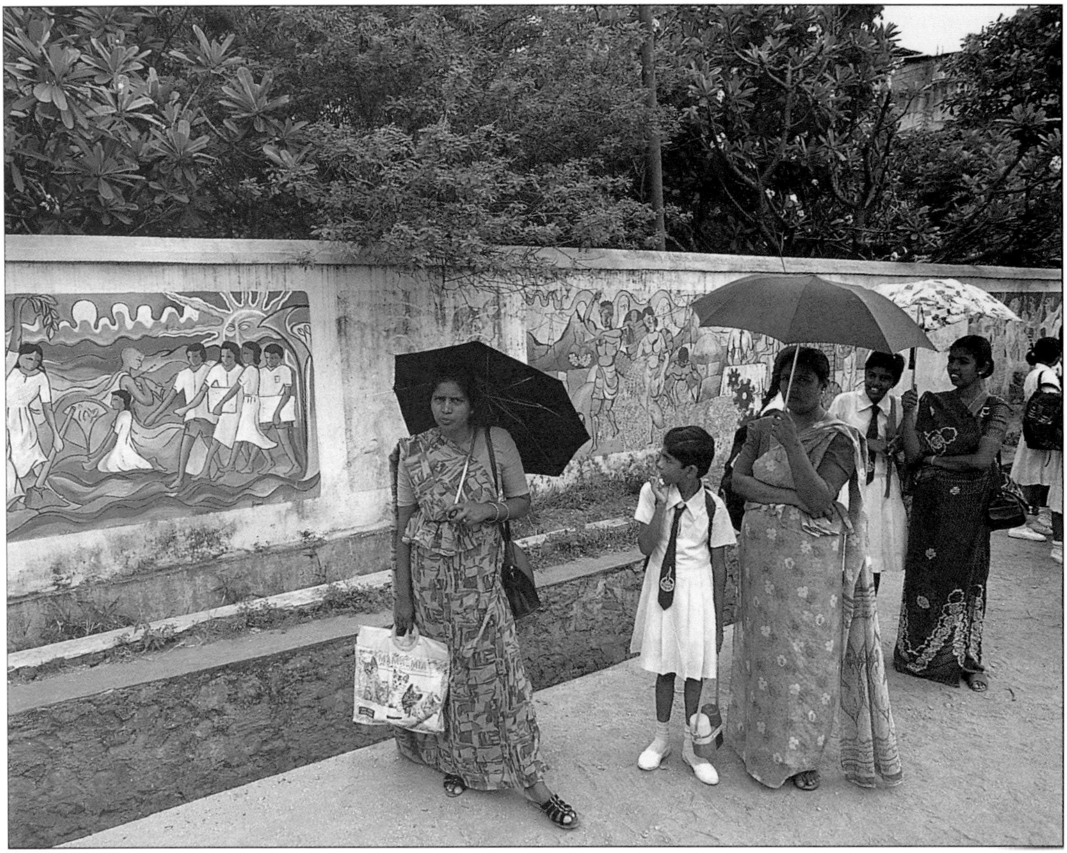

JEREMY HORNER / HUTCHISONLIBRARY

practitioners who will fulfil three equally important sets of needs:

- the needs of individual women,
- the needs of the nation, based on epidemiological data, available resources, etc.,
- the demands of society for professional competence.

The educational process must ensure that the students following the curriculum will have the appropriate competencies, i.e. the knowledge, skills and attitudes to practice midwifery safely. These will include not only technical competencies, but also relevant community developments skills, inter-personal skills, confidence and assertiveness, commitment to empowering women and working with the community, and the skills to identify, interpret and utilise research findings.

The fitness-for-purpose curriculum must be competency-based and meet agreed professional norms. This means that midwifery-trained practitioners must be inculcated in professional values and norms based on a sense of duty and the ethical obligation to carry out their work in a certain way. For example, the International Confederation for Midwives (ICM) expects all midwives to: 'use their professional knowledge (and skills) to ensure safe birth practices in all environments and cultures', and 'to respond to the psychological, physical, emotional and spiritual needs of women seeking health care, whatever their circumstances'.[28]

The 'Fitness-for-purpose' curriculum model for midwifery takes all the factors which influence the curriculum into account. If designed and implemented correctly, it will ensure the training of competent midwives who are capable of providing appropriate and cost-effective maternity care, which in turn will result in improved health indicators. In all, theywill have been enabled to make a positive impact on maternal and neonate morbidity and mortality.

The curriculum, to be effective, must be skills-based and taught by appropriately skilled and competent midwifery teachers, who have been specially prepared for this role. The essential content for such a curriculum was the subject of the ICM Pre-Congress workshop in Kobe, Japan in 1990. In the final report of the workshop it was acknowledged that, in many developing countries, the midwifery training was based on outdated curricula, frequently borrowed from other countries.[29] In addition, even when the content was appropriate, it was often taught by inexperienced teachers who themselves lacked essential midwifery skills and so perpetuated inadequate midwifery training.

In the years following the Kobe Congress, a great deal has been undertaken to reverse this situation. A great deal more material is now available to assist in the teaching of midwifery. For example the ICM with the assistance of WHO, UNICEF and others, has done a great deal to advocate for change. WHO commissioned the production of the popular and well-used Midwifery Education Modules,[30] which have undergone extensive field-testing and are a useful tool.

ICM have also developed a provisional set of midwifery competencies, launched at its 1999 Congress in Manila, which are now undergoing rigorous field-testing. WHO headquarters in Geneva are developing tools to assist midwives and midwifery teachers to define quality maternity care; in addition, they will soon be launching an essential maternity care package for use at District level.

The Technical Consultation for Safe Motherhood held in Sri Lanka in 1997 resulted in the reaffirmation of the central role of the midwife for Safe Motherhood. At the Consultation, there was also agreement that standards for maternity care for all service providers should be developed. The WHO/SEARO prototype Midwifery Practice Standards give countries a set a essential tools that they can use – if they have the political willingness to develop well educated midwives who can assist them to achieve the goals of Safe Motherhood.

There is still much left to do, but it is heartening to report that at the WHO/SEARO Inter-Country Regional Consultation for the Prototype Standards of Midwifery Practice for Midwifery-Trained Personnel, held in the region in November 1998, all South East Asian countries agreed to adopt the Prototype Standards as the basis of their work in-country. It is to be hoped that this indicates recognition of the value and worth of midwifery skills, and therefore of midwives, to assist in achieving the goals of Safe Motherhood goals. Only time will tell.

Conclusion

All societies (and therefore all governments) have an ethical duty to ensure that the needs of women in childbirth are met and that systems exist to protect their citizens from harm. In the case of childbearing women, this can best be achieved by ensuring that those who provide pregnancy and childbirth care can and do practise effectively and cause no harm to the public. This requires insisting that all workers have the necessary education and training and comply with a defined code of conduct, professional principles and standards that have been well-evaluated.

The definition of a midwife was first agreed in 1972 and is revised periodically to keep up with changes in the field. Essential maternity services packages have been agreed, and in South East Asian countries, basic standards of maternity practice for Safe Motherhood, which include some essential life-saving skills, have been developed and field-tested. Frameworks and tools currently exist to permit these to be put into place.

It is my belief that until there are sufficient numbers of trained midwives in society to enable all women to give birth under the care of someone who is competent, the goals of safe motherhood cannot be achieved. This is an enormous challenge for many countries. However, in the future, if midwives are appropriately prepared and allowed to practise the skills and duties described here, there is no doubt that they can and will make a significant contribution to achieving Safe Motherhood goals.

Acknowledgements

Some parts of this paper are based on the background paper prepared by the author with the assistance of Anne Thompson of the Department of Reproductive Health and Research, WHO, Geneva for the International Confederation of Midwives Mid-Triennial Regional Workshop, New Delhi, India, February 1998.

Correspondence

Della R Sherratt, Centre For Development Studies, School of Social Sciences & International Development, University of Wales, Swansea, UK. E-mail: d.r.sherratt@swansea.ac.uk

References

1. WHO, 1996. *Revised 1990 Estimates of Maternal Mortality: A New Approach by WHO and UNICEF*. World Health Organization, Geneva.
2. Hurdley VA, Cruickshank FM, Long GD et al, 1994. Midwifery-managed delivery unit: a randomised controlled comparison with consultant care. *British Medical Journal*. 309(Nov 26):1400-04.
3. Maine D, Akalin MZ, Chakraborty J et al, 1996. Why did maternal mortality decline in Matlab? *Studies in Family Planning*. 27(4):179-87.
4. World Health Organization, 1997. *Coverage of Maternity Care. Listing of Available Information*. 4th edition. WHO Family and Reproductive Health Division, Geneva.
5. Safe Motherhood: Ten Years of Lessons and Progress Technical Consultation. Colombo, SRI Lanka 18-23 October 1997.
6. Fortney J, 1997. *Ensuring Skilled Attendance at Delivery: The Role of TBAs*. The Family Health Research Triangle Park, NC.
7. Blanchet T, 1984. *Women, Pollution and Marginality. Meanings and Rituals of Birth in Rural Bangladesh*. University Press Limited, Dhaka.
8. Jeffrey P, Jeffrey R, Lyon A, 1988. *Labour Pains and Labour Power: Women and Childbearing in India*. Zed Books Ltd, London.
9. WHO WPRO, 1997. *Women's Health in a Social Context in the Western Pacific Region*. World Health Organisation Regional Office for the Western Pacific, Manila.
10. de Silva D, 1993. Impact of the development of a comprehensive system for community midwifery services on national maternal health in Sri Lanka. Paper presented at Inter-Country Consultation on Training and Utilization of Health Personnel with Midwifery Skills. World Health Organization South-East Asia Region Office, New Delhi, India, 6-10 December.
11. Simmons R, Koenig MA, Zahidul Huque AA ,1990. Maternal child health and family planning: user perspectives and service constraints in rural Bangladesh. *Studies in Family Planning*. 21(4):187-96.
12. Sherratt DR, Hancock M, 1993. *Evaluation of 4th Year Nurse-Midwifery Curriculum*. Project Report, British Council, Dhaka.
13. WHO SEARO, 1995. *National Programme Managers For Safe Motherhood. Report on an Inter-Country Workshop, India, 27 February-3 March 1995*. New Delhi.
14. UNICEF, 1993. Reduction of Maternal Mortality in Bangladesh during 1995-2000. A Concept Paper. UNICEF, Dhaka.
15. WHO SEARO, 1998. Inter-Country Consultation on Implementation of Standards of Midwifery Practice for Safe Motherhood in SEAR Countries. World Health Organisation Regional Office for South-East Asia, New Delhi, 24-26 November.
16. Bhatia J C, Cleland J, 1996. Obstetric morbidity in South India: results from a community survey. *Social Science and Medicine*. 43(10):1507-16.
17. WHO SEARO, 1996. *Utilisation of Midwifery Trained Personnel in SEAR countries: Standards for Midwifery Practice for Safe Motherhood*. Working Paper 1. An inter-country consultation. World Health Organization South-East Asia Region Office, New Delhi, India November 1996.
18. WHO, 1994. *Mother-Baby Package: Implementing Safe Motherhood in Countries*. Maternal Health and Safe Motherhood Programme, Division of Family Health, World Health Organization, Geneva.
19. World Bank, 1993. *World Development Report 1993: Investing in Health*. World Bank/Oxford University Press, New York.
20. WHO, 1996. *Care in Normal Birth: A Practical Guide*. Maternal and Newborn Health Safe Motherhood Unit Family and Reproductive Health World Health Organization Geneva.
21. AbouZahr C, Vlassoff C, Kumar A, 1996. Quality of health care for women: a global challenge. *Health Care For Women International*. 17(5):449-67.
22. Bruce J, 1990. Fundamental elements of the quality of care: a simple framework. In *Studies in Family Planning* .21: 61-91.
23. WHO/ICM/UNICEF, 1993. *Midwifery Practice: Measuring,*

Developing and Mobilising Quality Care. Report of a Collaborative Pre-Congress Workshop. Vancouver, 7-8 May.

24. Dickenson V, 1998. Moving audit into midwifery practice. *Practicing Midwife*. 7/8(July-Aug):12-16.
25. Gorzanski C, 1997. Raising the standards through supervision. *Modern Midwife*. 7(2):11-14.
26. WHO SEARO, 1998. *Inter-Country Consultation on Implementation of Standards of Midwifery Practice for Safe Motherhood in SEAR Countries*. World Health Organization South-East Asia Region Office, New Delhi 24-26 November 1998.
27. Morrow R, 1996. Concepts and methods assessing the quality of essential obstetric care. *International Journal of Health Planning and Management*. 6(3):119-34.
28. ICM, 1993. *International Code of Ethics for Midwives*. International Confederation of Midwives, London.
29. WHO/ICM/UNICEF, 1991. *Midwifery Education: Action for Safe Motherhood. Report of a Collaborative Pre-Congress Workshop. Kobe, Japan 5-6 October 1990*. World Health Organization, Maternal and Child Health & Family Planning Division of Family Health, Geneva.
30. WHO, 1996. *Midwifery Modules for Safe Motherhood*. Maternal Health and Safe Motherhood Programme, Division of Family Health, World Health Organization, Geneva.

Resources

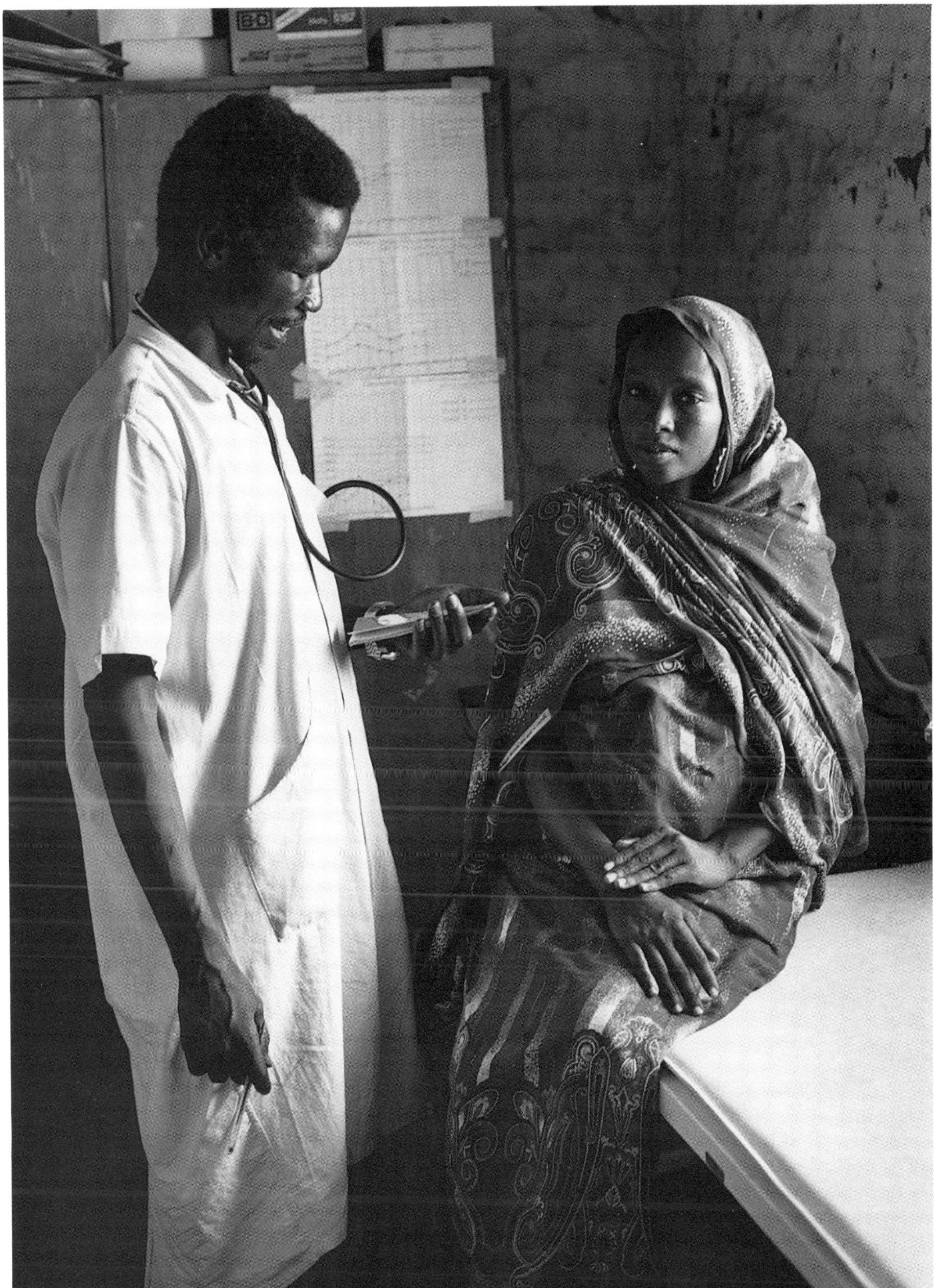

GIACOMO PIROZZI / PANOS PICTURES

Resources

Resources on the following list were selected because they advance understanding of Safe Motherhood; contain guidelines for best practice or practical advice for the development of policies, programmes and services; are international or regional in scope; or, in the case of journals and newsletters, because they are special editions covering new developments in the field.

Prepared by *Amy Kapczynski*

Books and Booklets

Beck D, Buffington ST, McDermott J, Berney K, 1998.
– **Healthy Mother and Healthy Newborn Care: A Reference Guide for Care Givers.**
– **Healthy Mother and Healthy Newborn Care: A Guide for Care Givers (Pocket Manual)**. American College of Nurse Midwives, Washington, DC.
Both available online at:
www.jsi.com/intl/mothercare/PUBS/Healthy%20Mother/guide.pdf or /reference.pdf

Berg C, Danel I, Mora G (eds), 1996.
Guidelines for Maternal Mortality Epidemiological Surveillance. PAHO/WHO/UNFPA.

Campbell O, Filippi V, Koblinsky M, Marshall T, Mortimer J, Pittrof R, Ronsmans C, Williams L, 1997.
Lessons Learnt – A Decade of Measuring the Impact of Safe Motherhood Programmes. London School of Hygiene and Tropical Medicine, London.

Department for International Development, 1997.
Time for Action: Reducing the Dangers of Pregnancy in Poor Societies. Options Consultancy Services, London.

Family Health Service Project, Nigeria, Mother Care/John Snow Inc, Johns Hopkins University, PCS, 1993.
Interpersonal Communication and Counseling Curriculum for Midwives. MC/JSI, Arlington VA.

Feuerstein M-T, 1993.
Turning the Tide: Safe Motherhood, A District Action Manual. Macmillan Press/Save the Children, London.

Fortney JA, Smith JB (eds) with the Maternal Morbidity Network, 1996.
The Base of the Iceberg: Prevalence and Perceptions of Maternal Morbidity in Four Developing Countries. December, Family Health International.

Fortney JA, Smith JB, 1997.
Training of Traditional Birth Attendants: Issues and Controversies. December, UNICEF/Family Health International.

Fortney JA, Smith JB, 1997.
Methodological Issues in Research on Traditional Birth Attendants. December, UNICEF/ Family Health International.

Graham WJ, Ronsmans CCA, Filippi VGA, Campbell OMR, Goodburn EA, de C Marshall TF, Shulman C, Davies JL, 1995.
Asking Questions about Women's Reproductive Health in Community-Based Surveys: Guidelines on Scope and Content. MCEU. London School of Hygiene and Tropical Medicine, London.

Howson CP, Harrison PF, Hotra D, Law M (eds), 1996.
In Her Lifetime. Female Morbidity and Mortality in Sub-Saharan Africa. National Academy of Science Press.

Maine D, 1990.
Safe Motherhood Programs: Options and Issues. Center for Population and Family Health, Columbia University, New York.

Maine D, Akalin MZ, Ward V M, Kamara A, 1997.
The Design and Evaluation of Maternal Mortality Programs. Center for Population and Family Health, School of Public Health, Columbia University, New York, June.

Maine D, Wardlaw T, Ward V, McCarthy J, Birnbaum A, Akalin MZ, Brown JE, 1997.
Guidelines for Monitoring the Availability and Use of Obstetric Services. UNICEF/WHO/UNFPA, New York.

Marshall MA, Buffington ST, 1998.
Life Saving Skills Manual for Midwives. 3rd edition. American College of Nurse Midwives, Washington DC.

Marshall MA, Buffington ST, 1998.
Life Saving Skills Manual for Policy Makers and Trainers. American College of Nurse Midwives, Washington, DC.

McGinn T, Maine D, McCarthy J, Rosenfield A, 1995.
Setting Priorities in International Reproductive Health Programs: A Practical Framework. Center for Population and Family Health, Columbia University, New York.

Measham DM, Kallianes VD (eds), 1995.
Issues in Essential Obstetric Care. Report of a Technical Meeting of the Inter-Agency Group for Safe Motherhood. Population Council, New York.

Mercer J S, Glatleider P, Bacci A, 1998.
Family-Centered Maternity Care: Training of Trainers Curriculum. American College of Nurse Midwives, Washington DC.

Murray SF (ed), 1996.
Baby Friendly, Mother Friendly. Mosby Press, London.

Nachbar N, Baume C, Parekh A, 1998.
Assessing Safe Motherhood in the Community: A Guide to Formative Research. John Snow Inc, Arlington VA. Available online at: www.jsi.com/intl/mothercare/cd_manual/index.htm

Sloan NL, Quimby C, Winikoff B, Schwalbe N, 1995.
Guidelines and Instruments for a Situation Analysis of Obstetric Services. Robert H Ebert Program on Critical Issues in Reproductive Health and Population. Population Council, New York.

Smith JB, Fortney JA, 1997.
Birth Kits: An Assessment. May, UNICEF/ Family Health International.

Starrs A, 1987.
Preventing the Tragedy of Maternal Deaths. A Report on the International Safe Motherhood Conference, Nairobi, Kenya, February 1987. World Bank/World Health Organization/ UNFPA.

Starrs A with Measham D, 1990.
Challenge for the Nineties. Safe Motherhood in South Asia. World Bank/Family Care International.

Starrs A, Inter-Agency Group for Safe Motherhood, 1997.
The Safe Motherhood Action Agenda: Priorities for the Next Decade. Report on the Safe Motherhood Technical Consultation, 18-23 October 1997, Colombo, Sri Lanka. UNFPA/UNICEF/World Bank/ WHO/ IPPF/Population Council/ Family Health International, New York.

Tinker A, Koblinsky MA, 1993.
Making Motherhood Safe. World Bank, Washington DC.

Tinker A, Daly P, Green C, Saxenian H, Lakshminarayanan R, Gill K, 1994.
Women's Health and Nutrition. Making a Difference. World Bank, Washington DC.

World Bank, 1994.
A New Agenda for Women's Health and Nutrition. World Bank, Washington DC.

World Health Organization, 1994.
Midwifery Practice: Measuring, Developing and Mobilizing Quality Care. Report of a Collaborative WHO/ ICM/UNICEF Pre-Congress Workshop, Vancouver, Canada. WHO/FHE/MSM/94.12. WHO, Geneva.

World Health Organization, 1994.
Clinical Management of Abortion Complications: A Practical Guide. WHO/FHE/ MSM/94.1. WHO, Geneva.

World Health Organization, 1994.
Mother-Baby Package: Implementing Safe Motherhood in Countries. WHO/FHE/ MSM/94.11. WHO, Geneva.

World Health Organization, 1996.
Safe Motherhood Needs Assessment. WHO/ FHE/MSM/96.18. WHO, Geneva.

World Health Organization, 1996.
Care in Normal Birth: A Practical Guide. Report of a Technical Working Group. WHO/ FRH/MSM/96.24. WHO, Geneva.

World Health Organization, 1996.
Studying Unsafe Abortion: A Practical Guide. WHO, Geneva. WHO/RHT/SMS/ 96.25.

World Health Organization, 1996.
Education Material for Teachers of Midwifery. WHO, Geneva.
- **Foundation Module: The Midwife in the Community**. WHO/FRH/MSM/96.1
- **Post-Partum Haemorrhage Module**. WHO/FRH/MSM/96.2
- **Obstructed Labour Module**. WHO/FRH/MSM/96.3
- **Puerperal Sepsis Module**. WHO/FRH/MSM/ 96.4
- **Eclampsia Module**. WHO/FRH/MSM/96.5

World Health Organization, 1998.
Unsafe Abortion: Global and Regional Estimates of Incidence of and Mortality Due to Unsafe Abortion with a Listing of Available Country Data. WHO, Geneva. WHO/RHT/MSM/97.16.

World Health Organization, 1998.
Post-Partum Care of the Mother and Newborn: A Practical Guide. WHO, Geneva. WHO/RHT/ MSM/98.3.

World Health Organization, 1999.
Emergency Obstetrics Manual. WHO, Geneva (in press, 1999).

Newsletters

International Midwifery Matters. International Confederation of Midwives, London.

MotherCare Matters. MotherCare Project/ John Snow Inc, Arlington VA.

Safe Motherhood: A Newsletter of Worldwide Activity. World Health Organization, Geneva.

Journal Supplements

Reproductive Health: The MotherCare Experience.
International Journal of Gynecology and Obstetrics. Vol 48 (Suppl), 1995. Guest Editors: T Türman, C AbouZhar, M Koblinsky.

Prevention of Maternal Mortality Network.
International Journal of Gynecology and Obstetrics. Vol 59 (Suppl 2), 1997. Guest Editor: D Maine.

A Randomised Controlled Trial for the Evaluation of a New Antenatal Care Model.
Paediatric and Perinatal Epidemiology. Vol 12, (Suppl) 2, 1998. Guest Editors: P Lumbiganon, P Bergsjø, H Ba'aqeel, J Villar.